EMDR and the Art of Psychotherapy With Children

Robbie Adler-Tapia, PhD, is a licensed psychologist who has worked with traumatized children and their families for more than 25 years. Dr. Adler-Tapia is EMDRIA certified in EMDR, an EMDRIA approved consultant, an EMDR Institute Facilitator, and an EMDR HAP trainer-in-training and has volunteered for EMDR HAP in New Orleans. Dr. Adler-Tapia has extensive training in developmental psychology and working with children 0–3 years of age. Dr. Adler-Tapia has served as clinical director for several nonprofit agencies and is currently in private practice in Tempe, Arizona, and has taught graduate-level classes on counseling and consultation. Dr. Adler-Tapia provides counseling, consultation, and psychological services for children and families referred by Arizona Child Protective Services and works with local police departments providing counseling and CISD services at her private office in Tempe. Dr. Adler-Tapia has provided training internationally on psychotherapy with traumatized children, including specialized trauma treatment with EMDR at several EMDRIA conferences, and she is conducting research on EMDR with young children. With her colleague Carolyn Settle, MSW, LCSW, Dr. Adler-Tapia is coauthor of *EMDR Treatment Manual: Children's Protocol* and has coauthored several studies on EMDR with children.

Carolyn Settle, MSW, LCSW, is EMDRIA certified in EMDR, is an EMDRIA approved consultant, an EMDR Institute Facilitator, and an EMDR HAP trainer-in-training. Carolyn has been an EMDR facilitator for 11 years and has facilitated in Japan, as part of the HAP team in New Orleans, and for the psychiatric residents at the University of Pittsburgh. Carolyn also provides specialty training on EMDR for children and has presented at several EMDRIA conferences and on using EMDR with children at EMDR Europe. Carolyn is a clinical social worker with 30 years of experience working with children. Carolyn specializes in posttraumatic stress disorder, depression, anxiety, phobias, attention-deficit/hyperactivity disorder, and gifted counseling for children, adolescents, and adults in her private practice in Scottsdale, Arizona. Along with her colleague Dr. Adler-Tapia, Ms. Settle has conducted a fidelity study on using EMDR with children under 10 years of age.

EMDR and the Art of Psychotherapy With Children

Robbie Adler-Tapia, PhD
and
Carolyn Settle, MSW, LCSW

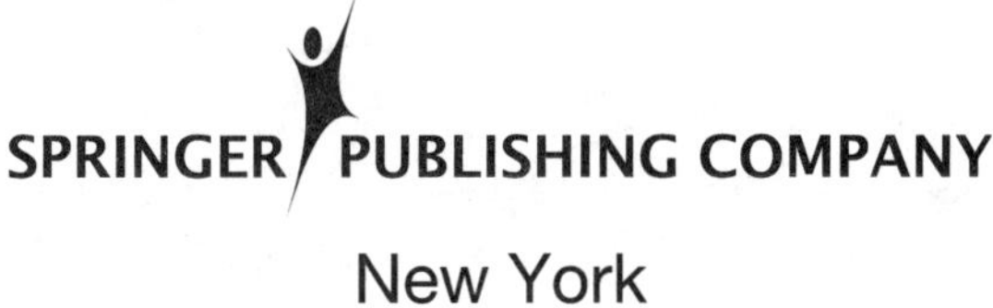
SPRINGER PUBLISHING COMPANY
New York

Springer Publishing Company, LLC
11 West 42nd Street
New York, NY 10036
www.springerpub.com

Acquisitions Editor: Sheri W. Sussman
Production Editor: Julia Rosen
Cover design: Joanne E. Honigman
Composition: Apex CoVantage

08 09 10 11 12/ 5 4 3 2 1

Library of Congress Cataloging-in-Publication Data

Adler-Tapia, Robbie.
EMDR and the art of psychotherapy with children / Robbie Adler-Tapia and Carolyn Settle.
p. ; cm.
Includes bibliographical references and index.
ISBN 978-0-8261-1117-3 (alk. paper)
1. Eye movement desensitization and reprocessing for children. I. Settle, Carolyn. II. Title.
[DNLM: 1. Desensitization, Psychologic—methods. 2. Psychotherapy—methods. 3. Child. 4. Eye Movements. 5. Professional-Patient Relations. 6. Psychotherapeutic Processes. WS 350.6 A237e 2008]

RJ505.E9A35 2008
618.92'8914—dc22 2007052665

Printed in the United States of America by Bang Printing.

This book is dedicated to our husbands—
Hugo Tapia and Ron Smith,

and our children—
Michael, Max, and Maura Tapia
and
Alex and Sara Smith

—our greatest joys, blessings, and accomplishments!

Contents

Foreword

It is an honor to write the foreword to *EMDR and the Art of Psychotherapy With Children*, which can serve as the Gold Standard for EMDR treatment with children and adolescents. The authors, with their combined talents as researchers and skilled mental health practitioners, have crafted procedures with age-appropriate language and modifications for the application of EMDR to young clients incorporating all the phases and steps of Dr. Francine Shapiro's standard protocol and underlying Adaptive Information Processing (AIP) model. They articulately provide an A–Z step-by-step approach for the application of EMDR to specific populations, including complicated cases with highly traumatized children.

The *Treatment Manual* that accompanies the book gives clinicians a clear road map to follow by providing examples and scripts to illustrate all 8 phases of Shapiro's model, forms with detailed instructions to assist in organizing and conceptualizing a case, and detailed procedural steps for applying each phase of EMDR to children.

In addition, Adler-Tapia and Settle have conducted research showing the efficacy of using each step of Shapiro's standard protocol to treat highly traumatized children, and contributed the resultant *EMDR Fidelity Treatment Manual for Children* to the EMDR Humanitarian Assistance Programs (see HAP Store at www.emdrhap.org).

I was fortunate to have met Dr. Shapiro at a time when I was becoming discouraged with how the school system was failing to respond to the emotional needs of so many children who struggled to survive academically and socially in the school environment. With EMDR treatment, children were able to overcome their low self-esteem; control their impulses; modify their behaviors in school; change their relationships with peers, teachers, and family members; organize their lives; and, essentially, change their low opinions of themselves. In each session every child would take one more step (and sometimes several steps at once) up the ladder toward positive growth. Needless to say, I became passionate about the EMDR methodology and its potential for treating children and adolescents.

Over the years, EMDR clinicians have discovered that the range of issues EMDR is able to treat with children is beyond the scope of what had originally been envisioned. Developmentally delayed, autistic, Down Syndrome, and ADHD children respond positively to EMDR. They are able to change their behaviors and beliefs about their self-worth once their fears and confusion are reprocessed. As a therapist, I worked with a developmentally delayed child, age 9, who learned to express herself more appropriately in her special education classroom and overcame her nightly bedwetting habits with EMDR treatment. I also used EMDR to help Ben, a Down Syndrome child, to process the sexual abuse of a nursery school teacher. In a follow-up session, Ben's mother, a trained EMDR therapist, reported to me that Ben would ask her to tap his hands (bilateral stimulation) to calm him when he was frustrated and agitated.

Learning EMDR in 1989 was a pivotal point and peak experience in my professional career. At this time I did not envision the impact EMDR would have on my life and the lives of millions of people around the world. Although I was inspired by the brilliance and creativity of Dr. Francine Shapiro, I underestimated her global intentions and far-reaching visions. To quote one of the EMDR Institute trainers as he was responding to Dr. Shapiro's comments at the conclusion of a trainers' meeting: "You plan to take on the healing of the entire world." To most of us, this seems like an impossible and lofty goal, but the impossible has never deterred Dr. Shapiro from pressing forward in her mission to bring EMDR to the far corners of the world in an attempt to stop the cycle of violence and suffering. Currently, her books have been translated into Italian, French, German, Serbian, Spanish, Flemish, Japanese, Korean, Chinese, Portuguese, and Russian.

Through the assiduous efforts of Dr. Shapiro and many devoted EMDR-trained clinicians, EMDR has become available to families and children in more than 80 countries in the world. EMDR Humanitarian Assistance Programs (HAP) send volunteer training teams, domestically and internationally, to underserved communities and those areas struggling to recover after natural or manmade disasters. The accomplishments of EMDR HAP, documented on their Web site (www.emdrhap.org), show that the power of EMDR goes beyond boundaries of racial and cultural differences. EMDR HAP has been instrumental in bringing together other nongovernmental organizations to collaborate in responding to cataclysmic disasters, and, specifically, organizations that serve children in underdeveloped countries. Not only is Shapiro's vision of global healing being implemented, EMDR is being recognized and utilized by children's hospitals and agencies worldwide.

The success of EMDR treatment with children is supported by research, which the authors have documented in chapter 1. Recently, two

Palestinian clinicians presented at the EMDR European Conference in Paris on their findings: Following initial treatment with EMDR, children showed resiliency when experiencing a second trauma (EMDR Humanitarian Assistance Programs, 2007). The group protocol developed by Jarero, Artigas, and Hartung (2006) for treating children traumatized by natural disasters is being successfully utilized by clinicians who have treated children after experiencing the traumatic effects of floods, plane crashes, hurricanes, earthquakes, displacement, and school shootings (see chapter 1).

Adler-Tapia and Settle in conjunction with EMDR HAP have conducted advanced specialized training in EMDR to clinicians working with children in the Gulf Coast in response to the aftermath of Hurricanes Katrina and Rita. The indefatigable efforts and numerous contributions of these two women are limitless. Their visions are as magnanimous as those of Dr. Shapiro. Their intentions in writing this book are to provide a standardized framework for successfully implementing EMDR with children, to encourage other therapists to use EMDR with children, and to promote the acceptance of EMDR as a psychotherapeutic treatment of choice for young clients. Each chapter emphasizes how to creatively adapt Shapiro's entire EMDR protocol, without eliminating any of the steps, to the treatment of children. Chapter 2 teaches not only how to get started but also outlines an overview of how to adjust the language and presentation of each phase to correspond with the cognitive ability of individual children. They include poignant case examples to demonstrate their teaching points and provide useful scripts to illustrate language appropriate for young clients.

In addition to making a significant contribution to the EMDR literature, the authors have provided a guideline for the basic principles, protocols, and procedures for research and treatment of children with EMDR. All practitioners of EMDR, regardless of the populations they treat, will find valuable information and solutions to challenging cases within the pages of this book. I foresee *EMDR and the Art of Psychotherapy With Children* as the first in a series of books by Adler-Tapia and Settle. Their expertise as clinicians, researchers, and writers warrant future books articulating the use of EMDR with advanced clinical applications.

The authors, with creativity, vitality, and passion, inspire readers to join them in their mission to bring EMDR treatment to the multitude of traumatized children regardless of their economic or cultural backgrounds.

Ultimately, the healing of one generation of children will impact the behavior and actions of future generations.

Robbie Dunton, MS
Coordinator, EMDR Institute

Preface

CAN WE LEARN TO USE EMDR WITH CHILDREN?

Why Not?

In 2000, I (R.T.) attended my first Part 1 EMDR training in Phoenix, where I listened to Dr. Sandra Wilson discuss using EMDR to treat traumatized children to expedite their healing. As a psychologist specializing in treating traumatized children, I was intrigued and thought of all the children in my practice that could benefit from EMDR. However, when I returned to my office, I struggled to find ways to implement the EMDR protocol with my child clients. Young children didn't understand the words of the EMDR protocol, and I needed to translate the protocol to try to make it work effectively. Even after searching the literature on EMDR with children, I still found that applying EMDR was challenging and frustrating for me as a psychotherapist. After a year, I decided to take the Part 2 training in EMDR, hoping that I would learn to more effectively use EMDR with children. Even after completing Part 2 training, I found that integrating EMDR into my clinical work with children and their families was problematic. My initial experience of trying to learn to use EMDR with children was so frustrating that I almost gave up trying to use it. I felt like the training that I had with EMDR left me unprepared to use EMDR with my child clients. I searched the literature on EMDR with children and was confused about how to use EMDR with children because what I read seemed to imply that the younger the child, the more the therapist omitted parts of the protocol. I also asked myself, "How many pieces of the protocol needed to be included to continue to call the treatment EMDR?"

How Can This Work?

This was the incredulous question I (C.S.) had in my mind as I started using EMDR. I'm really a skeptic, and EMDR was counterintuitive to my previous training in psychotherapy, but I kept getting good results.

Even so, I hesitated in completing the Part 2 training for 2 years. During those 2 years, I was using EMDR and making mistakes and trying things out and still getting pretty impressive results. I learned a lot, and it also made me realize the robustness of the EMDR treatment protocol. So by the time I completed the Part 2 training, I really learned the protocol the right way, and that's when my results became even more impressive. With precision and practice, I was using EMDR with kids with the whole eight phases. My mistakes were my best teachers, and even though I made mistakes with the protocol, the children still got better.

Tapping a Greater Expertise in the EMDR Community

The EMDR training manuals include a list of local EMDR facilitators with special training. In a quest for direction in effectively using EMDR with children, I (R.T.) sought direction and support through a free EMDR study group offered by certified consultants in the local EMDR community. I was excited to find that Carolyn Settle, MSW, LCSW, and Beverlee Laidlaw-Chasse, LPC, were not only using EMDR with children, but insisted that all eight phases of EMDR could be successfully implemented with even young children. With their support and direction, I gained confidence with using EMDR in my practice.

Soon after, I decided to attend the EMDRIA Conference in Denver to advance my skills with EMDR. Carolyn Settle and I met again at the EMDRIA Conference in Denver and discussed our passion for working with children. I also met another Arizona EMDRIA-approved consultant, Laurie Tetreault, who listened supportively to my excitement about using EMDR with children. She encouraged me to pursue my dream of having EMDR treatment available to all children.

After the conference, I decided to participate in an EMDR certification group with Carolyn and Beverlee. Through this group process I gained insight and confidence in using EMDR. Carolyn and I talked about how she had been trained in EMDR and began using the full protocol with children immediately, with tremendous results. Carolyn's ability to explain EMDR in very pragmatic terms was pivotal in my pursuit of expertise with EMDR. Carolyn's work with EMDR as a clinician and teacher has had an impact on many fledgling EMDR practitioners, and especially on me; therefore I was delighted when Carolyn agreed to collaborate with me on a research study on using EMDR with young children.

This Story Is Much More Interesting Than You Could Ever Possibly Imagine

Life is certainly more intriguing than fiction. That being said, it was exciting to meet Robbie, someone who was as interested in working with children as I (C.S.) was, and we were both curious about using the 8 phases with children. Robbie came to one of my study groups and discussed her pursuit of a research project. I was fascinated by her experience in doing research because that was something I was always interested in doing. At first, I thought I was just going to be doing research at the library and helping with the literature review, but in reality, it turned out to be an enriching and surprising adventure as well.

The Authors' Adventures

We began meeting to discuss the use of EMDR with young children and the process of conducting a fidelity study on EMDR with children. Since we started this adventure 3 years ago, we have spent hours talking about the use of EMDR with children and consulting about particular challenges in using EMDR with severely traumatized children. We have also met amazing clinicians who have shared their successes and challenges with EMDR. We have received incredible support and been given many opportunities from Francine Shapiro, Robbie Dunton, Andrew Leeds, Laurie Tetreault, and many others in the EMDR community.

THE VOICES OF THE BOOK

This book was written primarily in the voices of the two authors, Robbie Adler-Tapia and Carolyn Settle, who are practicing therapists, lecturers, and researchers writing about how we work with children and capturing how we think, play with, and treat children in a multifaceted and complex process. Sometimes words in black-and-white print lack the gestalt of the therapy. How do we capture our process and infuse this into the written word? Our task was to write about what we do with voices that carry context and tone, inflection and emotion with our entire selves that convey our passion for helping children. Making the words come alive with color, action, and emotion to help therapists experience what it is to use EMDR with children motivated our writing throughout this book.

Capturing and integrating the richness and diversity of the voices of therapists we have met in study groups, in consultation, and while facilitating during EMDR training sessions has also guided our descriptions of practicing EMDR. Incorporating what we have learned from training therapists to adhere to the EMDR protocol during our fidelity research study, and what we in turn gained from them, is also integrated into this book. Our experiences as practicing clinicians, and what we have realized from even our youngest clients, make up the richness of description from the voices of the children we have been honored to treat. To better illuminate some of our work, the children's stories are integrated into the case studies we discuss throughout the book. When we struggle with explaining what we actually do in our offices, we return to the children's stories.

Because we are at times one voice, and other times, we have different perspectives and cases, when we use the word *I,* we have identified which one of us is speaking by adding our initials (R.T. or C.S.) to provide clarification. We also use the terms *parent* and *caregiver* interchangeably throughout the book to refer to the child's primary caregiver. We use the word *child* and *client* interchangeably as well. Even though this book is written to instruct therapists on EMDR with children, most of the techniques and skills can be used with adult clients as well. Many therapists will say, "I only work with adults." We would encourage you to consider that when you work with adult clients, you are working with that client's entire set of life experiences and that, sometimes, the client's experience is from a child's perspective. No matter what the age of your client, we are many times working with maladaptively stored information that originated early in the client's life and thus is driven by a child's perspective.

WHY WRITE THIS BOOK?

As we began talking with each other and then providing training and consultation on EMDR, we found that we were trying to explain what we do in EMDR therapy with children, and we were often repeating what we had said many times before. Because we provided training at the EMDRIA conferences, advanced training on EMDR with children, and consultation with other professionals both together and individually, we wanted to have a tool to organize and guide therapists that was not yet available. Our goal with this book is to create a commonsense, written guide to provide support and direction for therapists to successfully use EMDR after completing basic training in EMDR.

We have also written a treatment manual that includes the protocols, scripts, and forms therapists will need to use EMDR in psychotherapy with children. The treatment manual, titled *EMDR and the Art of Psychotherapy With Children Treatment Manual,* can be purchased in addition to this book. The forms in the *Manual* are available to all purchasers. Please go to www.springerpub.com/adlerforms. After you download the file, you can access the forms by entering the password ADLER1.

Both this book and the accompanying treatment manual were written for two purposes. First, the book is focused on providing advanced training and support for therapists to be successful in using EMDR with child clients. We have written about the specific tools necessary for the therapist to implement the entire EMDR protocol and procedural steps in psychotherapy with children. This is taken from our professional experiences with our child clients and from the discussions in our EMDR study groups and research group. The second goal of this book is to document a standardized protocol for using EMDR with children for training and research purposes. This book includes a standard EMDR protocol for treating children, which is consistent with the eight phases of EMDR translated into children's language. By using the treatment manual, therapists have a convenient text to assist in practicing the EMDR protocol with young children in psychotherapy. With these two goals, in the following chapters, we will not only provide advanced training for therapists, but the framework for future studies on EMDR with children.

ORGANIZATION OF THE CHAPTERS

This book begins with a review of Adaptive Information Processing theory applied to EMDR with children and an abbreviated review of research on using EMDR with child clients. The second chapter explains how to get started using EMDR, before describing the steps in the EMDR protocol in case conceptualization with child clients. Chapters 3–9 explain the goals for the specific phases of the EMDR protocol, with directions for each session, instructions for the therapist, and finally, a script for therapists to use with child clients. Additional chapters describe advanced skills for using EMDR with special populations and innovative solutions to particular challenges with the EMDR protocol. This book will provide the assistance that therapists need to feel confident in learning to use EMDR successfully with young children.

Because this book was written to assist therapists in transitioning from training in EMDR to the actual implementation of EMDR with clients, we decided to organize chapters in a manner consistent with basic training and then bridge to detailed steps of how to really use EMDR. We have expanded the basic training in several directions. First, we have translated the EMDR standard protocol that is used for adults to effectively use with children. Second, the book instructs therapists on possible procedural considerations and clinical implications for decisions at each stage of the process. The chapters include subheadings of *procedural considerations* and *clinical implications,* where therapists are given options for deciding how to proceed with the EMDR protocol. Procedural consideration headings detail how therapists progress through the protocol, with recommendations for clinical decision making at different junctures in treatment. The clinical implication subheadings explore possible results arising from decisions made during the course of using the EMDR protocol. Finally, we have included case studies of EMDR with children; however, each child has been disguised in a manner that no case study represents the details of any individual child. We have included one complete transcript of an EMDR session with a 3-year-old, and his parents have consented for the transcript to be included in the book. We have also included pictures drawn by children, and we have parental consent for the drawings as well.

Even though this book is focused on specific skills for using EMDR with young children, many of the techniques are also effective with adolescent and adult clients as well. We use the word "client" to refer to tools for all clients and "child" to focus on tools specific to child clients.

We especially want to encourage practitioners to understand that the entire EMDR protocol can be used with child clients when therapists learn how to translate the protocol into both the verbal and nonverbal language of children. To do so, we wrote specific scripts for each piece of the protocol. Once therapists have acquired the confidence to use the entire protocol with young children, we then apply more advanced skills for clients with more complicated clinical presentations. These advanced skills do not deviate from the protocol but instead add specific tools for working with the specific symptom set.

Finally, the book includes specific language used in conducting EMDR therapy with children in the office. By having a manual, we provide a template for consistency across therapists using EMDR with children to standardize practice and document fidelity to the protocol. In this way, when a therapist says, "I am using EMDR with children," we are all speaking the same language. This is not to imply a rigid process but instead that there are common elements to EMDR that need to also be used with child clients. By establishing a common language and protocol for EMDR with children, we have a framework for both practice and research.

We have a dream that this book will not only provide the foundation to support therapists using EMDR with young children but also contribute to a paradigm shift in clinical work with children. We believe that one day, the mental health community will focus on providing more psychotherapy for children based on research that supports EMDR as evidence-based practice to decrease the use of psychotropic medications with children. Future studies on EMDR with children need to compare treatment with EMDR to treatment with psychotropic medications.

We hope to give each therapist a comprehensive framework to use EMDR in psychotherapy with children of all ages. We believe that someday, EMDR with children will be part of a standard of care in treatment to change the trajectory of the lives of many children toward a positive future for us all.

Acknowledgments

The authors are grateful to Dr. Francine Shapiro, Robbie Dunton, and Dr. Andrew Leeds for guidance and expert commentary on the information included in our research and in this book. We are also indebted to Dr. Kim Johnson for her tireless assistance and critical feedback in editing, and we want to thank Dr. David MacKinnon for his expertise in research methodology and humor in guiding us through our learning curve.

In addition, the authors are appreciative of the research therapists from Childhelp, including Dr. Bradley Crawford, Ana Gomez, Dr. Stephanie Vitanza, Jessica Whitacker, Mary Ducharme, Dr. Shefali Ghandi, Dr. Mario Lippy, and Amber Willocks, for dedication to the children and this study. The authors are greatly indebted to the staff, children, and families of Childhelp, and especially Mr. William Copeland, who advocated for the opportunity to conduct our study. We would like to thank the professionals who spent endless hours rating videotapes for adherence to the EMDR protocol, including Laurie Tetreault, Dr. Jonathon Brooks, Peggy Moore, Alicia Outcault, Dr. Shelley Uram, and Rosario Romero.

To our colleagues, Dr. Kim Johnson and Carol Kibbee, our thanks for their contributions of case studies.

And to our senior editor, Sheri W. Sussman, our appreciation for her guidance and support of two rookie authors.

Finally, we want to thank both our husbands and families for their support and patience, technical assistance, and hours of errands and housekeeping as we pursued this project. To Dr. Hugo Tapia and Michael, Max, and Maura Tapia, and Ron, Alex, and Sara Smith, for their love, support, and understanding, we love you all!

CHAPTER 1

Theoretical Underpinnings and Research on EMDR With Children

This book is based on the Eye Movement Desensitization and Reprocessing (EMDR) psychotherapy treatment methodology, as created by Francine Shapiro (1989a, 1989b) and the EMDR training program (Shapiro, 2007). EMDR is a comprehensive treatment approach that is based on the Adaptive Information Processing (AIP) theory. After reading Dr. Shapiro's books and completing basic training in EMDR, the professional is ready to return to the office and begin using EMDR with clients.

BASIC TRAINING IN EMDR

Prior to 2008, training in EMDR consisted of two parts before a psychotherapist completed the introductory training in EMDR. During this two-part training process, EMDR with children was offered as an overview, with recommendations for therapists to pursue advanced training. With this abbreviated training in EMDR with children, therapists returned to their offices to attempt to use EMDR with child clients. This is a daunting task, with little guidance and support for therapists to integrate EMDR into their clinical work with children.

Currently, basic training in EMDR consists of the therapist participating in two weekends of training and 10 hours of consultation regarding the use of EMDR in clinical practice. Both weekends include a brief overview of using EMDR with children; however, therapists who are interested in more in-depth understanding of EMDR with children now need to attend advanced training programs (Adler-Tapia & Settle, 2008).

Basic training in EMDR also includes discussion of the AIP theory that is the foundation for the EMDR treatment methodology.

ADAPTIVE INFORMATION PROCESSING AND EMDR IN CHILD PSYCHOTHERAPY

A comprehensive theory of psychotherapy with children needs to include an explanation of human development (along with hypotheses of how humans grow, learn, change, interact, and relate) as well as how psychopathology occurs. Throughout history, writers have attempted to explain the phases of human development, including cognitive, psychosocial, and psychological development, and at times, these theories have led to the development of models of psychotherapy. Yet many theories of human development have stopped short of explaining the development of psychopathology, much less creating treatment modalities for addressing when human development skews. For example, Piaget created a theory of cognitive development but did not expand his theory to explain how cognitive development goes awry or how cognitive development impacts mental health in children. In spite of the extensive work on human development, the majority of the models of psychopathology and psychotherapy are adult models.

Shapiro (2001) developed the AIP model to explain the mechanisms by which EMDR assists clients in moving disturbance to adaptive resolution. EMDR is a comprehensive treatment methodology, while AIP is the comprehensive theoretical approach to psychotherapy. In the AIP model, Shapiro theorized that the human organism is hard-wired to assimilate new information and to move to adaptive resolution when presented with experiences causing high arousal. In the event that the level of arousal is overwhelming and traumatic to the individual, the AIP progression is thwarted, and healthy processing does not continue. Instead, the event is stored with all the sensations and perceptions that the individual experienced at the time of the event. When the traumatic event is stored in its original form because the information processing system was not able to process the overwhelming event, that event does not continue processing through to adaptive resolution. With *trauma* defined as anything that negatively impacts the psyche, the event that is experienced as traumatic by the individual remains and continues to affect the individual's functioning. When a traumatic event occurs, the individual continues through life with dysfunctionally stored material manifesting in current symptomatology. The etiological event thus prevents the individual's natural healing process from functioning at full potential. With children, this traumatic event can also impact neurological development and all future experiences in the child's life. What experiences the child engages in or avoids is impacted by those previous life experiences.

The AIP model (Shapiro, 2001) concludes that emotional, behavioral, and mental health symptoms originate from the maladaptive storage of previous life events. In the future, as those stored experiences are activated, the client experiences disturbances and dysfunction in his or her current life.

For example, I (R.T.) treated a 5-year-old girl with moderate mental retardation who was nonverbal and medically fragile. This child had incurred many intrusive and painful medical procedures; therefore, each time she entered a doctor's office and saw a needle, she would faint. At times, the child would faint and experience additional injuries. This child also lived in a home with a family member with diabetes, and the family member regularly used insulin injections. The child would faint each time she saw a needle, an empty needle box, or anything remotely associated with needles. The parents brought the child for psychotherapy to address the child's fear of needles and medical care in general because the child needed ongoing medical interventions to stabilize her health. Physiologically, this child's system identified needles as threatening and as signifying that she was in danger, even though the needles had been used on many occasions to save the child's life. As the therapist (I) used EMDR to treat the fear of needles and medical procedures so that the child would be safe and be able to access the needed medical care with minimal further traumatization. The child's AIP system was accessed through EMDR, and the EMDR treatment process desensitized the child's association of needles and medical care as life threatening.

How does this occur? The AIP model proposes that the brain processes trauma much like the body processes physical injury. The physiological processing of injury occurs when the body automatically searches for the mechanisms for healing. The body continues with this healing process unless there is interference to the healing process such as infection or foreign bodies preventing healing. Under these circumstances, the natural healing process is thwarted. The natural healing process then requires intervention to resume the process of healing.

Shapiro (1989a, 1989b) devised a therapeutic process by which the therapist guides the client through a series of procedural steps to access the maladaptively stored information. By accessing those memory networks, the EMDR protocol focuses on reprocessing the accessed information so that the client can proceed with the healing process.

Because AIP theory postulates that the information must be accessed, stimulated, and then moved toward adaptive resolution (Shapiro, 2007), the client must be able to access and communicate this information, which is often difficult for children because children have not developed sufficient emotional literacy to report the experience to the therapist. Because children are at different stages developmentally, therapists must assess development in the client prior to proceeding with the EMDR protocol. The therapist then adjusts the EMDR protocol to meet the developmental needs of the client. Children often store memories in sensory/motor format, and therefore children may not have a coherent narrative to describe to the therapists; however, children can report sensations that arise when neuronetworks are probed. This is when the use of play therapy and art therapy techniques are indicated to facilitate the treatment process.

AIP theory concludes that memories are a combination of sensory input, thoughts, emotions, physical sensations, and a belief system but may actually have metacognitions instead. *Metacognitions* are the ability to have cognitions about cognitions, or the ability to think about thinking. Children have not fully developed a belief system with which to understand and process an event or experience because children have not yet developed cognitively to the point where they are able to think about their own thought processes; therefore accessing and processing of neuronetworks is different. In spite of the fact that children have not developed the same cognitive processes and do not have as expansive language skills as adolescents and adults, the AIP model still explains personality development as well as the development of dysfunction and pathology in children.

If, according to AIP, the assimilation of events into the associative memory network and accommodations of the client's previous identity to encompass it can be considered the basis of personality development (Shapiro, 2007), the earlier the intervention, the more positive the impact on the personality and the individual's overall health. AIP suggests that for individuals with extensive abuse and neglect histories, this learning and adaptive resolution cannot take place because they have insufficient internal resources and positive experiences to transform the initial dysfunction. When working with children in psychotherapy, the therapist also has a unique opportunity to provide opportunities for developing internal resources and positive experiences through resource development and mastery skills as part of the EMDR process.

ASSESSING THE LITERATURE ON EMDR WITH CHILDREN

When we began our pursuit of EMDR research with children, we found that the majority of publications that focused on EMDR with children suggested significant modifications to the eight phases of EMDR, if not eliminating steps in the protocol completely. The books on EMDR with children suggested that modifications to the eight phases of the protocol were necessary to treat children (Greenwald, 1999; Lovett, 1999; Tinker & Wilson, 1999). One of the only outcome research studies on EMDR with children, by Chemtob, Nakashima, and Carlson (2002), suggested that EMDR was successful with children. Yet what we read suggested that the younger the child client, the more steps in the protocol were eliminated, therefore decreasing adherence to the eight phases of EMDR. How could it be that we both thought we were using all eight phases of the EMDR protocol, yet there was no written documentation to support our clinical experiences?

We wondered about what conclusions we could then draw from the training and publications we reviewed on using EMDR with children. Was it really true that fidelity to the EMDR protocol was not possible with children, especially those under 10 years of age? Or was it that with more advanced training and support, therapists could find just as much success with EMDR with child clients as was being reported with adult clients? With this question in mind, we set out to document what we were finding in our clinical practices with even the youngest and most severely abused clients.

RESEARCH ON EMDR

The research on EMDR with adults is extensive, and because of that, EMDR is considered best practice for treating adults with posttraumatic stress disorder (PTSD). Unfortunately, the same body of research currently does not exist for treating children with EMDR. Since Shapiro (1989, 1995) introduced EMDR in 1987, a significant body of research has developed to support the efficacy of using EMDR as a treatment for PTSD with adult clients. The American Psychiatric Association (2004) and the U.S. Department of Veterans Affairs and U.S. Department of Defense (2004) endorsed EMDR as one of the treatments of choice for adult patients with PTSD. The National Institute of Mental Health has also endorsed EMDR as an effective form of therapy for trauma. In addition to the support of professional organizations, there is a substantial body of research that demonstrates the efficacy of using EMDR with adults; however, EMDR as a treatment of choice for adolescents, and especially children, has not been sufficiently documented.

RESEARCH ON EMDR IN PSYCHOTHERAPY WITH CHILDREN

In contrast to the research on EMDR with adult clients, published studies documenting the efficacy of EMDR with young children is limited. Research is necessary to establish EMDR for children as evidence-based practice. As shown in Tables 1.1 and 1.2, 16 studies have reported using the EMDR treatment protocol with children and adolescents (Ahmad, Larsson, & Sundelin-Wahlsten, 2007; Chemtob, Nakashima, & Carlson, 2002; Cocco & Sharpe, 1993; Fernandez, Gallinari, & Lorenzetti, 2004; Greenwald, 1994; Jaberghaderi, Greenwald, Rubin, Dolatabadim, & Zand, 2002; Jarero, Artigas, & Hartung, 2006; Korkmazlar-Oral & Pamuk, 2002; Muris, Merckelbach, Holdrinet, & Sijsenaar, 1998; Oras, Cancela De Ezpeleta, & Ahmad, 2004; Puffer, Greenwald, & Elrod, 1997; Rubin et al., 2001; Soberman, Greenwald, & Rule, 2002; Tufnell, 2005; Wilson, Tinker, Hofmann, Becker, & Marshall, 2000; Zaghrout-Hodali, Alissa, Dodgson, in press). These studies include the implementation of both individual and group protocols with child subjects.

EMDR Individual Studies With Children

Studies published on the use of EMDR in individual psychotherapy with children (Table 1.1) include single case designs, controlled studies, and comparative studies. Although these studies have analyzed the efficacy of EMDR with children and adolescents, of the 11 studies of individual EMDR treatment of children, a total of 162 children of the 216 children included in the research studies were provided a range of 1–12 sessions of EMDR. Eleven of the studies reported the use of less than six sessions of EMDR (mean 3.1 sessions per child) with only the Jaberghaderi and colleagues (2002) study reporting up to 12 sessions of EMDR; however, in this study, the EMDR treatment group of seven girls received eight or less sessions of EMDR (mean 6.1 sessions per child). The children in the studies ranged in age from 4 to 17 years. The EMDR treatment reported in all 12 studies ranged from 0.5 to 1 hour sessions provided by Part 2–trained therapists in all but three of the studies where the therapists had only Part 1 training.

Of the 11 published studies on individual EMDR treatment with children, six were controlled studies (Ahmad et al., 2007; Jaberghaderi et al., 2002; Muris et al., 1998; Puffer, Greenwald, & Elrod, 1997; Rubin et al.,

TABLE 1.1 Studies of Individual Treatment of EMDR With Children

Year of study	Studies	Number of subjects	Subject age range	Setting	Pre/Post-measures	Fidelity assessed	Tx manual used	Total EMDR sessions	Post-tx follow-up	Findings	Therapist training
2007	Ahmad et al. Controlled study EMDR vs. WLC for children diagnosed with PTSD	33 17 EMDR tx group 16 WLC	6–16 years	Child psychiatric outpatient clinic for traumatized children	25	No	Yes with "child adjusted steps."	8 sessions of EMDR (Range 1–8 sessions of EMDR, mean 5.9)	2 months after completing treating	Children in EMDR tx improved on re-experiencing symptoms	No information
2002	Chembtob et al. Brief therapy with disaster-related PTSD	32	6–12 years	School	1, 2, 3, 4, 5, 6	Yes	No (written step-by-step protocol)	3 EMDR	6 months	Substantial sustained improvement	4 PhD clinicians, 2 with PI EMDR training, 2 with PII
1993	Cocco & Sharpe Case study using auditory variant of EMDR	1	4 years, 9 months	Office	7, 8, 9	No	No	1 EMDR	1 month, 6 months	Both symptoms and behavior changed	No information
1994	Greenwald 5 case studies of treatment of traumatized children	5	4–11 years	Office	10, 11	No	No (child EMDR technical manual)	1–2 EMDR	1 week and 4 weeks	Substantial sustained improvement	1 PII trained PhD

(*continued*)

TABLE 1.1 Studies of Individual Treatment of EMDR With Children (continued)

Year of study	Studies	Number of subjects	Subject age range	Setting	Pre/Post-measures	Fidelity assessed	Tx manual used	Total EMDR sessions	Post-tx follow-up	Findings	Therapist training
2002	Jaberghaderi et al. CBT vs. EMDR for sexually abused Iranian girls	147 EMDR 7 CBT	12–13 years	University	12, 13	No	No	Up to 12 sessions of EMDR or CBT (mean 6.1)	2 weeks	A decrease in PTSD symptoms	1 psychologist PII trained
1998	Muris et al. EMDR vs. exposure therapy in spider phobias	26	8–17 years	University	14, 15, 16, 17	No	No	1 session of EMDR, in vivo exposure or computerized exposure	Timeline not reported	No significance	1 PII EMDR therapist, 1 behavioral therapist
2004	Oras et al. Traumatized refugee children treated with EMDR in psychodynamic approach	13	8–16 years	University hospital	24, 25	No	No	Range 1–6 sessions of EMDR	Timeline not reported	Significant improvement in functioning and PTSD symptoms, especially in re-experiencing	1 PhD, EMDR training not noted
1997	Puffer et al. Single session EMDR study with traumatized children	20	8–17 years	Office	18, 19, 20	No	No	1	1 week and 1–3 months	Significance on IES; less significant on CMAS	1 limited-licensed psychologist with PI training

Year of study	Studies	Number of subjects	Subject age range	Setting	Pre/Post-measures	Fidelity assessed	Tx manual used	Total EMDR sessions	Post-tx follow-up	Findings	Therapist training
2001	Rubin et al. Effectiveness of EMDR in Child Guidance Center	39 (TOTAL); 23 EMDR 16 No EMDR	6–15 years	Guidance center	7	Yes	No	5	6 months	No significance	8 MSWs, 3 MA psychologists, 1 PhD—all PII trained
2002	Soberman et al. Boys with conduct problems	29 boys 14 Standard of care plus 3 sessions EMDR 15 control	10–16 years	Residential treatment facility or day treatment facility at same facility	21, 22	No	No	3	2 months	Less distress, decreased PTSD symptoms, large reduction in behavior problems	1 Pre-doc intern, PII trained and used 100 sessions of EMDR
2005	Tufnell Case studies of PTSD	4	4–11 years	Mental health center	23	No	No	Range 2–4	6 months	PTSD symptoms resolved, results maintained	Child psychiatrist and psychotherapist—both PII trained

Pre- and post-measures key: (1) Kauai Recovery Inventory; (2) Child Reaction Index; (3) Revised Children's Manifest Anxiety Scale; (4) Child Depression Inventory; (5) Visits to school nurse; (6) Child Ratings of Helpfulness; (7) Achenbach Child Behavior Checklist Form; (8) Thought Problem Subscale; (9) Parent monitor; (10) Parent interview; (11) Problem Rating Scale; (12) PTSD symptom interview; (13) Problem behavior assessed; (14) DISC-R interview; (15) Spider Phobia Questionnaire; (16) Self-Assessment Manikin; (17) Behavior Avoidance Test; (18) Children's Manifest Anxiety Scale; (19) Impact of Events Scale (IES); (20) Subjective Units of Disturbance (SUD), Validity of Cognition (VOC); (21) Child/Parent Report of Post-Traumatic Symptoms (CROPS/PROPS); (22) Trauma Symptom Checklist for Children (TSCC); (23) Therapist Interview; (24) Post-Traumatic Stress Symptoms Scale for Children (PTSS-C); (25) Global Assessment of Functioning (GAF).

TABLE 1.2 Studies of EMDR Group Protocol With Child Clients

Year of study	Studies	Number of subjects	Subject age range	Setting	Pre/Post-measures	Fidelity assessed	Tx manual used	Total EMDR sessions	Post-tx follow-up	Findings	Therapist training
2003	Fernandez et al. Group protocol with elementary school treatment for disaster trauma	236	6–11 years	Italy School	1	No	No	2 psycho-educational groups using butterfly hugs	30 days & 4 months	Call from teacher, all but 2 had no symptoms at 30 days	3 PII trained PhDs
2006	Jarero et al. Group protocol with children who experienced a flood in their hometown	44 22 girls 22 boys	8–15 years	Pedras Negras, Mexico Temporary Shelters	2, 3	No	No	Two 50–60 minute groups	4 weeks	Significant decrease in CRTES scores and SUDS scores	1 lead therapist and emotional protection team (EPT)
2002	Korkmazlar-Oral & Pamuk Group EMDR with child survivors of earthquake in Turkey	16 13 girls 3 boys	10–11 years	Tent city in Adapazari	None	No	No	3.5 hours total for all activities of EMDR plus other activities	None	Children evidenced reduced SUDS	2 therapists Training not noted

Year of study	Studies	Number of subjects	Subject age range	Setting	Pre/Post-measures	Fidelity assessed	Tx manual used	Total EMDR sessions	Post-tx follow-up	Findings	Therapist training
2000	Wilson et al. EMDR group protocol with children in Kosovar-Albanian Refugee Camp	2 groups	17 6–10 years, 9 11–13 years	Refugee camp, Hemar, Germany	4, 5	No	Butterfly Hug Protocol	Each group received 2 hours on 3 consecutive days for total of 6 hours	Younger group 1 month and 1 week pre; 1 week and 2 months post		2 PhD EMDR facilitators
In press	Zaghrout-Hodali et al. Group EMDR with children in who experienced a shooting	7 3 girls 4 boys	8–12 years	Aida refugee camp in Bethlehem, Israel	SUDS Parent report	No	Butterfly Hug Protocol (Wilson et al., 2000)	5 total sessions: 4 group sessions; 1 follow-up session	5 months	SUD reduced to 0–1 per child report Parent report symptom reduction	2 therapists Training not noted

Pre- and post-measures key: (1) Teachers' pre- and post-behavioral observations; (2) Child Reaction to Traumatic Events Scale (CRTES); (3) Simplified Impact of Events Scale; (4) Saigh Children's PTSD Inventory Measure; (5) Children's Brief Psychiatric Rating Scale.

2001; Chembtob, Nakashima, & Carlson, 2002). Of the six studies, five were comparative studies of EMDR versus other methods of psychotherapeutic treatment for children or wait list control (Ahmad et al., 2007), and one study (Chemtob et al., 2002) used a randomized lagged group design to specifically treat children with posttraumatic symptoms.

EMDR Group Studies With Children

Five published studies (Fernandez et al., 2004; Jarero et al., 2006; Korkmazlar-Oral & Pamuk, 2002; Wilson et al., 2000; Zaghrout-Hodali et al., in press) have documented field studies on the use of the EMDR Group Protocol with children who had experienced a shared traumatic event due to either a manmade or natural disaster (Table 1.2). The EMDR Group Protocol or the Butterfly Hug Protocol was created by Jarero and colleagues (1999) to treat groups of children sharing a common traumatic event. Due to the need for trauma treatment during disaster situations with high numbers of victims and limited resources, the EMDR Group Protocol has been studied in the field as therapists have attempted to aid victims and reduce the impact of trauma especially on groups of children who have experienced the same natural or manmade disaster situation and/or shared a traumatic event. The field studies that have been conducted have occurred internationally in disaster areas where resources are limited and there are many child victims. In the five published studies of the EMDR group protocol with children, 342 children participated in one to six group sessions lasting from 50 minutes to 3.5 hours. Outcome measures and posttreatment follow-up assessments from these studies note that children have reduced symptoms and show resilience (Zaghrout-Hodali et al., in press).

As of the publication of this book, the 16 studies on EMDR with children suggest that EMDR with children is promising practice.

As with any treatment modality, the efficacy of the treatment intervention must be supported by research to justify the treatment modality as best practice. The 16 studies on EMDR with children suggest that EMDR is a promising practice in psychotherapy with children; however, the robustness of the methodology in these studies has come under scrutiny. Because of this, we have struggled to get EMDR authorized for children and have had grant applications denied. Not only is it difficult to get services authorized for children, but even when services are authorized, there are not many therapists trained to use EMDR with children. Many clinicians experience frustration and even abandon the use of EMDR because they lack confidence and support in successfully integrating EMDR with children into their clinical work. This is a travesty. But how do two clinicians convince the professional community that EMDR should be the treatment of choice for traumatized children?

Our First Research Study

Why would two clinicians pursue research? We have often asked ourselves this question. Ultimately, the reason we started using EMDR with children and why we are conducting research on EMDR with children is simple: We want EMDR to be available to all children. We began a fidelity research study at Childhelp (a national nonprofit for children who are victims of crime) and provided biweekly consultation for the therapists at Childhelp who were using EMDR with children. This research consultation group identified many training and clinical variables necessary to improve therapists' success in maintaining fidelity to the EMDR protocol in psychotherapy with young children. These findings are necessary in supporting and guiding therapists in using EMDR with even the youngest clients. The following conclusions are taken from the clinical experiences of the researchers, individual consultation with therapists who participated in the study, review of videotapes of therapy sessions, and documentation from research consultation group meetings.

Themes That Arose From the Qualitative Data. From this qualitative data, eight overarching themes emerged regarding using EMDR with children aged 2–10 years. Of these themes, five will be discussed including therapist-specific variables; variables specific to the unique characteristics of the individual child; variables specific to EMDR treatment with children; variables related to the treatment environment, including the therapist's office; and variables related to the parents of child clients and the home environment.

The following discussion will describe the initial conclusions about the variables that affected the therapists' ability to demonstrate fidelity to the EMDR protocol.

Therapist-Specific Variables. Therapist-specific variables include training and experience in working with young children; knowledge of child development; training and experience with using the EMDR protocol; confidence in the efficacy of EMDR; patience and creativity in teasing out the pieces of the EMDR protocol; and skill at developing rapport and attunement with the client.

In this study, all the therapists had at least Part-2 training in EMDR and had participated in biweekly consultation groups with feedback from Eye Movement Desensitization and Reprocessing International Association (EMDRIA)-Approved Consultants in EMDR. The consultants reviewed tapes and responded to questions from therapists regarding fidelity. Responses from the therapists were documented by the researchers and included in this study.

Therapists experienced in treating young children with training in child development and play therapy found it easier to adhere to the EMDR protocol with young children.

In addition to training and experience working with young children, therapists needed training in EMDR and experience using the eight-phase EMDR protocol. After Part 1 training in EMDR, therapists can practice using the EMDR protocol with children with minor traumas (Shapiro, 2001); however, the therapists in this study who were Part 2 trained struggled to use EMDR with highly traumatized children without additional consultation, training, encouragement, and experience. As therapists in the study practiced using the EMDR protocol, therapists reported greater success adhering to the EMDR protocol.

In a study on the effectiveness of EMDR with adult clients, Edmond, Sloan, and McCarty (2004) reported that "one of the therapists was positively biased toward the method, one was extremely skeptical to the point of being negatively biased against the method and the other two therapists were viewed as neutral" (p. 262). Therapists' bias toward the EMDR methodology also was evident in the data collected from research group meetings at Childhelp. The therapists' bias toward the EMDR methodology strongly contributed to the therapists' willingness to use EMDR with children. Therapists with a positive bias to EMDR were more likely to incorporate play therapy, art therapy, and other nondirective techniques in using EMDR with young children. Therapists who had been using play therapy, art therapy, and other nondirective therapeutic techniques prior to being trained in EMDR presented with a neutral or more cautious use of EMDR with children. This made it more difficult for some therapists to transition to the more directive procedures included in the EMDR protocol. However, when therapists used play therapy, art therapy, and child therapy techniques to elicit aspects of the EMDR procedural steps, therapists became more easily acclimated and then reported greater success in eliciting all phases of the protocol.

In addition, fidelity to the protocol was significantly affected by the therapists' confidence in their own clinical skills in treating young children, along with the therapists' confidence in their own skills adhering to the EMDR protocol. The most effective therapists had excellent clinical skills, especially with young children, had in-depth understanding of child development, and felt confident using the EMDR protocol. Therapists who read from the manual when they were first learning the EMDR protocol struggled to use the manual in therapy sessions. Once the therapist gained confidence in his or her own skills at using the EMDR protocol and knew the protocol without using the treatment manual, the therapist had greater opportunity to use play therapy, art therapy techniques, and creative tools in eliciting the steps of the EMDR protocol with young children. Discussion of the specific techniques and tools therapists created to elicit the steps of the protocol with young children is beyond the scope of this book. In general, therapists who used techniques beyond traditional talk therapy were most successful in eliciting all the steps of the EMDR protocol with children 2–10 years of age. For example, therapists often struggled to elicit negative and positive cognitions with children. Instead of using the language written in the adult treatment manuals, therapists in this study asked children to identify bad thoughts and good thoughts.

Rapport building and relationship development are foundations for any successful treatment (Dworkin, 2005). These variables became even more significant with the application of the EMDR protocol to severely traumatized children. In fact, the rapport and relationship between the therapist and the child were significant predictors of the ability of the therapist to engage the child in the reprocessing that occurs during the Desensitization Phase of EMDR. The relationship between the therapist and the child client was also affected by the attunement of the therapist to the child and by attachment issues.

Variables Specific to the Unique Characteristics of the Individual Child. Besides therapists' specific variables, the individual child client also brought unique challenges to the treatment provided in this study. The children in this initial fidelity study were all clients of Childhelp, USA, where the children are all identified victims of crime. In addition to experiencing significant trauma, the children's unique personalities and life experiences affected this study. The children ranged in age from 3 to 10 years, and many children were bilingual in Spanish and English.

In addition, the children were from various cultural and religious backgrounds. Therapists had to incorporate issues related to the child's culture into therapy. The specific religious affiliations of several children required adjustments to the therapeutic environment. For instance, one child belonged to a religious organization that did not allow certain holidays and figures; therefore the therapist had to move to a different office because certain figures in the office were disturbing to the child because of her religion.

Furthermore, children in this study were often involved in the legal process of prosecuting adults; therefore the therapist had to assess current stressors and provide resourcing to the child before proceeding with reprocessing targets.

Finally, the therapist had to assess the distress in the child's family environment as well as in his or her home and school settings to most effectively use psychotherapy with EMDR.

Variables Specific to EMDR Treatment With Children. As EMDR was originally designed as a treatment protocol for adult clients, translating EMDR into language children can understand is even more complicated with severely and chronically traumatized children. Because of this, the severity of trauma experienced by the child obviously has a significant impact on the child's willingness to participate in treatment. Therapists in this study often reported experiencing clients' resistance or avoidance of reprocessing. It was necessary to explore factors that were contributing to clients' avoidance. As cases were staffed and videos reviewed, factors were identified as fueling resistance. Variables that emerged included engaging the child in the treatment process; improving the child's ability to tolerate intense affect; child developmental tasks, including children's current focus and emotional literacy; the impact of child languaging, including translation of the EMDR protocol into terms appropriate for children; and the use of BLS with young children.

Variables Related to the Treatment Environment, Including the Therapist's Office. The therapist needed to invest time, especially during the Preparation Phase of EMDR, to successfully engage the child in the clinical process and ultimately convince the child that participating in therapy would be valuable to the child. One variable unique to this study was location. At a large facility like the Childhelp, USA, Children's Center, therapists needed to understand that children needed time to play, explore, and ultimately trust the therapist to be convinced that reprocessing trauma would lead to positive and desirable outcomes. Because the Childhelp, USA, Children's Center is an advocacy center that includes law enforcement, forensic interviewers, forensic medical facilities, and the clinical environment, the children in this study had been interviewed by detectives and often had participated in medical assessments prior to being referred for therapy. Unlike children participating in therapy in a private office or community mental health center, children in therapy at Childhelp, USA, had already associated stressful experiences with the facility prior to being referred for therapy. This required therapists to desensitize the child to the therapy environment for treatment with EMDR to proceed. Once the therapist recognized that the child's reticence to participate in therapy with EMDR sometimes was due to contamination of the facility environment, rather than difficulties with the EMDR protocol, the therapeutic process continued more successfully.

Variables Related to the Parents of Child Clients and the Home Environment. These variables included the parents' current emotional functioning, the stability of the home and school environments, the recency of the trauma, and unfolding secondary traumas such as changes to the family and home environment and forensic involvement. The emotional functioning of the child's parents often had a direct impact on treatment outcomes for children. The parents' own anxiety and trauma history had to be assessed and treated to improve the child's success in treatment. It was evident that the stability of the home and school environments posed significant challenges to EMDR with children. Often, when the home environment was destabilized or had been dysfunctional when the crisis/trauma occurred, the child's progress in therapy was stymied or halted. When this occurred, the therapist needed to stabilize the home and school environments for progress in therapy to continue. In addition, the recency of the trauma and co-occurring or secondary trauma to parents often contributed to the parents' own mental health issues and tendency to become more protective of the children. With several clients, the perpetrator was a sibling or parent, which profoundly destabilized the child's environment. Progress in treatment was prolonged and required patience and commitment from the therapist. In these cases, the child's participation in the EMDR fidelity study was difficult because therapists had to spend a significant amount of time during the Preparation Phase with the child and his or her family. This issue also delayed data collection for the fidelity study as therapy became lengthy. Several clients had to withdraw from the study because of new allegations that required forensic or legal involvement.

The research conducted on EMDR with children (Chemtob et al., 2002; Cocco & Sharpe, 1993; Fernandez et al., 2004; Greenwald, 1994; Jaberghaderi et al., 2002; Jarero et al., 2006; Korkmazlar-Oral & Pamuk, 2002; Muris et al., 1998; Oras et al., 2004; Puffer et al., 1997; Rubin et al., 2001; Soberman et al., 2002; Tufnell, 2005; Wilson et al., 2000), along with the fidelity study that we have conducted, form the foundation for documenting EMDR with children as a promising practice.

Of the eleven studies published on EMDR in individual therapy with children, a total of 185 children aged 4–17 years were reportedly provided from 1 to 12 sessions of EMDR (mean 3.8 sessions). Eight studies reported that therapists offered six or less sessions of EMDR. The EMDR treatment in all of these studies ranged from ½ hour to 1-hour sessions provided by therapists fully trained in EMDR in all but three of the studies, where the therapists had not completed basic training in EMDR.

SUMMARY

As with any treatment modality, the efficacy of the treatment intervention must be supported by research to justify the treatment modality as best practice. Conducting research on therapeutic processes is challenging and requires that specific criteria be met to establish the methodological robustness of the research study. More research studies need to be conducted on using EMDR to treat young children, yet how do you conduct studies if there are few therapists specifically trained to use EMDR with young children? What a difficult predicament. Where do you start? To demonstrate fidelity to the EMDR protocol, therapists must first receive standardized training in using EMDR and then advanced training in using EMDR with young children. This training starts with a written manual, with directions for the therapist to adhere to the protocol. In addition to using a manual, the therapists still need ongoing consultation and skill development to effectively implement the EMDR protocol. The purpose of this book is to document and attempt to standardize the use of EMDR with young children in an effort to provide a document that will assist educators and researchers in standardizing the EMDR protocol for use with young children.

The book began with a review of the theoretical underpinnings from the AIP Model and a brief summary of the published studies on EMDR with children. In this chapter, we also reviewed the research on EMDR in general, with a focus on the current research on EMDR with children. The next chapters of the book provide specific written instructions for therapists to use EMDR with children, with explanations for using each piece of EMDR protocol with even the youngest client.

We then provide specialty protocols for using EMDR with children with symptom presentations and diagnoses.

Future studies on EMDR with children are necessary to assess the efficacy of using EMDR to treat children. Currently, EMDR with children has the foundation for a promising practice, and with additional studies, EMDR with children can become recognized as evidence-based practice.

CHAPTER 2

Getting Started With EMDR

Integrating EMDR into your practice of psychotherapy can be challenging after returning from the first weekend of training. We found that it is common for therapists to hesitate using EMDR because the protocol can initially feel awkward and unfamiliar. This can be even more challenging for therapists who provide psychotherapy for children, particularly if they are used to a more nondirective approach to therapy. With a second weekend of training, the therapist has completed the basic training in EMDR, but still, many therapists struggle to implement EMDR into their practices, especially if they are working with children. What can we do? Well, some therapists may feel like EMDR can occasionally be used as a tool for treating children, while unfortunately, other very skilled therapists cannot find a way to get started, so they never use EMDR. This is disappointing because of the significant efficacy of EMDR in psychotherapy. In an effort to supplement the training on EMDR with children, we decided to write this book.

In this book, we present an overview of how therapists can get started in conceptualizing psychotherapy with the EMDR methodology through AIP theory. The focus of the book is to teach therapists to effectively use the entire EMDR protocol with young children.

This chapter provides a comprehensive overview of how to get started with EMDR after completing basic training. The book continues with chapters that detail the basic skills in using EMDR with children and then transitions to more advanced skills in using EMDR with children with specific diagnoses and presenting issues. Finally, we conclude this book with goals for the future of EMDR with children, while encouraging therapists to consider conducting research to compel the practice of EMDR with children into the mainstream of child psychotherapy. It is our hope to inspire therapists to begin thinking about conducting research and how important research is to therapists to validate and advance our practice of psychotherapy.

In the end, the most significant goal of this book is to provide best practice for children who are in need of expert psychotherapy to change the trajectory of their lives. Our hope is to provide guidance and support to therapists to launch them in their practice of EMDR. This is the art of treating children with EMDR.

GETTING STARTED WITH EMDR

Ongoing support through consultation, study groups, and advanced training clearly enhances a therapist's confidence in his or her clinical ability to effectively use EMDR in psychotherapy. Throughout the remainder of this chapter, we make practical suggestions for getting started with EMDR with clients of any age. We have collected the nuggets of wisdom we have heard from other EMDR experts, including trainers and facilitators; what we have gleaned from study groups and consultation groups; and what we have learned from our research study groups, which we led for 2 years as we conducted our fidelity study. We summarize the instructions we offer students of EMDR each time we present specialized training or facilitate during EMDR training to encourage therapists to take the risk to get started using EMDR when they return to their offices and work with clients. We review the books we recommend that students read, explain the unique challenges of each phase of the protocol, describe the techniques and tools for bilateral stimulation (BLS), and develop an approach for case conceptualization with various populations of children. It is with this knowledge that therapists can learn the art of treating children with EMDR.

Books on EMDR

First, to learn the EMDR protocol and understand the theoretical underpinnings of the AIP model, we suggest that you acquire several seminal books to guide your practice of EMDR. We also summarize the current books on EMDR with children.

It is important to read Shapiro's (2001) book *Eye Movement Desensitization and Reprocessing* to get in-depth direction and explanation for each piece of the protocol. It is important for the therapist to have a foundational knowledge of the EMDR protocol before trying to use

EMDR with children. We have taken Shapiro's book and then translated the protocol into a language that is usable with child clients. As you integrate EMDR into your psychotherapy practice, it will be helpful to refer to Shapiro's book for clarification on a regular basis.

We also suggest you read the *Handbook of EMDR and Family Therapy Processes* (Shapiro, Kaslow, & Maxfield, 2007), which includes several chapters in which Shapiro expands her explanation of the AIP model and the eight phases of EMDR. This is an edited book, in which the authors discuss how to conceptualize psychotherapy cases from an AIP model as an "integrative psychotherapy approach" (p. 28).

In *Through the Eyes of a Child*, Tinker and Wilson (1999) provide a scholarly overview of psychotherapy with children, detail the history of EMDR with children, discuss the theoretical underpinnings of EMDR with children, and finally, include many case examples of EMDR treatment with children.

Greenwald (1999) provided techniques for the treatment of children that are especially focused on working with adolescents, with an emphasis on treating oppositional–defiant clients, in his book *Eye Movement Desensitization Reprocessing (EMDR) in Child and Adolescent Psychotherapy.*

Lovett (1999) described the parent narrative and how to use this process in psychotherapy with children in her book on using EMDR with children, titled *Small Wonders*. The parent narrative can be very useful for children who are nonresponsive, and we have used the parent narrative for children with traumatic brain injuries who are unable to participate on their own.

Each book on EMDR with children provides a different foundation for working with children. There are important tools and skills included in each book that can benefit the therapist who is trying to learn to use EMDR effectively with children.

Research on EMDR

In chapter 1, we reviewed the research on EMDR. Even if you are a therapist who typically avoids reading research studies, we suggest reading published articles on the efficacy of EMDR. It is imperative that practitioners refer to research to guide their practice and prepare them to better explain EMDR to clients and to third-party payers. Because there is a trend in public health and community mental health to use evidence-based practices, it behooves the therapist to be able to defend the use of EMDR through references to studies that document the efficacy of EMDR. To simplify the overview of EMDR with children, we compiled a table listing all the studies on EMDR with children and unique characteristics of each study (see Tables 1.1 and 1.2).

In chapter 1, we described the research we have conducted on using EMDR with children 2–10 years of age. This research study began as an effort to document that the entire EMDR protocol could be used with even very young children if therapists had the tools and confidence to implement the entire protocol. We also summarized the challenges of using EMDR with young children and what therapists can do to gain confidence and expertise with EMDR based on the qualitative data we collected during the fidelity study.

THE EIGHT PHASES OF EMDR

We organized the remainder of this chapter by using the eight phases of the EMDR protocol as headings. This organization in no way suggests that the protocol is linear and sequential. On the contrary, the psychotherapy process with actual clients is often circular, with the therapist needing to return to earlier phases of the protocol as more information arises during the desensitization process, when new memory networks are accessed. For example, after taking a thorough history and creating a treatment plan, the therapist may learn new and more detailed information about the client's history during the Assessment Phase of the protocol. With this new information, the therapist may determine that the client needs additional resources to tolerate reprocessing the new information.

It is common to start desensitization and realize the client needs additional preparation skills with which to process a particular memory network. The EMDR therapy process is often unpredictable and surprising, as the therapist and client learn together how the client has experienced and stored the traumatic event. We have found there is often a missing piece arises that explains why the event has become encapsulated and not completed by the individual's natural healing process.

At each phase of the EMDR protocol the therapist needs to be aware that clients process in unique ways, and it is the client's unique healing process that needs to be followed by the therapist using EMDR. This is where the previous tools you have learned as a therapist can be integrated into the phases of the EMDR protocol.

Your ability to listen, be attuned, and use your own skills to listen and facilitate the process and provide translation from adult language to child language is essential to the treatment process throughout the eight phases of EMDR.

Client History and Treatment Planning Phase

The EMDR model is a comprehensive template for case conceptualization in mental health treatment. The significant pieces of many other therapies can be integrated into the eight phases of the EMDR protocol. Consider the purpose of Phase 1 of EMDR, Client History and Treatment Planning. Most therapies begin with taking a client's history and then proceeding to treatment planning. Therapists, in most treatment modalities, are trained to collect a client's history and identify treatment issues to aid in the treatment planning process. With EMDR, the unique addition to the client history–taking process is that the therapist listens for the client's negative self-perceptions, beliefs, and cognitions as well as emotions and unique body sensations as the client describes his or her presenting issues. The therapist notes aspects of the client's presentation in each of these areas, whether in thought process (cognitions), affect (emotions), or body sensations, as reported by the client, or body language, as observed by the therapist, all to be further explored in latter phases of the EMDR process. The themes with which clients present, including negative self-perceptions, beliefs, and cognitions, would be typically presented in any psychotherapy intake process by clients and included in treatment planning for psychotherapy; however, the significance of these issues is at the root of symptom manifestation from an AIP theoretical perspective and is what guides the therapist through the eight phases of case conceptualization in EMDR. The therapist is also watching the client's affect, expression of emotions, and reported body sensations as evidence of maladaptively stored information and clues to how the client might process. Sometimes the affect, emotions, and body sensations are even symptoms of the earlier event that has remained frozen in the client's neurobiological system. With children, we are not just listening and observing for these areas, but also eliciting information from parents, including a detailed description of how the child responded to a particular situation or event. Our observations as therapists as well as the data collected from the child and the child's parents offer data to guide the development of working hypotheses about the child's treatment needs and the direction for therapy.

During this first phase of EMDR, we are also assessing for affect management, affect tolerance, emotional regulation skills, self-soothing skills, and other needed skills that are important processes to any type of therapy. We note the skills with which the child enters treatment and make a determination as to what skills the child will need to learn during the Preparation Phase to continue through the phases of the EMDR protocol.

Explaining EMDR to Both Parents and Children. It is important to explain EMDR to both parents and children in terms that all family members can understand. Client understanding of the EMDR methodology is imperative in engaging the child and family in the therapeutic process. This can be a simple process, with specific examples of how to explain

EMDR to adults and children included in chapter 4. Once the child and family have consented to the treatment process, the therapist then gathers information to aid in case conceptualization.

Case Conceptualization in EMDR With Children. Therapist case conceptualization in treating children with EMDR includes integrating both the parent input and child input in the process of collecting a client history and writing a treatment plan for psychotherapy. It is our experience that what parents identify as issues and what children identify may be very different.

Not only do children and parents often identify different targets for therapy, they may also present different symptom manifestations. Symptoms that are of concern to parents may not seem as important for children. Parents will often identify external symptoms, while children will often report internal symptoms. For example, parents will often bring children to therapy for temper tantrums or "meltdowns," while children may be more concerned about getting in trouble for the temper tantrums.

The difference between what children present and what parents present is also important in treatment planning because it guides the therapist to ask the parents how they will know the child is progressing in therapy. What are the parents' goals for their child's therapy? Ask the parents how they hope the child will be acting, behaving, and feeling when therapy is completed.

Remember that it is critical to also ask the child for his or her goals for therapy. The therapist needs to ask the child how he or she wants to think, feel, and behave or what he or she wants to be able to do instead of what he or she is doing now.

In chapter 3, we will explain in detail how to explore both parent input and child input throughout the EMDR treatment process to capture a comprehensive treatment process for the child.

From a case conceptualization perspective, the therapist is attempting to listen for how the trauma is stored for the child. A child's experience of a traumatic event is frequently stored in unusual and surprising ways. Children may identify a traumatic event in an imaginative manner such as a ghost or a monster. A child may explain that he or she cannot sleep in his or her own bed because there is a monster in the closet, when the therapist knows from the parent that the child has had difficulty sleeping since being in a car accident. This is the beginning of the process of examining how the child experiences the world and manages the distressing and traumatic events that have brought the child to therapy.

Once the therapist has conducted the intake and written an initial treatment plan, therapy then proceeds with the Preparation Phase of EMDR.

Preparation Phase

During the second phase of EMDR, the therapist's primary goal is to prepare the child for reprocessing during the remaining phases of EMDR by teaching *Safe/Calm Place, Metaphor, BLS,* and the mechanics of EMDR. In addition, the therapist is providing psychoeducational and skill-building activities for the child.

Most therapies assess the client's resources and then facilitate the client learning needed skills to improve the client's functioning. Any previous skill-building activities that the therapist had typically used in psychotherapy can be implemented in the Preparation Phase. Guided imagery, systematic desensitization, assertiveness training, pieces of trauma-focused cognitive behavioral therapy, or any other interventions the therapist had found beneficial to clients are equally important to consider teaching a client during the Preparation Phase or at any other time that the therapist assesses that the client needs particular skills to be successful in therapy. For example, children often benefit from learning how to take deep breaths for self-soothing and from progressive muscle relaxation exercises. With EMDR, we often teach children resource skills and install mastery experiences to provide the scaffolding from which children can build healthy experiences and reprocess traumatic events.

During the Preparation Phase it is important to teach clients the ability to titrate the impact of intense emotions. We have found that the more the client feels capable of managing intense affect and self-soothing, the more effective the therapeutic process. Children especially need to feel powerful and competent in therapy to actively participate in the healing process. It is our experience that when children are feeling overwhelmed by their intense emotions, they are much more likely to be reluctant to participate in therapy.

Stop Signal and Safe/Calm Place. Clients of all ages also need to have resources, including a *Stop Signal* to communicate to the therapist that the client is too overwhelmed to continue with reprocessing and a Safe/Calm Place for titrating intense affect. The child needs to be able to metaphorically go to a Safe/Calm Place during reprocessing with EMDR if the affect becomes overwhelming and the client cannot continue. Teaching Stop Signal and Safe/Calm Place will be discussed in detail in chapter 4. No matter what the age, all clients need to have identified a Safe/Calm Place and a Stop Signal with which to communicate with the therapist. Safe/Calm Places and Stop Signals with children are important and can be elicited from even very young children with adjustments to the directions the therapist uses. For example, young children may need to draw a picture or several pictures of a Safe/Calm Place that can be used in sessions.

Variations of working with Safe/Calm Place with children will be included throughout this book.

During the Preparation Phase it is also important for the therapist to be able to provide psychoeducational information to both parents and children that explains the AIP model and psychotherapy with EMDR. We will give you examples of how to do this later in the book.

Bilateral Stimulation (BLS). One of the hallmarks of using EMDR is learning how to implement the different types of BLS. BLS is any external movement that produces alternating stimulation of the two sides of the client's body to get alternating activation of the two sides of the brain. In EMDR treatment, the primary form of BLS is eye movements (EM), where the therapist has the client follow either the therapist's fingers or some other type of stimulation that creates eye movements that go back and forth, while crossing the midline of the client's body. There are other kinds of BLS, including tactile, auditory, and combined types. In EMDR training, therapists are encouraged to use only eye movements because the research on EMDR is almost entirely based on eye movements as BLS. There are many types of BLS that can be used with clients of all ages.

Eye movements can be elicited by the therapist by moving your fingers as taught in EMDR training. I (R.T.) have been known to put stickers on my fingers or to draw happy faces on my fingers for the child to track. Therapists can also use penlights on the floor or wall for the client to follow or purchase specialized equipment for eliciting eye movements. Children will track with their eyes and enjoy the use of puppets or finger puppets, stuffed animals, or other toys selected by the child to increase the child's focus on the eye movements.

It is not uncommon to notice a client stop tracking the eye movements or to see eye movements that are not always fluid. This may happen for several reasons. The client may have difficulty tracking the stimulus. The therapist can slow down the eye movements and tell the client to "Push my fingers with your eyes." Sometimes it may be necessary for the therapist to stop and wiggle their fingers in order to make sure the client is still tracking. Sometimes the client may be processing a memory and the therapist will notice jumpy eye movements or the client's eyes may flutter. You can always check in with the client in order to see what is happening. In addition to assessing the client's ability to track the type of bilateral stimulation, the number of saccades also impact the client's ability to track the stimulus.

It is important to determine the number of saccades (passes back and forth) that are necessary when working with a particular client. Dr. Shapiro and the research suggest that eye movements should move as fast as the client can tolerate in order to activate processing rather than just tracking. The therapist can tell the client that, "I'm just guessing at the speed and number of passes, but you can tell me to stop or continue." By giving the client the power to continue or stop the saccades, the therapist becomes more attuned to the individual client's unique manner of processing.

Therapists can also provide bilateral stimulation through tactile stimulation such as tapping on the clients hands or using a device especially designed for therapist use during EMDR. There are many different ways to use tactile forms of BLS with clients and some creative and fun ways to engage children with BLS. This too will be discussed in detail in a future chapter.

Therapists can provide auditory stimulation by using technological equipment that can either pulse in the client's ears or by attaching a CD player or IPOD to the equipment in order for the client to use music as bilateral stimulation. Some therapists use remote speakers that can be placed on either side of a play area or sand tray and then use a pre-programmed CD that provides alternating auditory stimulation. It is important to monitor that actual bilateral stimulation is occurring because children are active and may not stay in between the two speakers.

When using a device that provides bilateral stimulation, it is helpful to start by turning all contro ls including auditory and tactile volume and speed to the lowest level of the control. Proceed by slowly increasing the speed, intensity or volume until the client chooses a setting that is most comfortable.

For a more in-depth discussion of BLS, the reader is referred to chapter 4.

Once the client has been taught EMDR and the mechanics of EMDR, and the client has learned the skills to manage intense affect and participate in the remaining phases of EMDR, the treatment process continues with the Assessment Phase.

Assessment Phase

The Assessment Phase includes the procedural steps of the EMDR protocol. In Phase 3 of EMDR, the therapist and client formally identify targets for reprocessing. Identifying targets for reprocessing is one of the significant goals of the Assessment Phase. Even though targets have been identified in a targeting sequence during the Client History and Treatment Planning Phase, it is during the Assessment Phase that the therapist identifies a specific target for reprocessing. This is also where the EMDR protocol is unique from other types of therapies. If you remember, the Assessment Phase is the focus of several of the practicum experiences in basic training in EMDR, when the therapist is learning the procedural steps.

Identifying Targets. There are many ways to identify targets with clients. When working with children, we have created some imaginative ways to identify targets that tap into a child's way of processing. After the target is identified, the client is asked to pinpoint the worst part of the memory. Children may identify the worst part of the memory by drawing pictures, working in the sand tray, using puppets, and utilizing many other types of art and play therapy techniques.

Selecting the Image. The target and the image are not the same thing. This is often confusing for therapists learning EMDR. A *target* is an issue, incident, experience, or memory from the client's life. An *image* is a picture that represents the worst part of the target.

Negative and Positive Cognitions. When the image of the target is identified, the Assessment Phase continues with the art of distilling the child's core beliefs in the form of negative cognitions. This process requires patience, creativity, and attunement to the client. The therapist needs to invest time in identifying a negative cognition that resonates for the client. Clients may initially offer several negative cognitions. If the client offers several cognitions, it is important for the therapist to explore which of the client's negative cognitions feels the strongest when associated with the specific image. When a negative cognition resonates for a client, the client will quite often exhibit an emotional and physical reaction to hearing the negative cognition. Our experience is that when the negative cognition resonates for the client, there is an obvious reaction that validates the negative cognition. With adult clients, a significant amount of time may be spent on distilling the negative cognition that represents the client's core negative belief about himself or herself. With children, this process can be as simple as asking the child about the bad thought that is associated with the target and image. Children are not as likely to exhibit the telltale reaction to the negative cognition that we have observed in adolescent and adult clients.

A negative cognition for an adult is a presently held belief that is irrational, self-referencing, and able to be generalized. But for children, their negative cognitions may be trauma-specific and more concrete, and may be a feeling word or sound like fantasy to the therapist.

Once a negative cognition has been identified, the therapist has essentially connected to the client's memory network. Along with a negative cognition, the therapist then identifies the positive cognition. The positive cognition is what the client would like to believe about himself or herself, instead of the negative cognition. The positive cognition also needs to be realistic, self-referencing, and generalized for an adult client. For a child, again, the positive cognition may be trauma-specific, presented in a feeling, and appear to be in imaginary or fantasy terms. For example, a child might say, "John bad." And the positive cognition or good thought might be "John better now." We will discuss the impact of child development on processing cognitions in chapter 5.

With the positive cognition, having the client identify what he or she wants to believe is very important because it is an educational process of having the client consider possibilities. What is it that the client wants to be able to believe about himself or herself instead now?

Validity of Cognition. Continuing in the EMDR process, the therapist next assesses the validity (VoC) of the positive cognition. The VoC is measured on a 7-point scale, ranging from 1 (*completely false*) to 7 (*completely true*). Measuring the VoC is often confusing for adult clients as well as children. Even therapists may get confused while explaining the VoC. Consequently, in a later chapter, we have included a detailed explanation of how to explain and obtain the VoC from clients. Although measuring the VoC is somewhat challenging, it is possible and important to attempt to obtain a VoC from even the youngest clients. Children often need to have the VoC measured in concrete terms. There are many playful and creative ways to elicit a VoC from a child.

Once the therapist has asked the client how true the positive cognition feels to the client now, the process has moved from a cognitive level to a feeling level.

Therapists often will ask the client what the client thinks, rather than what the client feels, when eliciting a VoC. This may become problematic as the therapist is trying to get the client to move to a feeling level. It is important to remember that the therapist is asking for a feeling, not a thought.

Expressing the Emotion. After the VoC, the therapist asks the client for the emotion associated with the target. Whatever emotion the child reports, the therapist notes it and continues with the procedural steps. Many therapists will probe the client for more emotions; however, one emotion is sufficient to continue with the process. If the therapist asks the client for more emotions, the client will most likely report additional emotions due to demand characteristics of pleasing the therapist. In psychotherapy, a *demand characteristic* occurs when the therapist asks the client a question that implies the expected answer, outcome, or result. It is important to be aware of demand characteristics while conducting psychotherapy because the client may respond with the answer that the client believes the therapist wants to hear. This is especially true with children. The therapist needs to use clinical judgment to determine if the client is providing the answer that the client believes will please the therapist or an answer that would allow the client to avoid an uncomfortable therapeutic topic. If the client is responding from this position, a demand characteristic exists.

Subjective Units of Disturbance. Once the client has identified an emotion that is connected with the target, the therapist immediately asks the client to assess how disturbing the emotion feels to him or her now on a scale from 0 (*no disturbance*) to 10 (*most disturbing*). This is a measurement of the subjective units of disturbance, or SUD.

Body Sensation. As soon as the client chooses SUD, the therapist asks the client for the body sensation. Once the therapist connects the image and negative cognition together, the therapy process moves into the Desensitization Phase of EMDR. Children are often quite able to follow the steps of the Assessment Phase when the therapist can use age-appropriate language and explain the process to the child. More in-depth explanations for eliciting each step of the protocol with children will be provided later in the book.

Desensitization Phase

The Desensitization Phase begins when the therapist links together the image, the negative cognition, and where the client feels it in his or her body and starts BLS. The length of the Desensitization Phase can be only minutes within a single session or expand over several sessions that could take months, depending on the number of channels associated with the chosen target. If the negative cognition is connected to many experiences in the client's history, the links between memories can be extensive. The connections may be clear or may appear to be tangential and irrelevant. This is when the therapist's patience and attunement is vital. The therapist's ability to hang in there and stay out of the client's way is crucial to the desensitization process. Many therapists will return to the original target even though the client is continuing to process. It is only necessary to return to the original target if the therapist believes the client has completed a memory channel and the therapist is reevaluating the original target. The therapist asks the client to return to the original target to assess where the client is in reprocessing the target during desensitization. The therapist simply asks the client to bring up the original incident and then report what the client gets now. Whatever the client reports, the therapist instructs the client to "go with that" and continues with desensitization. If the client identifies any disturbance at all, the therapist continues with desensitization.

If, in the clinical opinion of the therapist, the client's target appears to have been completed, the therapist then takes a SUD measurement. The therapist may suspect that the target has been reprocessed when the client's responses are neutral or positive. For example, the client may begin to make statements approximating the positive cognition. A client may say, "I was only a kid, I couldn't have stopped him." Even children have an observant part of themselves that gives them a different perspective of when they are young and helpless. This perspective indicates client movement and the possibility that the target no longer has emotional value.

One of the things we have noticed in our discussions with clinicians is that there is often a surprising amount of reprocessing to be completed between SUD of 1 and 0. We have discussed at length what the clinician should do when the SUD is at a 1 or less, but not at a 0. What does *ecologically sound* mean? This is what is taught in the EMDR basic training, but we encourage therapists to consider that they need to take the time to reprocess to a 0. We will discuss in depth when a SUD of 1 is ecologically sound and when this needs to be clinically explored in chapter 6.

In our experience, being aware of the client's nonverbal presentation is just as important as listening to what the client verbally reports. Some clients may overfocus on doing the desensitization process perfectly. They stare, hold their breath, or try to memorize everything they notice during BLS. This is when it is important to repeat the directions to just noticing what is happening. For example, clients may stop blinking as they try to stare at the eye movements, and then the clients' eyes may begin to tear. This can cause a client to struggle with eye movements. Clients may need to be reminded that it is fine to blink while following the eye movements.

Client breathing is a significant factor in any type of therapy. As the therapist remains attuned to the client's nonverbal signals, breathing can mean many different things. Watching the client's breathing during reprocessing is critical. Anxious clients may take very shallow breaths. When clients are reprocessing a target, the client many initially hold his or her breath and then may take a shallow breath and then a deep breath when he or she has reprocessed through the target. Clients may also stop breathing while reprocessing a memory, and the therapist may need to remind the client that it is very important just to notice their breathing. Other clients may think that they are supposed to hold their breath during BLS. These clients again need to be instructed just to notice their breathing.

Clients may also try to remember everything that comes up during BLS to report this to the therapist. It is helpful to tell the client that the therapist only needs a brief report of the last thing the client noticed when the therapist paused the BLS. Although many clients like to report everything they become aware of during BLS, encouraging the client to only report the last thing he or she noticed facilitates the process. If the client appears distracted, confused, reports that nothing is happening, or that he or she is not noticing anything, the therapist can simply instruct the client to just go with that. This may just be part of the client's progression.

Children may become very still as they are reprocessing or may become very agitated. What is important to notice is that either behavior reflects a significant change in behavior that was not evident prior to beginning the Desensitization Phase and reprocessing of an identified target. It is imperative to learn each client's unique presentation. Encouraging the client just to notice what is happening during reprocessing and go with whatever comes up is a hallmark of effective reprocessing in EMDR. It is important to know that it is during the Desensitization Phase that a lot happens in EMDR. We will expand on possible challenges and clinical decision making in the remaining chapters.

Completing a Target. When therapists first start using EMDR, we have found that many therapists struggle with determining when a target is complete. Therapists will need to use clinical judgment when deciding that the client has completed the Desensitization Phase. When the therapist has had the client return to the original incident and the SUD is 0, the therapeutic process is moving from the Desensitization Phase to the Installation Phase. The therapist may decide to continue with the desensitization process if the VoC remains 5 or less. We are recommending that the therapist consider a VoC of 5 or less as indicative of the need to continue with desensitization. By moving to the Installation Phase, the protocol calls for the VoC to be measured with each successive set of BLS, which can be very distracting. During the Desensitization Phase the therapist does not need to evaluate the VoC as frequently as during the Installation Phase.

The EMDR protocol suggests that once the therapeutic process has moved to the Installation Phase, the therapist should evaluate the VoC with each successive set of BLS, which has the potential to increase the likelihood of demand characteristics. If the therapist continues with desensitization until the client begins to report successive positive statements, it is then clinically indicated that the client is ready for installation of the positive cognition. It is our recommendation for therapists to consider during case conceptualization, when determining the flow of the EMDR protocol, that the therapist continue with the Desensitization Phase until the VoC reaches a 6, and then the process can move to the Installation Phase. It is our assessment that the process flows much more effectively, and this decreases the likelihood of demand characteristics, when the therapist continues with desensitization until the child repeats positive responses that are essentially the same for several sets. For example, the child may say, "I *am* a good kid." The therapist responds, "Just notice that," and continues with BLS. The child then repeats, "I am a *good* kid," and the therapist responds, "Just notice that." If it is evident that the child is presenting with the positive cognition or a close approximation, the therapist can then consider that the client is ready to move to the Installation Phase of EMDR.

Installation Phase

Once the SUD is at a 0, the therapist begins the Installation Phase by combining the original incident and the positive cognition and checking the P.C. If the P.C. fits, continue with Installation. With each successive set of saccades, the therapist evaluates the VoC. Installation continues as long as the VoC strengthens. When the VoC reaches a 7 or greater and holds, the process moves into the Body Scan Phase of EMDR.

During installation, it is important to continue with the same number of passes of BLS as used with the individual client during desensitization because it is necessary to ascertain if any unprocessed material remains.

Children will progress through the Installation Phase very quickly. In chapter 7, we provide a detailed description of how to implement the Installation Phase of EMDR with even very young children.

Body Scan Phase

After desensitizing the target and installing the positive cognition, the EMDR protocol continues with the body scan. The client is asked to hold the original incident together with the positive cognition and to scan his or her body from head to toe for any disturbance. If any disturbance is noted, the client is asked to focus on the disturbance and is instructed to "go with that." Sometimes the client will report nothing and that the client is feeling fine or calm, and the process proceeds to closure. If the client reports some type of physiological disturbance, this disturbance is desensitized. This may be a link to another channel or memory, or sometimes clients may just notice things in their bodies. Once a clear body scan is achieved, the process continues to closure.

With children, the body scan may require education, instruction, and demonstration. Children may notice an external cut or bruise and need to be redirected to internal sensations such as headaches or tummy aches. Teaching children how to scan their bodies can involve explaining that scanning their bodies is like an X ray, where we are looking inside their bodies from the tops of their heads to the tips of their toes. Sometimes it is useful to use some type of toy to demonstrate how to scan one's body.

Children may report unusual body sensations in their arms or legs and can then be instructed to "go with that." Specific instructions for body scan with children will be discussed in chapter 7. It is important to note that the Body Scan Phase often moves quickly for children, and then children are ready to play.

Closure Phase

The progression of the Closure Phase of EMDR is dependent on the status of the EMDR session. If the client has completed all previous phases, closure continues with future template. If the session is an incomplete session, closure continues with stabilization of the client with instructions for in-between sessions.

Closure of a Completed Session of EMDR. With a completed session of EMDR, the SUD is 0, the positive cognition has been strengthened and installed to a VoC of 7, and there is a clear body scan. This is where some confusion exists for therapists. If the past events and current issues have been reprocessed, it is then beneficial to continue with the future template, if session time allows. Otherwise, the therapist can choose to continue with the future template in the next session. The decision to process all past events and all current triggers before moving to a future template has to be driven by case conceptualization and clinical judgment. We have found that by processing one target through to future template, the client then leaves the therapy session empowered with the belief that he or she can handle the presenting problem that initially brought the client to treatment. The positive results that emerge from completing the EMDR protocol leave the client with a positive association with therapy and the motivation to continue with EMDR, even when the process is distressing. This is especially true with children. When children experience the positive benefits of EMDR by experiencing mastery and successfully reprocessing a target through to future template, many children will return and initiate reprocessing of additional, and sometimes even more difficult, targets.

In case conceptualization with children, the therapist may consider reprocessing a more current target with a child as a mastery experience. With some children, going after the most disturbing target may be overwhelming and create a resistance to reprocessing in therapy. If the child seems to struggle and balk at desensitization, it is helpful to target an incident that is less disturbing to demonstrate for the child the benefits of reprocessing. Once the child experiences mastery of an incident, the child may be willing to tackle more difficult and complicated targets.

Future Template. This entire part is symptom driven, and if you think case conceptualization along the lines of symptom manifestation, this will help guide the choice of the future template. The symptoms with which the client presented at the initial intake guide the selection of the future template. If the parents brought the child into therapy due to the child's refusal to go to school, the future template would focus on the child imaging getting ready and going to school tomorrow, and then continue with the protocol for the future template until the child can imagine going to school with positive outcomes. This is a positive template for the future related to the symptoms that initially brought the child into treatment. Future template is the opportunity to rehearse future desired behaviors and outcomes.

An example is a child who has anxiety after being in a car accident. The original assessment would be on the car accident and then float back to the earliest time when the child thought or felt "I'm not safe." Then the therapist processes the earliest memory, comes to the current trigger of the car accident, and then moves the therapy to the future template of "I'm OK," as the client imagines riding in the car.

Another example for future template is test anxiety. The child presents with anxiety regarding a future examination. The therapist could identify the negative cognition of "I'm dumb" and have the client float back to the first time the child thought or felt "I'm dumb." Once that earliest memory is identified and reprocessed, the therapist then processes current symptoms and then has the client focus on the positive cognition of "I'm doing the best I can" when imagining taking that future examination.

Another possible future template is when a client has processed a history of sexual assault. In such a situation it is extremely important to focus on the current symptom manifestation. For example, if a child has been molested, the future template is not "I can handle it," but a more symptom-related template such as "I can sleep in my bed because I'm safe now" or "I can speak up now and tell adults, who will take care of me." The origins of the symptoms' manifestation are from the molestation, with current symptom manifestation involving difficulty sleeping in bed or being assertive. Future template can focus on the client imagining being able to sleep in his or her own bed.

Three-Pronged Approach. All three examples illustrate the three-pronged approach of EMDR, which includes past–present–future. With case conceptualization, the approach depends on the length of time remaining in the session. A brief time remaining requires closure to end the session and help the client return to his or her life without significant distress; with time available, the therapist continues with future template to complete the EMDR protocol for the specific target.

Clear, concrete future events are important when conducting a future template process with a child. For example, one child was brought to therapy by her parents because she was unable to sleep in her own bed. The therapist (C.S.) asked about the most horrible time that the child had struggled with related to sleeping in her own bed. The therapist attempted to have the child float back to the first time she remembered not being able to sleep in her own bed, and the child recalled not being able to sleep in her own bed after getting ill and throwing up in her bed. At that time, the little girl's parents allowed the child to sleep with them. Following this incident, the child worried about getting sick and her parents not hearing her, so she wanted to sleep with her parents every night. The therapist first targeted this memory in the past that was driving the current symptoms of the child experiencing difficulty falling asleep. Once the child had processed the past memory and current symptoms had abated, the therapist had the child imagine sleeping in her own bed in the future. The child imagined herself sleeping in her own bed and even getting sick, but being able to call her parents if she needed them. Following this future template process, the child reported that she was able to sleep comfortably in her own bed. This experience of the future template not only created a success experience for the child, but engaged her in the efficacy of EMDR and laid the foundation for the child to process more difficult traumatic events from her past.

Closing an Incomplete Session. In addition to the variations for closure of a completed EMDR session, there are treatment interventions necessary following an incomplete session of EMDR. With an incomplete session of EMDR, it is essential for the therapist to stop the reprocessing in time to ground the client in the office and contain any disturbing materials, if necessary, before the end of the session. With adults, the therapist (C.S.) reminds the client that he or she has done work during therapy and then uses the analogy of a train by explaining to the client that in this trip from California to Miami, the therapist has estimated that she believes that in this session, the client has made it to Dallas. The therapist then reminds the client that between sessions, the client may continue on the train trip to Miami and even end up in the Bahamas, which often elicits a laugh because it is not possible to take a train from California to the Bahamas.

The goal of closure following an incomplete session is to stabilize the client so that the client may leave the therapist's office firmly grounded in the present, with skills to manage any additional processing or distress that may arise.

With children, it is important to teach children self-calming and self-soothing techniques to use between sessions. It is also important to explain to children and parents that reprocessing may continue between sessions and what children and parents can do to assist the child in coping with the continued reprocessing. It is necessary to teach techniques such as *containers,* relationship skills, and other tools for children to use to cope with intense emotions. We will expand on techniques we have found helpful in detail in chapter 6 on desensitization.

Reevaluation Phase

The final phase of EMDR is the Reevaluation Phase. There are actually two different times that the therapy protocol may necessitate reevaluation: at the beginning of the next session, and when evaluating the treatment process to aid in discharge planning.

The first type of reevaluation occurs at the beginning of the next session following a session in which a target has been desensitized. The therapist asks the client to return to the original incident and asks the client, "When you bring up that original incident, what do you get now?" Clinical judgment guides how this process unfolds and will be explained in detail in chapter 8.

The second type of reevaluation occurs when the therapist and client review all targets to make sure that no additional disturbance exists and that all targets have been reprocessed. Once the therapist and client have agreed that all targets have been reprocessed successfully and the symptoms identified at the beginning of treatment have been addressed, the therapist and client together can plan for treatment discharge following their successful treatment process. This is the goal for all clients.

FIRST CLIENT CONSIDERATIONS

During Part 1 of EMDR training, participants are encouraged by the EMDR trainer to consider clients in their practice who may be appropriate candidates for EMDR treatment. Some EMDR trainers and facilitators may suggest that the EMDR model is a tool for the therapists' toolbox but do not encourage therapists to develop their use of EMDR as a template for all therapy. We have met with therapists who are confused as to the application of EMDR and cannot decide if EMDR is just a treatment tool for trauma or, as we believe, that the EMDR methodology is a comprehensive template for case conceptualization with all clients.

For your first client, we recommend that the therapist consider choosing a client with whom you have established a therapeutic relationship. This first client would ideally have a relatively minor trauma for the therapist to address when first using EMDR. The therapist will explain that he or she has learned a new procedure that is supported by research and, after receiving training in this type of therapy, believes that EMDR would be beneficial to the client. We suggest that you explain to the child client that you will be reading the protocol from a script and will be writing down the client's answers because we are old and forgetful, and what the child reports is very important.

Typically, we will provide a brochure or article on EMDR and offer to have the parent watch Donovan's (1999) educational video *Looking Through Hemispheres,* which can be purchased from the EMDR Humanitarian Assistance Project. This video is for adults and is not applicable to child clients; therefore we may choose to have parents watch the video, but the video does not offer any information on EMDR for children.

Since there is no video or brochure specifically for children, we suggest that therapists write a description of EMDR to be shared with children.* This is very simple, and in age-appropriate language, it will give

---

* Therapists can purchase the book, *Dark Bad Day, Go Away* (Gomez, 2007) to read to children.

the reader some examples we have used to explain EMDR to children as well as what we have learned from the children with whom we have had the honor to work in our respective offices.

For example, during a session with a young boy, in which he had just reprocessed his scary target, the little boy reported with surprise, "You know those buzzies [tactile stimulation] are like a vacuum. They just suck out the dirt and leave the good stuff behind." Feeling comfortable explaining EMDR to children and parents is one area that is very important for therapists. If the therapist feels confident in explaining EMDR, the child and parents will tend to feel more comfortable with the process.

After educating the client about EMDR, the therapist can then proceed with the Assessment Phase.

THE THERAPIST'S ROLE IN EMDR

One of the most difficult parts of getting started with EMDR is for the therapist to get out of the way. After practicing therapy either in graduate classes or in professional settings, therapists may be trained to rephrase clients' statements or somehow respond verbally to the client. It is important to learn when the therapist should stay quiet and only say, "What do you get now?" and "Go with that." This feels awkward at first and typically causes the therapist to be initially uncomfortable with the EMDR protocol. Because of this, many therapists struggle with staying out of the client's process. During the Desensitization Phase, it is particularly important to stay out of the client's process as the client reprocesses memories, to permit the client to reprocess without interruption, influence, or guidance. Many therapists are tempted to rephrase the client's statements, offer insights, or make suggestions to the client. While reprocessing with EMDR, this is not necessary, and actually slows the client's reprocessing.

With children, it may be even more difficult for the therapist to stay out of the way because the therapist may need to help the child focus and keep on track. Clinical judgment is required for the therapist to determine if the child is losing focus or if what appears to be losing focus is actually the child's unique way of reprocessing. Getting attuned to the individual child's processing and being able to patiently follow the child's processing requires practice and experience with EMDR.

SETTING UP THE OFFICE FOR EMDR, AND ESPECIALLY FOR WORKING WITH CHILDREN

With adult clients, the therapist really needs to create an office atmosphere that is comfortable for the therapist and the client. It may be necessary to arrange seating so that the therapist can prop his or her arm in a manner that will be comfortable for the therapist to do ongoing BLS. It is also necessary to arrange seating so that the therapist can arrange for "ships that pass in the night," as is taught in EMDR basic training (Shapiro, 2007).

From a basic office setting for working with children, it is helpful to have floor space and a large tablet and drawing tools like crayons or markers. This can be a simple process. It is not necessary to have many toys or anything specific for EMDR. Therapists can use any play therapy and/or art therapy activities, but these are not necessary. It is important to differentiate between what is necessary and what is fun to have in the office. The sand tray and dollhouse and other toys can assist the child in creating a scene of the incident and worst image, and even the bad thought/negative cognition. There are also tools that can assist in teaching the child about emotional literacy and problem solving. We will discuss this in a later chapter.

We both use the NeuroTek Advanced Audiotek Device® with auditory and tactile stimulation and find that children particularly enjoy using the device as a means for BLS (http://www.neurotek.com).

INTEGRATING PLAY THERAPY INTO THE EMDR PROTOCOL

Since children process and communicate through play, we integrate play therapy tools and techniques within the EMDR protocol as we conceptualize the treatment of children. Throughout the book, we have included play activities in all aspects of the art of using EMDR with children.

EMDR PROGRESS NOTES

When first using EMDR in psychotherapy, it is beneficial for the therapist to use a detailed progress note to ensure adherence to the EMDR protocol. With children, we use a clipboard that we can juggle while moving around the office shadowing children.

At the EMDR trainings, participants are given a practice worksheet for the practicum exercises. This worksheet is for practice during EMDR training; however, the procedural steps outline from the Part 1 and Part 2 EMDR Training Manuals (Shapiro, 2007) is a more comprehensive document, containing in-depth instructions and added dimensions to the EMDR protocol.

The procedural steps outline document also assists therapists in conceptualizing the EMDR treatment process through each step of the protocol and helps with clinical decision making. With EMDR clinical decision making, the therapist must decide when the client may be at the end of a memory network channel, and the therapist must go back to reevaluate the target. In addition, the practice worksheet from the EMDR trainings does not suffice for a progress note because it does not include all the phrases needed to continue in the EMDR protocol.

COGNITIVE INTERWEAVES

If the client encounters blocked processing, the therapist has tools to assist the client in continuing to reprocess, including *cognitive interweaves*. Therapists may decide to use cognitive interweaves; however, it is important for therapists to use other, more subtle interventions for blocked processing before using cognitive interweaves. The goal is to jump-start the processing with as little therapist intervention as possible. It is important to read chapter 10 on blocked processing and attempt the procedures for blocked processing before using cognitive interweaves. Because cognitive interweaves are taught at the second weekend of training, therapists tend to use cognitive interweaves without attempting other techniques first to assist the client with blocked processing. This does not mean that cognitive interweaves are the first choice of techniques that therapists should use when the client encounters blocked processing; rather, learning to use cognitive interweaves is challenging, which is why they are taught in the second weekend of training.

ADDITIONAL TOOLS FOR GETTING STARTED WITH EMDR

As therapists learn to case conceptualize with the AIP model and the comprehensive treatment process of EMDR, they can benefit from additional skills used by experienced EMDR therapists. This is why we strongly encourage therapists learning EMDR to participate in study groups and seek consultation. In addition, it is extremely helpful to read publications on using EMDR and even participate in a Listserv specifically for EMDR therapists.

Study Groups

It is valuable to participate in an EMDR no-fee study group. Check in the back of your Part 1 manual for a list of no-fee study groups in your area or at http://www.emdria.org. These are great places to network with other EMDR therapists, ask questions, and also make referrals. There may also be an opportunity to connect with other child therapists who are using EMDR.

Listservs

You can also join the EMDR Listserv. This is an online community of EMDR therapists who share information about using EMDR with clients. You can find out more about the Listserv at http://www.emdria.org. At the EMDR International Association (EMDRIA), there are also specialty Listservs for specific populations, including the EMDRIA Children's Special Interest Group (SIG). Therapists can learn how to become part of the Listservs at the EMDRIA Web site (http://www.emdria.org). Also on the EMDRIA Web site, there are links to worldwide EMDR organizations and Web sites.

SUMMARY

In addition to the nuances in getting started with EMDR, there are additional skills and solutions for clinical work when using EMDR in psychotherapy with children. This book will give the practitioner step-by-step details to begin using EMDR with children. Integrating these skills into clinical practice requires patience and a commitment to learning EMDR. This entire book offers practical directions for therapists to use to improve their practice of EMDR with all clients, but especially with young children.

There is minimal research on EMDR with children. This in no way suggests that EMDR with all ages of children is contraindicated. In fact, even very young children respond well to all the phases of the EMDR protocol. So after the initial weekend of EMDR training, using EMDR with a child client requires, first, experience and training in working with children. Then, the therapist must use clinical skills especially designed for children to process the pieces of the EMDR protocol within a developmental framework appropriate to the individual child. Distilling the pieces of the protocol with play therapy or art therapy techniques is effective with all clients, and especially with young children. This chapter summarizes the basic skills therapists will need to get started with EMDR, with the remainder of the book written specifically to give practitioners the tools needed to use EMDR with children of all ages.

CHAPTER 3

EMDR Phase 1: Client History and Treatment Planning

Common to most mental health treatment approaches, the process of psychotherapy begins with the psychotherapist conducting a thorough client history to aid in case conceptualization and planning treatment. Case conceptualization from the Adaptive Information Processing (AIP) Model begins with client history and treatment planning as well. A comprehensive intake needs to have been completed for every client. Eye Movement Desensitization and Reprocessing (EMDR) therapists are also listening for themes, possible targets, trauma history, attachment history, and potential negative cognitions. Once a comprehensive intake has been conducted, the therapist can continue with an EMDR-focused Client History and Treatment Planning process. What is unique to the Client History and Treatment Planning Phase of EMDR is that the therapist is listening for possible targets, negative cognitions, and core beliefs that may be driving the client's current symptomatology. When working with child clients, this process includes information gleaned from the child, the child's caregivers, and possibly, the child's educational environment. Assembling a thorough client history from all available resources is pivotal in effective treatment planning for children.

Once the client's history has been gathered from both the parent and the child, the therapist then uses clinical assessment to write a treatment plan to guide the client's therapeutic process. This chapter will provide resources to augment any client intake and treatment planning a therapist is already using in practice.

With Phase 1 of EMDR, Client History and Treatment Planning begins the process of becoming attuned to the client's unique concerns and issues, physical and emotional capacities, while creating the safety necessary for the client to process trauma. Pacing the use of EMDR is an important part of the therapist's clinical responsibility. The therapist needs to become attuned to both the client's physical and emotional presentation and unique needs to prepare the client for the desensitization process. Getting in sync with the client's distinctive experiences of living and processing sensory input is a foundation for effective therapy. This is another ongoing clinical process that underlies all clinical interventions and the therapeutic relationship.

The Client History and Treatment Planning Phase is focused on creating a targeting sequence for EMDR. The targeting sequence begins with identifying a negative cognition or belief and having the child attempt to identify the touchstone event first associated with the negative cognition. After identifying the touchstone event, the therapist then identifies a progression of events for reprocessing with EMDR. This progression encompasses the child's life experiences that are driving the current symptom presentation with which the child presents for therapy along with future desired experiences that will create the clustering of events around a specific negative cognition. This creates an EMDR targeting sequence for each negative cognition identified for the individual child. Pursuing this initial intake process is dependent on the child's ability to tolerate the exploration of the targeting sequence. If the child becomes overwhelmed by this process, the therapist may need to move to the Preparation Phase of EMDR to provide resources and stabilization skills for the child before continuing to explore targeting sequences. In this way, Phase 1 and Phase 2 of EMDR are interwoven processes, rather than a sequential process. Clinical decision making is driven by the child's ability to participate comfortably in the Client History and Treatment Planning process without being overwhelmed and retraumatized by the process in therapy. We will further discuss clinical decision making regarding this issue throughout this chapter.

CLIENT HISTORY

Conducting a thorough intake process that includes client history and assessment of client functioning aids in effective treatment planning. In our practices, we use standard intake forms and a second EMDR form. At the end of this chapter, we have included an example of our Client History and Treatment Planning Form, which is focused on EMDR (see Exhibits 3.1 and 3.2).

Exhibit 3.1 EMDR Client History/ Treatment Planning Form

(This form is completed in addition to the clinician's standard intake form.)

1. What are the parent's current concerns and goals for treatment? *("I know my child will have been successful in treatment when_______.")*

2. Themes: (What themes are presented by child/parent related to responsibility, safety, control/choice?)

3. Symptom Assessment: (Does child/parent have any indication as to precursor of symptoms? How long have symptoms been present? Are there any times when symptom(s) are not present?)

EMDR Client History/ Treatment Planning Form (Page 2)

4. Identify traumatic experiences as reported by parent only. The therapist asks the child to wait in playroom while interviewing the parent regarding targets: (What is the worst trauma experienced by the child per parent report? Assess for currently activated traumas including traumas/triggers most closely related to current distress or symptoms. Note any additional traumatic experiences spontaneously reported by the child. List triggers, that is, people, places, things, and so on that activate traumatic memories, cause distress or symptoms, or lead to avoidance.)

5. Identify traumatic experiences as reported by the child. (The therapist asks the child to rejoin the session and interviews the child per the target identification script. The child may not identify any of the responses that the parent has identified.) The therapist also completes assessment tools (for a child 8 years or older) during this process. (The parent is asked to wait in the waiting room and complete the assessment tools if child is comfortable with the parent leaving.)

EMDR Client History/ Treatment Planning Form (Page 3)

6. Identify mastery experiences presented by the child. ("Tell me something that you are proud of that you have done. Tell me a time when you felt really good about yourself.")

____

Notes:

____

Clinician's name: ____________________ Date: ____________

Clinician's signature: ______________________________

Exhibit 3.2 Child/Adolescent Symptom Monitoring Form

Date______________ *Child's Name* ____________________________

Parent Completing Form ____________________________________

Therapist ____

Symptoms	Day by Day (Following Therapy)						
	Day1	Day2	Day3	Day4	Day5	Day6	Day7
Stomach aches							
Diarrhea/Constipation							
Sleep Disturbance							
Behavioral Problems							
Tantrums/Acting Out							
Crying							
Avoidance Behaviors							
Agitation							
Urination/Bowel Problems							
Refusal Behavior							
Anxiety							
Change in Eating Habits							
Headaches							

Note: 1 = minimal, 2 = moderate, 3 = severe

Other symptoms possibly related to treatment:

Symptoms Positive Changes	Day by Day						
	Day1	Day2	Day3	Day4	Day5	Day6	Day7

Note: 1 = minimal, 2 = moderate, 3 = severe

Additional Comments/Concerns:

____

____

____

____

____

____

____

____

Please complete this form and bring it to your child's next session. Thank you!

Initial assessment of the client includes assessing the client and the client's life. Special emphasis should be on the child's age, developmental level, and understanding of the context of the child's life experiences. We recommend that both parents and children be interviewed to conduct a thorough client history.

Interviewing Parents and Children

The therapist can decide whether or not the child will attend the first session based on the clinical judgment and practice of the therapist. We typically do a brief phone interview with parents when they call to schedule a first appointment. During the phone interview we ask the parent to describe their concerns about the child and how the parent came to decide that the child was in need of psychotherapy. We also assess for appropriateness of the referral and how to structure the initial sessions in the office. It is during this phone interview that we decide how to proceed with organizing the initial sessions and determine when it would be most appropriate for the child to first visit the office.

Some therapists may choose to have the parent attend an intake session alone to gather history without the child present. If the child attends the session, we recommend that when it is time for the parent intake interview, the child be asked to wait in the playroom or waiting room while the parent is interviewed. We make this decision based on our assessment of how much the parent report will influence what the child reports. The child's age is one determining factor in this decision.

There are several reasons to decide not to have the child in the office while interviewing the parent. First, the parent may have his or her own issues and unresolved affect related to the incidents, which will be identified for the child. Second, the parent's targets may be different from the child's, and we do not want the parent's statements to contaminate what the child may report. If the child listens to the parent's statements, the child may echo the parent's statements, rather than reporting the child's own issues/targets. Third, the child may not volunteer targets that are embarrassing, or the child may have forgotten a target that needs to be addressed in treatment. All of these issues need to be considered by the therapist, yet ultimately, the target selected in the Assessment Phase for reprocessing must resonate for the child. All of the targets identified during the client history are noted as a targeting sequence for further exploration during the Assessment Phase.

After interviewing the parent, the therapist can either schedule a second session to interview the child or bring the child into the session if the child has been waiting during the parent interview. The therapist may choose to have the parents sit quietly in the room while interviewing the child to make the child more comfortable in the office. While meeting with the child, the therapist should also attend to the child's nonverbal communication, including changes in breathing, mannerisms, skin tone, and so on.

Script. The following script can be used when interviewing the child:

"What did your mom/dad/caretaker tell you about why you came here today?" If the child does not respond, then the therapist continues with the following script.

"Your mom/dad/caretaker told me that you had some worries, thoughts, or feelings that are bothering you." If there is no response from the child, the therapist offers some symptoms presented by the parent, for example, "Your mom/dad/caretaker said you have bad dreams. I'm wondering if there are other things that are bothering you that your mom/dad/caretaker doesn't know about that we should talk about today." On the basis of therapist attunement with the child, the therapist first attempts to have the child verbalize the target, but the child may need alternative options.

"If you want to, we can draw a picture or put all those things that are bothering you on my whiteboard so we don't miss any." Allow the child to select the therapeutic tool to use in identifying targets for desensitization. The therapist can use sand tray, toys, or other activities to engage the child in identifying targets.

During the intake process, the therapist is also noting possible negative cognitions that may be themes for what the client reports as current symptomatology. For example, does the client repeatedly weave in statements that indicate the child feels "I'm bad" or "My friends don't like me"? This negative cognition is one piece of evidence of underlying conflict in the child's life that leads to memory networks that require reprocessing to adaptive resolution.

Procedural Considerations

The therapist is noting themes that the client is presenting that can be clustered together under similar negative cognitions, beliefs, emotions, and/or body sensations. By clustering targets, the therapist's goal is to organize the targets for greater efficiency during reprocessing in the Desensitization Phase. Symptom presentation initially drives the exploration for *Touchstone Events*. For example, if the client presents with a behavioral issue, then the therapist is considering when this behavioral issue first started and what incident or memory is driving the current behavioral issue. This is true for negative cognitions, beliefs, emotions, and body sensations as well.

AIP theory suggests that by clustering the targets, the therapist can then better manage goals for treatment planning and with succinct exploration of the Touchstone Event. Shapiro (2001) developed the AIP model to explain the mechanisms by which EMDR assists clients in moving from disturbance to adaptive resolution. EMDR is a comprehensive treatment methodology, while AIP is the comprehensive theoretical approach to psychotherapy. (The reader can refer to chapter 1 for a discussion of AIP theory.) The Touchstone Event is defined by Shapiro (2001) as the initial event that was maladaptively stored that is driving the current symptomatology. During the Client History and Treatment Planning Phase, the therapist is listening for touchstone events and may be able to probe for touchstone events if the client is able to tolerate the process. If the client is fragile, clinical judgment is necessary to determine if additional preparation is necessary before probing for touchstone events. If the client needs additional resources to cope with questioning about touchstone events, it is clinically indicated to proceed with the Preparation Phase. If the child is coping with this process continue with once the standard Client History and Treatment Planning process is completed; this will be discussed in the remainder of this chapter.

With children, the therapist is listening both for concerns identified by the parent as well as symptoms presented by the child. (Questions for target identification are also included during the Assessment Phase, see chapter 5.) We believe we cannot emphasize strongly enough how important it is to remember to ask the child as well as the parents. Children will frequently manifest sleep disturbances; somatic complaints; behavioral issues; separation anxiety; regulatory challenges, including emotional regulation; and various types of fears. It is especially important to ask children about their fears, worries, and/or problems. Parents may readily identify symptoms, while children may require additional therapeutic intervention to elicit the child's perspective. Young children especially may present symptomatology in Metaphorical terms such as a fear of monsters. The therapist can ask a child directly to verbalize concerns, or the therapist can ask the child to draw a picture of the thing that scares the child or bothers him or her the most.

The focus of treatment may not always be obvious. The presenting problem may indicate underlying issues that are stored maladaptively. The overlay of the presenting problem can suggest that additional probing is necessary to identify core issues. In addition to probing for core symptomatology, the therapist can use more formal assessment tools for evaluating children and to identify core issues. Specific tools for evaluating children are discussed later in this chapter.

In this process, the therapist is striving to understand what it is like to live in that child's world and what the child's experience is of being in the world. What is it like to walk in that child's bare feet? Who is important in the child's life? As part of case conceptualization, the therapist is developing attunement to the child to get to know the client by having a sense of wonder and curiosity about the child. As a therapist, I (R.T.) imagine what it is like to be with that child. Where does the child struggle? When is the child happy and fun and delightful? It is not only important to become attuned to the child, but also to imagine what it would be like to parent the child, so as to speculate on the parent–child relationship and how that relationship is impacting the client's presenting issues.

Listening for Targets

Targets are representations of unresolved pieces of the child's history that manifest in current symptomatology. Beginning with the first session with the child and continuing through the entire EMDR eight phases, therapists are listening for possible targets that may require reprocessing. This does not mean that the therapist has identified the specific targets for processing at this point, but only that he or she is making notes, mental or written, to explore the possible target issues and negative beliefs as the therapist proceeds. Targets may include memories, images, negative cognitions, unresolved feelings, behaviors, and body sensations. Any disturbance reported by the child or parent may indicate unresolved issues that lead to potential targets.

The following areas to be addressed in the Client History and Treatment Planning Phase are included because of the particular significance these areas have on case conceptualization with EMDR.

Presenting Problem

Clinical assessment will guide the process of identifying the presenting problem, with the therapist asking the client simple questions like "Why now? What do you want to get out of being here? How will we know when we're done?" Depending on the client, the therapist may or may not gather a significant amount of information during this process. This is when the therapist is first conceptualizing the course of treatment. The therapist must also evaluate the stability of the child's home environment; school experience, if applicable; significant relationships; health/medical history; affect tolerance; and possible trauma history.

Psychosocial History

In this section we review the child's family history and ask with whom the child currently lives and about custody issues. We also explore the child's history of positive and negative experiences and relationships. It is important to ask about significant people in the child's life, including day care providers, schoolteachers, friends/playmates, and siblings. What births and deaths have occurred in the family that have affected the child? What positive and negative changes have occurred in the child's life, including moves, changes in schools, and so on?

Parent–Child Attachment/Attunement

In assessing the child's attachment experiences, we explore the history of the child's caregivers and explore any disruptions to the relationship between the child and primary caregiver, including periods of separation due to changes in caregivers, parent or child illness or injury, parent military deployment, and so on.

During the initial contact with parents and/or caregivers, the therapist is also listening for the parents' own attachment and developmental history and its implications for parenting their own child. The therapist is assessing the parents' attunement to the child and how the parents' mental health and attachment history may be impacting the child's current symptom manifestation. One way to observe the parent–child relationship is to notice the family in the waiting room or during other opportunities to observe the parent and child interact without intruding. Another way to observe parents and children is to have a playroom with an observation window. I (R.T.) have a playroom with a window that allows unobtrusive observation of the child and family. This process also allows for assessment of how children separate from parents.

Separations, disruptions, and insults to the parent–child relationship may be conceptualized as attachment trauma and be one focus of EMDR reprocessing. The parent–child relationship and the parents' marital relationship are typically significant issues that impact the child. Working with children who present with attachment trauma and/or reactive attachment disorder will be discussed at the end of this book.

Educational History

What educational experiences has the child had? What impact have those educational experiences had on the child, both as possible resources and mastery experiences as well as possible distressing and/or traumatic experiences? Many children will report stressful school events that, through the eyes of a child, are experienced as traumatic. One child presented with school phobia after she threw up when asked to read in front of the class. This event was targeted with EMDR in order that the child could return to school.

Religious Affiliations/Cultural Dynamics

What is the family cultural identity? What language does the family use in the home? Understanding the child and family cultural dynamics impacts the resources and limitations that may be accessed during processing with EMDR. For example, one child with whom I (R.T.) worked came from a religion in which angels could not be used for resources because of the religious interpretations of angels.

Developmental History

The assessment of the client should include prenatal and perinatal experiences; cognitive functioning; expressive and receptive language skills; self-help skills; social development; emotional development, including emotional literacy; and sensory integration issues. It is especially important to understand the child's unique characteristics and current developmental accomplishments to understand how to translate EMDR for the individual child. Each chapter of this book will provide examples of how to translate EMDR into a child's language, depending on the child's unique developmental levels.

Medical History

What was the child's birth experience? What current medical conditions does the child have? What medical interventions has the child experienced in his or her lifetime? Are there any family members with significant medical issues? There may be experiences that have impacted the child's mental health functioning, including a history of high fevers, head injuries, surgeries, intrusive medical interventions, chronic medical conditions, and incidents that may be unique to the area in which the child lives. For example, in Arizona, where we both live, children may have experienced scorpion stings, which can be both traumatic and a neurological insult. For example, bark scorpions are common in the Phoenix metropolitan area, and the bark scorpion venom includes a neurotoxin that can cause significant medical problems for a child. When I (R.T.) explored the history of a child who presented with distress and anxiety, the medical history included a near-death experience due to a bark scorpion sting. The neurological impact of the bark scorpion's venom, along with the traumatic experience of almost dying, were both targets for EMDR with this particular child.

It is also important to explore recent illnesses that the child may have experienced. I (R.T.) had a child who presented with recent onset of hallucinations and bizarre thoughts. The child had previously been diagnosed with ADHD but had functioned very well in school and at home within a structured environment. After experiencing an illness with a high fever, the child began to hallucinate and became more aggressive and noncompliant. After referring the child for a psychiatric evaluation, the psychiatrist diagnosed the child as having Pediatric Autoimmune Neuropsychiatric Disorder (PANDAS) and prescribed medication to treat the illness. The child returned for psychotherapy to process the trauma of suddenly experiencing hallucinations and having difficulty explaining what was happening to his parents.

Assessment of Current Stability

The therapist should assess the child's current stability, including a minimental status exam. Clinical judgment regarding the child's stability should include evaluating specific issues such as the child's risk of displaying suicidal behaviors, any history of juvenile offenses, sexually reactive or trauma-reactive behaviors, emotional volatility, or physical complications that would make the child particularly fragile.

Children with single-incident traumas may not require significant preparation for reprocessing the traumatic event with EMDR, while children with cascading traumas may need a much greater degree of skill building and resourcing to work through the EMDR process. The client's trauma history and current stability are both integrally related to case conceptualization and pacing with EMDR.

The treatment of children living in unstable environments must focus primarily on frontloading in the Preparation Phase, where the therapist works on assisting the child to develop both internal and external resources, containment skills, affect management, and survival skills. We will discuss the Preparation Phase in the next chapter, but it is important for therapists working with children living in fragile environments to be aware that it may take a significant amount of time to ever move into the Assessment Phase of EMDR. Clinical judgment is, again, extremely important in case conceptualization with children living in unstable environments and must include pacing and titration skills for the child. The therapeutic process must proceed at a pace that allows the child to stabilize in the environment, without causing such disruption that the child deteriorates. However, even children who are living in foster care or unstable or dangerous environments can benefit from EMDR. Case conceptualization must focus on a therapeutic process that is manageable for the child given the child's current life situation.

Affect Tolerance

The child's ability to tolerate intense affect needs to be assessed to determine what affect tolerance skills the child may need to learn during the

Preparation Phase of EMDR. Explore with both children and caregivers how the child expresses anger. How does the child respond to fear? How does the child cope with frustration? In the office, it is important for the therapist to observe how the client responds to questions. Does the child become more anxious or active in discussing certain issues? What does the child do to avoid a specific topic that the child may not want to discuss? How does the child handle distress?

Trauma History

As part of the trauma history, the therapist needs to assess the child's symptomatology and possible dissociation. Trauma is loosely defined as anything that negatively impacts the child's psyche. It is imperative that therapists remember that children may be traumatized by experiences that would not be considered traumatic from an adult perspective. The exploration of a trauma history must be from a child's perspective of life.

Current Resources, Innerpersonal, and Interpersonal Skills

The therapist should attempt to assess what current resources and skills the child has and focus on child strengths. The child should be asked to talk about times when the child felt particularly successful or accomplished. This allows for relationship building between the child and the therapist, while providing an opportunity for the therapist to gather vital information that can be used to help the child in the future. Installation of mastery experiences and the benefit to the child during treatment will be explained at a later time.

Potential Targets

Targets are identified from child reports, parent reports, and/or by the child's symptom presentation. One of the issues the therapist needs to explore with targets is to understand how the child has stored the particular experience in the child's memory networks. Targets can be stored in the brain as cognitions, emotions, body sensations, beliefs, pictures, images, sounds, smells, and other sensory input. Children may often store traumatic events Metaphorically or in unusual and unexpected ways. Children often create their own narrative from pieces of a memory that the child has formed in a manner that might not make sense to an adult. Children will often identify traumatic experiences by talking about monsters or aliens. Children naturally seek out explanations for things they do not understand. It is not important that the therapist understand what exactly happened to the child, but instead that the therapist is able to understand that the child has created an explanation to attempt to cope with the distressing or traumatic event. I (R.T.) encourage children to identify traumatic events by letters or symbols or drawings, without exploring the details of what occurred. It is not necessary for the therapist to probe into the child's experience, but instead to understand that the child has experienced the event as problematic.

Listening for Negative Cognitions

The EMDR theory is based on organizing negative cognitions and beliefs into the three categories of responsibility, safety, and choices. Listening for misattributions of responsibility for traumatic experiences is very important, especially when treating children. Children will often assume responsibility for a traumatic experience because this allows the child to retain some power in the traumatic situation and a false sense of control over future potential victimization. As the therapist is listening for these negative cognitions, the therapist is exploring a possible targeting sequence of events, as much as the child can tolerate. There are several ways to explore the targeting sequence, as long as the child can tolerate the processing without becoming overwhelmed. The goal is to start with the negative cognition and first ask the child, "When was the first time you remember thinking, 'I'm bad'?" If the child can identify an earlier time, that earliest memory becomes the touchstone event, and then the therapist can explore other times that the child remembers thinking, "I'm bad." Those other memories then become past events that are part of the progression of events in a targeting sequence that are arranged as much as possible in a chronological order, starting with the touchstone event, then past events and more recent events that the child can recall. This can be explored in more detail as part of mapping targets, which is explained in chapter 5, on the Assessment Phase of EMDR. In this manner, the therapist is clustering events around a negative cognition or belief to most effectively organize maladaptively stored events for assessment and reprocessing during later phases of EMDR.

Attempting to identify a touchstone event by using some type of floatback technique is often difficult with children who tend to be more present oriented and concrete. It is important for therapists working with children to recognize that the therapist may need to use additional skills, which are described in chapter 10, on blocked processing and cognitive interweaves, to assist children in becoming aware of previous events. We recommend the use of a cognitive interweave floatback as one technique to help children with touchstone events, as is discussed in chapter 10. With younger children, we sometimes create a targeting sequence, focused on how the child's symptoms developed, rather than on specific events.

We will ask the child and/or parent to identify when the symptom began and create a map of the child's symptoms and associated experiences.

Again, if the child cannot tolerate the direct exploration of the targeting sequence, the therapist may need to move to the Preparation Phase of EMDR to focus on developing resources for affect tolerance. This targeting sequence then becomes part of a comprehensive treatment plan.

TREATMENT PLANNING

Gathering data pertaining to the client's life is an ongoing process that continues throughout therapy, even after a formal client intake is completed. As the psychotherapist continuously listens for new and changing experiences in the client's life, an initial treatment plan is generated to guide treatment. Treatment planning is a fluid process that is evaluated in each session, as goals are accomplished, added, or changed. With children, there are multiple voices contributing to the child's treatment plan.

The therapist may ask the parents and the child their goals for treatment; however, the parents' goals, the child's goals, and the therapist's goals may or may not overlap. The therapist should make note of all the goals identified by each individual and then write the treatment plan with the client. Treatment planning identifies the symptom and/or issue to be treated, the treatment process, and the outcome goal for therapy.

Effective treatment planning includes the therapist's ability to conceptualize the client's case. As with any type of mental health treatment, assessing how the child may have stored the traumatic memory is a significant part of the treatment planning process. The therapist must ask specific questions about events that were happening in the client's life at the time that symptoms began and what negative cognitions originated as a result of the client's history. Oftentimes, client's symptomatology is driven by unresolved trauma that is associated with concurrent pieces of the client's history. To effectively conceptualize treatment planning with the individual client, the therapist needs to ask what other events were happening at that time. The therapist is often looking for the missing piece. For example, if the child experienced a traumatic medical procedure at the same time the child's parents were going through a divorce, the therapist will most likely need to target the traumatic medical procedure and any difficulties the child experienced related to the parents' divorce. With one child, I (R.T.) targeted the child's sexual abuse by a neighbor; however, after the child disclosed the abuse, the child's father no longer felt comfortable touching the child. Neither the father nor the child reported this to me; however, the child's distress from the sexual abuse did not decrease until we explored how the child's family had changed after she had disclosed. This was the missing piece in the child's treatment. We have experienced many situations in children's lives when it appeared that treatment had come to an impasse, when in fact, there was a missing piece from the past or present that was continuing to drive the child's distress that was not known to the therapist.

In addition, treatment planning is not always sequential, nor is it completed during this part of therapy. Treatment planning is an ongoing and fluid process that occurs throughout therapy, as goals arise and are teased out, and others are completed. In working with children in a forensic environment, I (R.T.) often work with stabilizing children in order that the child can testify to the assault. With these children, it is difficult for the child to process the traumatic experiences until the perpetrator is arrested and the criminal/legal process is concluded. I have found that many children are unable to discuss their abuse until the perpetrator is incarcerated and the child feels some level of safety in the community. To explore the child's current situation, we offer the following script for therapists to consider in working with children. As with any script we have included in this book, we encourage therapists to adjust the script to meet the individual needs of the child.

Therapist Script for Client History and Treatment Planning

After interviewing the parent, bring the child into the session and utilize the following script when interviewing the child: "What did your mom/dad/caretaker tell you about why you came here today?" (if the child does not respond, then the therapist continues with the following): "Your mom/dad/caretaker told me that you had some worries, thoughts, or feelings that are bothering you" (if no response from the child, the therapist offers some symptoms presented by the parent, for example, "Your mom/dad/caretaker said you have bad dreams" or "I'm wondering if there are other things that are bothering you that your mom/dad/caretaker does not know about that we should talk about today."). Based on therapist attunement with the child, the therapist first attempts to have the child verbalize the target, but the child may need alternative options: "If you want to, we can draw a picture or put all those things that are bothering you on my whiteboard so we don't miss any." (Allow the child to select the therapeutic tool to use in identifying symptoms and concerns for treatment planning. The therapist can use sand tray, toys, or other activities to engage the child in this experience.)

With some children, this would be an opportune time in therapy to begin the mapping process that is described in detail in chapter 5. It is important for the therapist to focus on rapport building with the child and on beginning the process of encouraging the child's confidence in the therapy process. Some children may feel overwhelmed by this process, or intimidated or embarrassed. We assure children that what they share in the therapy office is private and will only be shared with the therapist and the child's caregivers. This is also a time when we will explain to children and parents that the therapist's job is as a helper to the child and his or her family, and if the therapist is concerned that the child is in danger, the therapist will take steps consistent with the laws of the state to protect the child. The therapist must weave the issues of informed consent into the therapy process during this initial client history and treatment planning process. I (R.T.) explain to children that I am a worry doctor for children and that I help children and their families with things that are bothering the child. And I (C.S.) tell children that children come to see me to talk about their worries or bothers, sometimes about school, sometimes about home, sometimes about other stuff.

Informed Consent

Therapists can continue to use the informed consent forms (at the end of this chapter), consistent with the agencies and statutes of the therapist's professional ethical and legal requirements. We also will ask the child to sign an assent for treatment. This assent for treatment asks the child to also agree to participate in the therapy process. This assent for treatment from the child is not a requirement, but rather an intervention focused on engaging the child in the process and empowering the child to be an active participant in his or her own treatment process.

Establishing the Therapeutic Relationship and Engaging the Client in Therapy

The process of establishing a therapeutic relationship with the child begins the moment the child enters the therapy office. Engaging the child in therapy requires establishing a healthy working relationship with the therapist. One of the ways to do this is by making therapy as playful and fun as possible because play is the tool for children to understand and process the world and to communicate their experiences and interpretations of their world to others.

Developing the child's sense of safety and security in the office and with the therapist is also important. The therapist needs to take the time to stabilize the child and to make the therapy office a safe place. Depending on the individual client, the therapist may need to use additional skills and techniques to engage the client in the EMDR process and to assist the client in establishing a sense of safety in the office and with the therapist. The child's attachment history can impact this process, and it is important to be aware of the fact that when children have trauma in their attachment relationships, this can also complicate the therapeutic relationship. The therapeutic relationship may be the child's first experience of a healthy and receptive attachment environment, where the child can heal and begin to learn to attach in positive ways. If the child is not attached in healthy ways, the child may be more active and harder to calm, and the child may have poor boundaries that will have to be addressed as part of therapy. The impact of attachment trauma on the therapeutic relationship and process will be further discussed in a later chapter.

Establishing a working relationship with the child will also augment the assessment process in order that the therapist can conduct a valid assessment of the child. Because many of the assessment tools are self-report measures, the child must be comfortable enough with the therapist to be able to engage in the assessment interaction.

ASSESSMENT TOOLS FOR EVALUATING CHILDREN

There are many self-report and parent report scales for assessing children that can be found free on the Internet or purchased by professionals. Some tools are translated into several languages. We have included an overview of assessment tools (in the reference section of this book) we use in assessing children during treatment and how those specific types of assessment are integrated into comprehensive treatment planning.

Initially, the therapist should request copies of all previous assessment and testing of the child and then consider using the following scales for evaluating the child's current functioning and progress in treatment. In conducting comprehensive assessment of children, mental health professionals consider assessments of cognitive, academic, emotional, developmental, and mental health issues. If no previous assessments are available, the therapist may need to consider referring the child for a comprehensive psychological evaluation.

Mental health professionals in treatment roles need to consider referring children for evaluations and the ethical and legal issues that cover evaluating children.

Ethical and Legal Issues

There are legal and ethical issues that address the issue of mental health professionals having roles as both evaluator and treatment professional, and we refer professionals to their respective professional organizations regarding conducting assessments. Most cognitive, academic/achievement, and developmental evaluations require specialty training to administer and interpret the tests.

Cognitive/Intellectual Assessment

Therapists can request previous testing from schools and other professionals or refer families for cognitive assessments of children. There are standardized tools for assessing cognitive functioning in children, including the Wechsler Intelligence Scales for Children–IV (Harcourt Assessment, 2003) and the Stanford–Binet–5 (Roid, 2003), which are frequently used scales to assess the intellectual functioning of children.

Academic/Achievement Assessment

Academic and achievement assessments are conducted by schools or professionals in hospitals and private organizations. Cognitive and academic/achievement assessments are also used to evaluate children for learning disabilities, along with assessing for mental retardation, reading disorders, language disorders, and other developmental disorders.

Developmental Assessment

Conducting developmental assessments of children is important not only in treatment planning, but also in helping parents to understand the child's developmental level and to determine if the child is delayed in any areas of development. Common assessment tools for assessing children's development include the Alpern Developmental Profile–3 (DP-3), the Ages and Stages Questionnaires® (ASQ), and several sensory integration tools.

DP-3 (Alpern, 2007) assesses the child's functioning in five areas, including physical functioning, adaptive behavior, social–emotional functioning, cognitive functioning, and communication skills, for children from 0 years to 12 years and 11 months. This tool needs to be purchased.

The ASQ (Bricker & Squires, 1999) assesses for development in eight different age scales from 4 to 60 months of age. The ASQ assesses for communication skills, gross motor skills, fine motor skills, problem-solving skills, and personal–social skills and provides scores for each subscale. The ASQ is easily administered and can be used in understanding the child's development at various stages to assist in effectively guiding treatment. The ASQ is also an assessment tool that must be purchased.

In addition to developmental scales, it is helpful to assess for sensory integration issues, especially with young children. Even though sensory integration is a symptom of other mental health issues, including autism and Asperger's Disorder, sensory integration dysfunction (SID) is most often diagnosed by occupational therapists. Checklists for sensory integration concerns are available online at http://www.starcenter.us and can be used for screening children in therapy. There are many online resources for information on sensory integration and sensory processing issues that are available for download (http://www.incrediblehorizons.com/sensory-integration.htm). We also recommend, for therapists and parents, *The Out-of-Sync Child: Recognizing and Coping With Sensory Processing Disorder,* by Kranowitz (2005). These scales can assist the therapist in understanding how the child processes information and are especially important when selecting the type of bilateral stimulation that may be most effective with the child. The implications of sensory integration issues will be discussed throughout this book.

Most mental health professionals in a treatment role with children will use academic, cognitive, and developmental assessments conducted by other professionals; however, mental health professionals in treatment roles will often conduct emotional and behavioral health assessments of children as part of a comprehensive treatment plan.

Behavioral Assessment

Behavioral Assessment System for Children–II (BASC-II; Reynolds & Kamphaus, 2006) is a comprehensive assessment system for evaluating children's behaviors, with assessment forms that collect input from children, parents, and teachers. The BASC-II includes both clinical and adaptive scales to assist in identifying areas of concern and confirming diagnostic issues with children ages 2–21 years. The BASC-II must be purchased from Pearson's Assessment Group.

Emotional Assessment

In addition to intellectual, achievement, developmental, and behavioral issues, it is important for therapists to assess children for symptoms of trauma and dissociation. As mental health practitioners, we work under the hypothesis that most clients use some type of dissociative process to cope with trauma. For the purposes of assessing children for EMDR, we recommend the following scales:

The Children's Impact of Traumatic Events Scale–Revised, by Wolfe, Gentil, Michienzi, and Sas (1991), is a scale used to assess the impact of abuse on children, with questions focused on identifying symptoms consistent with posttraumatic stress disorder, and can be found online (http://vinst.umdnj.edu/VAID/TestReport.asp?Code=CITESR).

The Children's Reactions to Traumatic Events Scale–Revised (CRTES-R), by Jones (2002), has been used to assess children for symptoms associated with experiencing a traumatic event. The CRTES-R is frequently used in research studies to assess for pre/posttest functioning in children to assess for treatment effectiveness.

The Trauma Symptom Checklist for Children (TSCC), by Briere (1996), is an assessment tool that identifies symptoms of posttraumatic stress in children aged 8–16 years. The TSCC can be purchased from Psychological Assessment Resources (http://www.parinc.com).

The Traumatic Stress Symptom Checklist (TSSC), by Adler-Tapia (2001), was designed to assess symptoms of traumatic stress in young children aged 0–6 years. This checklist has not been normed or validated, but rather includes symptoms consistent with a diagnosis of posttraumatic stress disorder in children, which suggests the scale has face validity. This scale is available online (http://www.emdrkids.com).

The Children's Dissociative Checklist–3 (CDC-3), by Putnam, is available online (http://www.energyhealing.net/pdf_files/cdc.pdf). The CDC-3 is helpful for screening for dissociation in children. There is no scoring for this checklist, but rather, the questions are used to explore the presence of particular symptoms associated with dissociation.

Finally, a summary of scales is available online (Association for the Study and Development of Community, http://www.capacitybuilding.net/Measures%20of%20CEV%20and%20outcomes.pdf).

ASSESSING CHILDREN'S READINESS FOR THERAPY/SELECTION CRITERIA

The most significant issue in the successful treatment of children is engaging the child in the therapeutic process. To successfully engage the child in therapy, the therapist needs to first assess the child's readiness for treatment. Since the child is rarely the one who initiates therapy, it is necessary to assess the child's readiness for therapy and willingness to engage in the therapeutic process. The therapist can initially play with the child and ask the child, "What did your mommy or daddy tell you about why you came to play with me?" The therapist needs to ask some type of question that explores what the child has been told by the caregiver and the child's expectations for being at the therapy session. This initial discussion then leads the therapist to the opportunity to discuss therapy, the therapist's role, and the purpose for therapy. The therapist can also use this opportunity to explain mental health and psychotherapy in developmentally appropriate terms.

During this interaction, the therapist is continuing to become attuned to the child and is assessing the child's level of comfort and safety in the office. Will the child engage in a play activity with the therapist? What is the child's level of comfort in separating from the parent? What is the child's level of activity, and how does the child explore the office? A child with a secure attachment should gradually take greater interest in exploring the office, while either physically or visually checking in with the parent. This checking-in process should decrease as the child establishes a comfort level with the therapist and the office setting. Treating children with attachment issues requires more advanced clinical skills in using EMDR and will be discussed in greater detail in chapter 11.

During this interaction with the child, the therapist may have an opportunity to install mastery. If the therapist feels a level of attunement with the child, the therapist may determine that installing a mastery experience will benefit the child and engage the child in the therapeutic process.

Monitoring Child Symptoms

With this understanding of the goals for the Client History and Treatment Planning Phase of the EMDR protocol, the following session protocol provides the therapist with step-by-step procedures for the therapy session. We have included a Child Adolescent Monitoring Form (see Appendix III and p. 48.) for therapists to give parents to use to document the child's behaviors and progress between sessions. Some parents may need the form explained in more detail, depending on the parent's level of psychological awareness. We will give the parent several blank copies of the form and ask the parent to return the form at the next session.

Providing Psychoeducational Information

In addition to monitoring the child's behavior between sessions, we are also teaching parents about children's reactions to distressing and traumatic experiences. Explaining the etiology of children's symptoms and behavioral issues is extremely beneficial to parents and enhances parents' insights and understanding of their children as well as engaging parents in the therapeutic process.

We provide psychoeducational materials for several reasons. First, it is important to provide educational information about trauma, abuse, and other children's issues for parents and children to read between sessions. There are many books and Web sites to which one can refer children and parents for more information. Providing psychoeducational information and materials to children and parents is very important to assist in helping families understand how children deal with distress and to assist in gaining skills in relaxation, stress management, emotional literacy, and parenting. Second, it is important to allow families to ask questions in sessions and to practice new skills in sessions, with the therapist's guidance.

At the end of the Client History and Treatment Planning Phase, when the therapist has gathered all relevant information and created a working treatment plan, the therapist can explain the next step in the psychotherapy process to transition into the Preparation Phase of EMDR.

SUMMARY

The first phase of EMDR treatment is the Client History and Treatment Planning Phase, which is focused on gathering information about the child and family as part of developing a treatment plan. This forms the foundation for the next phases of treatment. The therapist may need to cycle through the Client History and Treatment Planning Phase and the Preparation Phase, depending on how stable the child is and how the child tolerates the discovery of past events that are driving current symptomatology. These past events are identified to develop a targeting sequence clustered around the child's negative cognitions and beliefs. If a child cannot tolerate the exploration of past events, the therapist may need to provide resourcing and affect tolerance skills, as discussed in the next chapter, on the Preparation Phase of EMDR, before proceeding with further investigation of past targets.

Along with the clinical tools discussed in this chapter and the integration of various techniques for working with children, we have included an outline of the progression of an initial EMDR session with children.

INITIAL EMDR SESSION PROTOCOL

1. Therapist greets and introduces self to child and parent.
2. Therapist reviews initial patient information packet and all informed consent forms and answers child and parent questions.
3. Therapist provides parent with self-report instruments and explains purpose of instruments. Parent is instructed to complete

standardized assessment forms, as determined by the therapist, which may include the BASC-II, the Children's Dissociative Checklist (CDC), the Sensory Integration Checklist, and the Traumatic Stress Checklist for Infants, Toddlers, and Preschoolers (if child is less than 8 years of age; if child is over 8 years, parent should complete TSCC with therapist in the first session), and return completed forms to therapist. Parent is also asked to have teacher/caregiver complete BASC-Teacher format and to return forms at the next session. Therapist has parent sign release of information form for teacher and caregiver.

4. Therapist completes client history and treatment planning using forms provided. (Client history and treatment planning process is completed with child and parent in session, except where indicated on form.) Therapist completes Children's Impact of Events Scale–Revised and TSCC with child in therapy session.
5. Therapist begins to note possible targets for EMDR based on presenting problems suggested by child and parent. This is the beginning of creating a targeting sequence for EMDR.
6. Therapist identifies general treatment goals with measurable behavioral objectives and completes treatment plan form, for example, "I know my child will have completed therapy when he/she has a 50% increase in successful school attendance."
7. Therapist explains child monitoring system forms for use between sessions and gives parent a copy of child monitoring system form for parent use.
8. Therapist reviews consent forms (see the Consent for Treatment of a Minor and the Child Assent Form at the end of this chapter) with child and parent and answers any remaining questions.
9. Therapist reviews treatment goals with child and parent and answers any questions before scheduling the next session.

CONSENT FOR TREATMENT OF MINOR

This is an authorization for (therapist name) to provide treatment and/or diagnostic services to my child/adolescent, ____________________ ______ (name). By signing this Consent for Treatment, I certify that I legally have custody or joint custody of my son or daughter and, thus, can legally consent for treatment of my child.

Parent/Guardian signature: ____________________ Date: __________

CHILD ASSENT FORM

I understand that my parent or guardian may consent for my treatment; however, I have also been asked to give my assent for my own treatment. By signing below, I realize that the therapist listed above has elicited my own assent for treatment.

Child's name: ______________________________ Birth date: ____________________

Sign your name here: ______________________________ Witness: ____________________

CHAPTER 4

EMDR Phase 2: Preparation Phase

The Preparation Phase establishes the foundation for continuing with the procedural steps of EMDR. This phase captures multiple areas that are the foundation for therapy, including establishing a therapeutic relationship and engaging the client in the therapeutic process; explaining EMDR; acquiring informed consent for treatment; assessing the client's resources and skills; assessing the client's home environment; determining what individuals will need to be included in the psychotherapy; and finally, teaching the mechanics of EMDR.

EXPLAINING EMDR AND INFORMED CONSENT FOR TREATMENT

During the Preparation Phase, therapists need to explain EMDR to both parents and children and document informed consent for the treatment process like any other type of psychotherapy. Informed consent for EMDR can be integrated into the therapist's intake process as part of the overall consent for psychotherapy, as was discussed in chapter 3. We do not recommend that therapists request a second consent specifically for EMDR. We have included an example of a consent for treatment form as Appendix I.

Explaining EMDR to Parents

Explaining EMDR to parents is a straightforward process of educating parents about EMDR: what it is, how it works mechanically, and what it can do for their child. The therapist can reference the research on brain functioning and the mind–body connection. The therapist can also explain that their child's behavior and symptoms may be the brain's and body's adaptive response to the child's life experiences. Even though there is no longer trauma, the child may be locked in a pattern of responding to anything that looks, sounds, smells, or feels like the original experience as if it is the regular experience happening all over again. The therapist can also explain trauma to parents using a broad definition, with emphasis on how their child will reprocess and integrate frightening, hurtful, or traumatic experiences.

The depth of this explanation needs to be appropriate to the parents' comfort level and needs. The therapist can offer handouts to the parents to read at their leisure and can make references to Internet resources and other written materials as well. The National Institute of Mental Health, in September 2001, published a document titled "Helping Children and Adolescents Cope With Violence and Disasters." This document is available from the National Institute of Mental Health (NIMH) Web site (http://www.nimh.nih.gov/publicat/index.cfm). The U.S. Department of Health and Human Services, Substance Abuse and Mental Health Services (SAMHSA), published a document titled "Tips for Talking to Children in Trauma" in September 2005. This document is available from the SAMHSA Web site (http://www.samhsa.gov). Finally, the American Academy of Child and Adolescent Psychiatry, in October 1999, published a document that reviews posttraumatic stress disorder in children titled "Posttraumatic Stress Disorder" (No. 70 of the Facts for Families series of articles). This document is available online (http://www.aacap.org/publications/factsfam/ptsd70.htm). The therapist can choose to refer the parents to these Web sites or download the handouts to give to parents as needed.

Explaining EMDR to Children

Since explaining EMDR changes for children of different ages, this section addresses how we might explain EMDR to children. We might discuss with children how therapy helps with worries or things that bother children, but we make this explanation simple and straightforward.

Typically, we will just explain EMDR to children by demonstrating how EMDR works and then allow the child to ask questions during the process.

Script. The following is an example of a possible script that therapists can use to explain EMDR to children.

"I want to show you something we call EMDR and see how it works for you" (therapist will utilize the language unique with the individual child).

"When we do the EMDR, we use these tools. We can use all kinds of things for EMDR, so let's find out which one works best for you." (Therapist starts with eye movements and then moves to other types of bilateral stimulations [BLS], as appropriate for the individual child.)

"I want to show you this thing that I have." (Therapist brings out EMDR NeuroTek machine [http://www.neurotekcorp.org] with buzzies.) "This thing tickles a little when you hold it in your hands. Do you want to try?" (Therapist teaches the child how to use NeuroTek and allows the child to experiment. Therapist will assess child's response to machine. If child is comfortable, therapist continues. If child appears uncomfortable with buzzies, then therapist explores other types of BLS with child. Therapist then will demonstrate audio BLS with NeuroTek machine.)

"It doesn't seem like you like the buzzies. I want to see if maybe you'd like to hear the sounds this machine can make instead?" (Therapist demonstrates audio BLS and allows child to experiment. If child is comfortable with audio BLS, continue. Once child is comfortable with some type of BLS, continue explaining EMDR.)

"With the _________ [BLS], we're gonna have you think about that _________ [target] and just see how that works for you."

"Do you have any questions about how this EMDR thing works?" (If child has questions, therapist responds to questions.)

During the discussion of EMDR, the therapist is also listening for the child's resources and skills to become attuned to the child and build the foundation for processing in EMDR.

ASSESSING THE CHILD'S RESOURCES

Children bring to therapy their own internal and external resources with which to deal with life. During the Preparation Phase, therapists are assessing the client's current resources and what resources and skills the client needs to learn to improve the client's mental health and overall functioning.

Assessing the Child's Internal Resources and Skills

Therapists can assess children's resources and skills through direct questioning, interactional activities, and observation. The child's responses from the client history and treatment planning phase can be incorporated and expanded during the Preparation Phase. For example, the child's responses to questioning about mastery experiences can provide evidence of the child's current resources and needs. If the child feels competent when playing baseball, baseball Metaphors and baseball activities in psychotherapy would be a good place to start in building rapport with the child.

Direct Questioning. Whatever tools or techniques you have used as a therapist can be incorporated at this point. In this part of the therapy process, the therapist is trying to identify resources, skills, skill deficits, and resource challenges as well as trying to become attuned to the child and develop rapport in the therapeutic relationship. The psychotherapy process with children is anything but linear. As the therapist is asking the child questions, the therapist is also making note of the child's nonverbal responses, arousal level, affect, activity level, and general comfort in interacting and responding to questions. The therapist is noting the child's thought processes, expressive language, and creativity as well as noting parent–child interaction when the parent is in the room. Whether or not the therapist chooses to ask the child the questions with the parent in the office is driven by many variables, which will be discussed later in this chapter.

Asking children direct questions in a nonthreatening manner can include asking the following questions, which are specifically designed to pendulate between simple questions and more probing questions to engage the child in the therapy process without overwhelming the child with emotionally laden topics. (We have also included a list of Child Interview Questions on pages 11–12 in the *EMDR and the Art of Psychotherapy With Children Treatment Manual*, Adler-Tapia & Settle, 2008.)

What school do you go to?
What's your teacher's name?
What's your favorite subject in school besides recess and lunch? (This usually gets a giggle from the child.)
If you had three wishes, what would they be?
What's your favorite color?
If you ruled the world, what would be two things you would change right away?
What's your favorite television program?
What makes you laugh?
What's your favorite sport or activity?
Tell me something that makes you sad.
What's your favorite animal?

Who lives at your house? (Explore people and pets.)
Who is your favorite superhero? (possible resource)
I ask children about their bedroom. Who shares your room? Who decorated your room? What's your favorite thing in your room? (This question extracts information about the child's position in the family. Who makes decisions in the family? Is the child allowed to make decisions about his or her own room, or did a parent decorate the room, and did the child have any input?)
What's your favorite movie? What's your favorite video game?
What do you do when you get really upset? Do you go to your room? Do your ride your bike, or play video games, or watch television?
Do you like to listen to music? What songs do you like the most? Do you ever listen to music when you're happy or upset?
Tell me something that is annoying to you. (If the child is someone who is bothered by tags in their clothing, this question may be more expansive.)
Who do you talk to when you're upset?
Who are your best buddies? What do you guys like to do together?
What do you do at recess?
Do you ever have headaches or stomach aches?

It is not necessary to ask all of the questions to all children or to ask all the questions in this particular order. These questions can be asked as a series during one session or over several sessions. As the therapist notes the child's responses to the questions, the therapist may choose to change the direction of the questioning or ask more in-depth questions in a particular area. While asking questions, the therapist also has the opportunity to make connections for the child and teach the child about the child's own process. The therapist may want to emphasize for the child what resources the child already possesses, for example, a child who plays the piano when upset is already using healthy self-soothing techniques. This is an opportunity to emphasize the positive behaviors and skills that the child already possesses.

This questioning process can also include the parent at some point. Asking a parent what the parent observes the child doing when the child is happy or upset is helpful. It is important to notice how attuned the parent is to the child. What does the parent actually notice about the child? How does the parent handle the child's challenging behaviors? Does the parent emphasize the child's strengths or problems? What does the child's behavior trigger in the parent?

Interactional Activities to Assess Children's Resources and Skills. We both have children use drawing as an interactional and diagnostic tool. We will frequently have a child draw a picture of his or her family. Some children will readily begin this task, while others may be reticent to draw the picture. Both decisions by the child are important information for the therapist. We will provide as much drawing material and tools as the child needs to complete this task and then engage in conversation with the child while the child draws.

If the child is receptive to drawing, we will also ask the child to draw a self-portrait, a picture of his or her family, and his or her favorite place, real or imaginary. Again, this provides a great deal of information and can be potentially diagnostic. Any type of projective activity allows for assessment of resources and skills as well as for discovery of possible targets for reprocessing during the desensitization phase.

Observation. Observation is a critical psychotherapeutic tool. The therapist is always observing the child, the child's interactions with and without the parents, and the child and parent's interactions with the therapist. We are always noticing how parents and children interact. Does the parent appropriately monitor the child's behaviors, or is the parent controlling or unaware of the child's behaviors? For example, if the child needs to use the restroom, does the parent assess the situation and facilitate the child safely using the restroom, as is appropriate given the specific details of the office situation?

It is important to note that what the child does not say is just as important as what the child does say in therapy. Observing the child during questioning and during interactional activities is equally as important. A great deal of data can be gleaned from these activities and interactions. At this point, clinical judgment will guide the process, as the therapist determines what skills the child currently possesses and what skills the child needs to continue through the next phases of EMDR. An important finding from the research study we conducted was that successful preparation and skill building prevented children from becoming resistant to EMDR. Skill-building techniques for children are included in chapter 9, on resourcing, coping, and mastery.

Assessing the Child's External Resources

One of the pivotal issues in utilizing EMDR in therapy with children is the home environment and parental influences, extended family resources, and friends, teachers, and school and community supports. To whom can the child turn to deal with difficulties?

Treatment challenges can arise due to instability in the home environment, including homes where there is domestic violence, divorce, and/or parental chemical dependency or mental health issues.

A child's resistance to EMDR is most likely to appear when the pieces of safety and security are missing, especially in the home environment. Resistance to EMDR can be avoided by adjusting the pace of therapy in order that the child has some sense of power over what happens in the therapy process.

It is also important to assess how these parental variables impact the child's treatment and to explore how parental variables will be addressed in the child's therapy. When is it beneficial to use a parent cotherapist model?

As professionals, we have had many discussions related to including parents in sessions with children, and we each have our own perspective on this subject. We have included Table 4.1 as a guide; however, we would like to encourage you to consider making an active decision about the parent's role in therapy and also remember that during the course of treatment, the decision can change. The decision about the parent's involvement in the session should be considered on a case-by-case basis, depending on the treatment goals for the child.

For me (R.T.), the issue is not when to include parents, but when to exclude parents. As a matter of professional practice, I only exclude parents from sessions when parents may be harmful to children such as would constitute a referral to child welfare professionals. Because I work with children in the foster care system and in adoption situations, in addition to working with seriously and chronically traumatized children, the opportunity to work with attachment issues and model healthy adult–child interactions is crucial. I will often work from the perspective of a parent as a cotherapist, especially with young children. A 4-year-old child cannot leave the therapy session and return home and teach parents about more effective parenting and about the child's experience in therapy. My view is that the therapy is often only as effective as my cotherapist, who is the parent who interacts with the child on a daily basis, when I may only see the child for an hour a week. By including the parent in the child's therapy, I can provide clinical interventions for the child, while also educating and modeling for the parent. At times, I may even engage the parent in the therapy process, such as when I have the parent hold the child while the child is reprocessing a traumatic event. With the parent as a resource, the child can feel supported, and the parent can learn how to be more supportive of the child. I can provide education and coaching for the parent in the office, instead of asking the parent to leave the office and attempt new skills with the child at home. This is a way to maximize the opportunity for therapeutic intervention into the family system.

Conversely, in my practice, I (C.S.) am more likely to work with children in intact families, where the child has experienced a single-incident

TABLE 4.1 The Implications of Including Parents in EMDR Sessions With Children

	Parent in Session	Parent Not in Session
Parent's mental health status/ Abusive parent	If the parent has identified and addressed their own mental health issues.	The parent's mental health issues have not been addressed and interfere with the child's processing in sessions.
Parent expectations	The parent has realistic expectations for the child and the progression of therapy.	The parent has expectations of the child and of the therapeutic process that stymie the therapy.
Parent's treatment history	The parent has addressed their own issues in previous/ current therapy.	The parent is currently in therapy and unable to participate in the child's therapy.
Parent's ability to tolerate affect	Is the parent able to tolerate the child's affect?	The parent is unable to tolerate the child's affect and will attempt to intervene.
Attachment	One goal of therapy is improving parent–child attachment.	The parent–child attachment is not a primary goal of treatment.
Sharing information	The parent is an observer and can assist the child.	The parent is unable to remain observer; therefore, the therapist shares information with the parent to assist between sessions.
Parent Cotherapist	If the parent can address issues listed above, the parent can serve as cotherapist.	The parent's own issues distract, and the child and/or therapist must care for the parent.

trauma. I (C.S.) always involve parents, but I tend to have the parents included in the session at the beginning and end of sessions. I will ask the parent to wait in the waiting room while the child is in therapy once the child is comfortable being alone with me. I find that the child is more likely to be more open and honest in therapy when the child does not have to be concerned about the parent. I also notice that parents may experience vicarious trauma from what the child reports, especially when the parent is experiencing trauma or the parent has his or her own mental health issues that have not been adequately addressed. My (C.S.) experience is that parents will often influence the child's target as well as the child's negative and positive cognitions. The child may report what the parent wants to hear, instead of staying with his or her own spontaneous process.

TEACHING THE MECHANICS OF EMDR

While continuing to enhance the therapeutic relationship, the therapist needs to explain the mechanics of EMDR, which includes explaining and demonstrating BLS, establishing the client's Safe/Calm Place for use during the desensitization phase, and teaching emotional literacy, self-soothing and calming techniques, Stop Signal, the EMDR Metaphor, containers, and resources and mastery.

Bilateral Stimulation (BLS)

Description. Shapiro (1995, 2001) reported that she discovered EMDR in 1987 after walking and while thinking about a traumatic event in her life; when she ended her walk, she felt significantly better. As Shapiro thought about what had happened, she realized that her eyes had been moving back and forth while she was walking, and the distress she was experiencing had decreased (Shapiro, 1995, 2001). A more detailed history of how Shapiro discovered the efficacy of using eye movements is detailed in her books (1995, 2001).

Because of the need for alternative forms of BLS, therapists began to experiment with other types of BLS, even though the majority of research on EMDR has consisted of BLS with eye movements. We strongly encourage therapists to attempt to use eye movements with clients first. It is important to find the type of BLS that works best for the client. As therapists experiment with using different kinds of BLS, it is important to explore whether the discomfort with eye movements is directly related to a physiological response from the client or whether the physiological response is a remnant of a memory that the client needs to explore. Furthermore, if a client begins to cry and cannot track the eye movements, the therapist may have to switch to a different type of BLS to continue reprocessing the memory.

Some clients even have two or three types of BLS, such as when a therapist uses the NeuroTek light bar. With electronic devices, it is possible to use eye movements, tactile stimulation, and auditory tones at the same time, or a combination of the three.

Types of BLS. BLS through eye movements, tapping, auditory stimulation, and other variations is a critical step in the desensitization phase of EMDR. There are several types of BLS, including eye movements; tapping; NeuroTek devices, which can provide visual, tactile, and auditory stimulation, depending on the type of machine; butterfly hugs (Jarero, Artigas, Mauer, Alcala, & Lupez, 1999) and lady bug hugs; and the Fonzy hug.

Eye Movements. Therapists can refer to original training in EMDR for details about eye movements; however, we have included specifics about using eye movements with children.

It is important to test eye movements with children, but the therapist must be creative and flexible. Some children are able to select one type of BLS and are very successful with just one type. Other children need frequent changes in the type of BLS to continue to reprocess the memory and stay focused.

Therapists simply have the child follow the therapist's fingers like is taught in EMDR training, or the therapist can draw faces on his or her fingers or put stickers on his or her fingers for the child to follow. Some therapists will have the child select a finger puppet, hand puppet, stuffed animal, or other type of toy for the child to track, while following the bilateral movements the therapist creates. Therapists can also use a magic wand or some type of pointer for the child to follow. This will also help with the therapist's arm if the therapist gets tired or is uncomfortable with the repetitions of eye movements. The therapist can use a penlight or a laser pointer on the floor or wall for the child to follow with his or her eyes. The therapist must be careful not to point the light at the client or in the client's eyes. There is really no limit to what therapists can use to create the BLS, as long as the stimulation creates the eye movements that evoke BLS of the brain.

Tactile Stimulation. Tactile stimulation can come in many forms and can be created by the therapist, the child, or electronic devices. The therapist can tap on the child's hands, shoulders, or knees, with the child's permission. The child can drum, clap, stomp, play patty cake, slap his or her knees, tap his or her feet while sitting in a chair, or use the butterfly hug, lady bug hug, or Fonzy hug. The *butterfly hug* (Jarero, Artigas, Mauer, Alcala, & Lupez, 1999) has the child cross his or her arms across the chest and alternatively tap on his or her own forearms. The *lady bug hug* has the child link his or her fingers together and move his or her hands, alternating the fingers back and forth. The *Fonzy hug* has the child cross his or her arms and tap on the outside of his or her hips. The lady bug hug and the Fonzy hug are variations of the butterfly hug. The butterfly hug has also been used in a group protocol that will be discussed later in this book.

Auditory Stimulation. Auditory stimulation can be created in many creative ways as well. Auditory stimulation typically requires some type of electronic device, such as using a prepared CD such as those marketed by David Grand (http://www.biolateral.com) or by using a NeuroTek device (http://www.neurotekcorp.com). The CDs from David Grand are CDs that can be used in any CD player, and the CD is preformatted to alternate sounds. These CDs contain many different sounds, but the speed of the alternating auditory stimulation cannot be adjusted.

In addition, any type of CD can be used with the specific NeuroTek device that allows for auditory stimulation. The NeuroTek device is a electronic tool that is used to create BLS. The NeuroTek device can provide auditory and tactile BLS. The auditory stimulation can be from tones that are created by the machine, which the client hears through headphones or a CD player, or from any type of audio player that can be attached to the NeuroTek device that allows for the client to select the type of sounds or music. It is our experience that children and adolescents prefer the audio stimulation and are particularly engaged when they can choose the music. I (R.T.) will allow the client to use any type of music that is preapproved by parents or caretakers, and I have even downloaded a specific song onto my iPod at a client's request.

Multiple Types of BLS. We both use electronic devices like the NeuroTek device for electronic BLS. We both believe that having an electronic device for creating BLS with children is well worth the financial investment. The NeuroTek company sells a device that creates tactile and auditory stimulation either directly from the device or by connecting the device to a CD player or an MP-3 player.

I (R.T.) use a video rocker for children to sit on in the office, with the NeuroTek device connected to the video rocker. In doing so, the child can hold the tactile wires that we often will refer to as "buzzies" because the device buzzes in the child's hands, and I will connect the audio wires to the speakers on the video rocker so that the child also gets bilateral auditory stimulation while sitting in the rocker.

Remote speakers can also be wired on either side of a play area or a sand tray to create the auditory BLS while the child is playing. I (R.T.) have put remote speakers on either end of the sand tray so that while the child is working in the sand tray, the auditory stimulation is on either side of the child's head to create the BLS. This may be cumbersome if the child is moving around a great deal, but I (R.T.) have found that children who are focused on working in the sand tray often benefit either from the bilateral auditory stimulation with the speakers or from having the buzzies in the child's socks while the child is creating a scene in the sand tray. The use of the sand tray for creating negative and positive cognitions or for reprocessing a memory will be discussed in several sections of this book.

Clinical Decision Making With BLS

The use of BLS, when to change types of BLS, and when to continue, even if the client is struggling with the BLS, are all based on clinical judgment and the therapist's attunement to the client.

Case Study: Savannah Becoming Assertive

I (C.S.) worked with a little girl who was traumatized after experiencing anaphylactic shock theoretically from an unknown food allergen. After we processed through the trauma from the experience, she continued to have anxiety and distress from a current situation in her life. Savannah processed some of the distress, but then began to cry, and it was evident to me that she needed some assertiveness skills and that the child was struggling with relationships. I allowed her to talk through her feelings about the situation and stopped using the BLS because my assessment was that this was a unique developmental experience for this child and not a memory that needed to be reprocessed. This type of situation is more common for children than adults because children are first experiencing life situations for which they may not have prior awareness or skills with which to deal with the situation. We continued the BLS in a subsequent session, after discussing the skills that she needed.

Differences Between Adults and Children Regarding BLS

If the therapist assesses that the client needs a specific skill to continue with reprocessing, the therapist may need to stop and return to the preparation phase to insert needed skills for the child. With case conceptualization, children may be missing the life experience with which to reprocess a specific incident or cope with a current situation. This is where clinical judgment is extremely important. The therapist should ask, "Does the client possess the needed skills with which to continue reprocessing, or does the client need to learn a new skill to continue?" In clinical decision making, the therapist may be aware that the client has skills with which to continue reprocessing and may need to use a cognitive interweave to help the client connect with the needed skill; however, if the therapist believes that the client is in fact missing a needed skill with which to continue, the therapist may need to take a break from the reprocessing and teach before the desensitization process can continue. This may be a difficult concept for therapists to grasp until therapists have had practice with more clients of different ages and life experiences.

The therapist must also determine if the client is avoiding the intensity of the situation and needs encouragement to continue, versus a client who is missing a skill that prevents continuation of the reprocessing.

Speed and Number of Saccades

As with any client, the speed of the BLS needs to be adjusted for the comfort of the individual client. It is important for the therapist to stay attuned to the client and make adjustments as needed for the client to continue working in therapy. The number of saccades (bilateral pass that encompasses both sides) also needs to be adjusted for the individual client's needs. We will tell the client, "I'm just guessing when to stop the bilateral stimulation and check in with you, so if you want me to stop sooner or keep going, just let me know." This is a place where the client can use the Stop Signal, which we will explain later in the chapter.

Demonstrating BLS to Clients

We have included a script for how therapists can explain BLS to children. We included a script for demonstrating BLS to children earlier in this chapter. We have also repeated information included in chapter 2 for teaching and organizational purposes.

Eye movements can be elicited by the therapist by moving one's fingers, as taught in EMDR training. I (R.T.) have been known to put stickers on my fingers or to draw happy faces on my fingers for the child to track. Therapists can also use penlights on the floor or wall for the client to follow or purchase specialized equipment for eliciting eye movements. Children will track with their eyes and enjoy the use of puppets or finger puppets, stuffed animals, or other toys selected by the child to increase the child's focus on the eye movements.

It is not uncommon to notice a client stop tracking the eye movements or to see eye movements that are not always fluid. This may happen for several reasons. The client may have difficulty tracking the stimulus. The therapist can slow down the eye movements and tell the client to "push my fingers with your eyes." Sometimes it may be necessary for the therapist to stop and wiggle his or her fingers to make sure the client is still tracking. Sometimes the client may be processing a memory, and the therapist will notice jumpy eye movements, or the client's eyes may flutter. You can always check in with the client to see what is happening. In addition to assessing the client's ability to track the type of BLS, the number of saccades also impacts the client's ability to track the stimulus.

It is important to determine the number of saccades, or passes back and forth, that are necessary when working with a particular client. Shapiro (2001) and other researchers suggest that eye movements should move as fast as the client can tolerate to activate processing, rather than just tracking. The therapist can tell the client, "I'm just guessing at the speed and number of passes, but you can tell me to stop or continue."

By giving the client the power to continue or stop the saccades, the therapist becomes more attuned to the individual client's unique manner of processing.

Therapists can also provide BLS through tactile stimulation, such as tapping on the clients hands, or by using a device especially designed for therapist use during EMDR. There are many different ways to use tactile forms of BLS with clients and some creative and fun ways to engage children with BLS.

Therapists can provide auditory stimulation by using technological equipment that can pulse in the client's ears or by attaching a CD player or iPod to the equipment in order for the client to use music as BLS. Some therapists use remote speakers that can be placed on either side of a play area or sand tray and then use a preprogrammed CD that provides alternating auditory stimulation. It is important to monitor that actual BLS is occurring because children are active and may not stay in between the two speakers.

When using a device that provides BLS, it is helpful to start by turning all controls, including auditory and tactile volume and speed, to their lowest levels. Proceed by slowly increasing the speed, intensity, or volume, until the client chooses a setting that is most comfortable.

Once the therapist has identified the child's preferred type of BLS and identified the settings that are most comfortable for the child, the therapist can proceed with using the BLS to install a Safe/Calm Place for the child.

Safe/Calm Place

Defining Safe/Calm Place. The goal of this Safe/Calm Place exercise is to assess whether or not a child can access a positive resource and create a Safe/Calm Place that the child can use at any time to self-soothe and contain intense emotional experiences. Safe/Calm Place for children is often a relaxed, calm, comfortable place. The Safe/Calm Place can be used during the session, at the end of the session, or between sessions for the child to self-soothe and calm himself or herself.

During the session, the child may need the Safe/Calm Place if reprocessing becomes overwhelming and the child is unable to proceed. The child may automatically go to the Safe/Calm Place, or the therapist may need to remind the child to use the Safe/Calm Place, if necessary.

The Safe/Calm Place can also be used at the end of the session to end the session in a positive manner. At the end of the session the therapist will remind the child of the Safe/Calm Place and may also use deep breathing and other techniques, such as the light stream, which is a relaxation technique that is taught in EMDR Basic Training, to end the session.

Finally, the child can be reminded to practice using the Safe/Calm Place between sessions to enhance the place and practice self-soothing. In addition, the child can be instructed to use the Safe/Calm Place if the child is anticipating a difficult situation such as the upcoming test of a visit with a noncustodial parent.

Additional Skills in Using the Safe/Calm Place Exercise With Children. In the process of teaching the Safe/Calm Place, the therapist is beginning to build trust with the child and become attuned to the child's experience of positive experiences, and especially with the child's response to BLS.

So, in the process of creating a Safe/Calm Place, the therapist is also teaching mindfulness in order that the child will notice what his or her emotions are and how his or her body feels. Sometimes, for younger children or children who have limited emotional literacy skills, this may be the time to teach skills. Some children may not have a vocabulary to describe emotions and/or body sensations. Children may also not know how to describe body sensations or associate those body sensations with emotional language.

Therapists may find that while trying to create a Safe/Calm Place with a client, the client will begin to report that the Safe/Calm Place has changed or become contaminated with stressful material or experiences. This is another section where the therapist's clinical judgment becomes important because the therapist has choices on how to proceed. If the Safe/Calm Place becomes negative in some way, the therapist can opt to contain whatever has happened and create a different Safe/Calm Place with the client. Or, if the therapist feels comfortable proceeding, the therapist may decide to continue with the information that has surfaced while attempting the Safe/Calm Place exercise and continue with the EMDR protocol. In general, Safe/Calm Place seems to be easier with children with single-incident traumas and more difficult with children with chronic and severe trauma.

I (R.T.) believe that the client's ability to create and sustain a Safe/Calm Place is directly related to the client's experiences of positive and consistent attachments. For example, I have worked with children living in foster care and group home settings who struggled with a Safe/Calm Place initially, but later, when the child was placed in a long-term foster home or in an adoptive home, the child was eventually able to create a Safe/Calm Place more successfully because of the experience of having a stable adult caregiver in the client's life. My (R.T.) belief is that the Safe/Calm Place exercise is diagnostic of the client's attachment experiences and the client's ability to even attach internally and sustain positive resources.

Challenges to Using the Safe/Calm Place Exercise. One of the things that we discovered in our research study is that the Safe/Calm Place exercise that one was taught to use with adults needs to be modified with children. This is especially true in the language therapists use. We will use words like *calm, happy, comfortable,* or *special place* with children because the word *safe* may have negative connotations or be contaminated for some children, especially severely traumatized children. We have worked with children who cannot recall ever having an experience of feeling safe; therefore we need to identify a word to which the child can relate.

We have also learned that the therapist may not need to use any BLS or very short sets of BLS with children to prevent the place from being contaminated or to prevent the child from linking with negative memory networks. One of the things that we noticed in our consultation meetings is that we spent an inordinate amount of time discussing the therapist's difficulty getting Safe/Calm Place for children. Some common themes we identified when the therapist struggled with creating a Safe/Calm Place were that (a) the child was not familiar with the therapist's office (intakes were done by an intake worker instead of the therapist, so a rapport had not developed); (b) the therapist had used too many saccades of the BLS during one set, or the therapist used too many sets of the BLS, and the child would go into a negative place and start processing; (c) the fear of the perpetrator came back; (d) the home environment was not safe; and (e) severely traumatized kids had a more difficult time.

To improve success with the Safe/Calm Place exercise, we ask therapists to consider the following:

1. The therapist needs to make sure the child has time to play in the office to become comfortable with the office before processing.
2. The therapist needs to remember to keep the number of saccades of the BLS at no more than two to three passes at a time.
3. The therapist needs to remember to only do one set of BLS before proceeding to the next step of the Safe/Calm Place. It is extremely important to keep the BLS short to enhance the Safe/Calm Place, but not move the client into reprocessing a distressing event.
4. It is important for the therapist to educate the family/foster parents on safety issues in the child's environment. The child may not be able to establish a Safe/Calm Place because the child's environment is not safe. This is one instance of where the Safe/Calm Place exercise may be diagnostic, and the therapist will have to explore the child's current situation and assess for safety.
5. It is possible for the therapist to focus on a mastery experience instead.
6. It is possible for the therapist to guide the child through creating an imaginary Safe/Calm Place. For example, I (R.T.) worked with a young boy who was preparing to testify in a criminal case, and

he could not identify a Safe/Calm Place. So instead, the boy imagined that his Safe/Calm Place was in the Mario Brothers video game, and he lived in the castle, where he was protected by many people and devices. Each week, the child fortified this Safe/Calm Place, until the day he testified.

7. It is important for the therapist to have some sense of the current genre that the child is using. I (C.S.) had a child who used Hogwarts from the Harry Potter books as a Safe/Calm Place, and the child chose the word Dumbledore as the cue word for the Safe/Calm Place. I knew that in the newest Harry Potter book, Dumbledore had died, and I was able to assist the child in selecting a different cue word to prevent the Hogwarts Safe/Calm Place from having a negative association.
8. It is also beneficial to ask the parents to assist the child in practicing the Safe/Calm Place at home. The parents should be instructed to have the child practice the Safe/Calm Place with the cue word when the child is feeling comfortable and not to practice when the child is feeling unsafe. Once the child has mastered the Safe/Calm Place with the cue word, it is possible for the child to practice using the Safe/Calm Place in situations where the child is feeling stressed.

Safe/Calm Place Protocol for Children

Instructions to Therapist. The client is taught a Safe/Calm Place to utilize as a tool for affect management. When clients cannot locate a Safe/Calm Place, consider that diagnostic and that the client is in need of additional resources before continuing with desensitization.

If the therapist continues with the Safe/Calm Place protocol, the therapist uses a maximum of two to four saccades of BLS at a slow speed so as not to bridge into trauma memories. If the child's identified Safe/Calm Place becomes unsafe, then the therapist asks the child, "Can we make this Safe/Calm Place feel safe again, or do we need to choose a different Safe/Calm Place?"

Script. The therapist can introduce a Safe/Calm Place in the following way: "OK, so I want to do something that's called the Safe/Calm Place. We can use Safe/Calm Place at the end of sessions or between sessions. I want you to learn how to use the Safe/Calm Place, so we're going to practice it."

Step 1—Picture (image). "Can you think about a real place, or imaginary place, that makes you feel safe, calm, relaxed, or happy? What place makes you feel this way the most? Do you have a picture of it?" (If appropriate, therapist allows child to draw picture of image.)

Step 2—Emotions and sensations. "Think about that safe/comfortable/relaxed place. What feeling do you have?" (Therapist pauses; if child does not respond, therapist provides examples of feelings to educate child.) "Do you feel relaxed, comfortable, safe, happy, excited? Where do you feel that _________ feeling in your body?" (Therapist pauses, and if child appears confused, therapist provides examples.) "Well, some kids feel it in their head, some people feel it in their tummy, and some feel it in their heart. Where do you feel it? Can you touch it?"

Step 3—Enhancement. Therapist then says, "Think about that __________ [picture], and that _________ [feeling], and where you feel it in your body, and let's turn on _________ [BLS] for a few seconds." Stop BLS and say, "Tell me what happened now?" (If the child feels better, the therapist should do several more sets of BLS. If the child's positive emotions do not intensify, the therapist can try alternative BLS, until the child reports improvement.)

Step 4—Cue word(s). "If we could pick one word that would help to remind me how you feel right now, what word would that be? OK, so when I say _________, what do you notice?" (Add set of BLS.)

Step 5—Self-cuing. "Now I want you to say the word _________, and when you say it, notice what you're feeling."

Step 6—Cuing with disturbance. "Now let's practice with your word. I want you to think about one little tiny thing that bothers you just a little bit and notice where you feel that in your body." (No BLS used at this point.)

Step 7—Self-cuing with disturbance. The therapist then asks the client to bring up a disturbing thought once again and to practice the Safe/Calm Place exercise, this time without the therapist's assistance, to its relaxing conclusion.

Step 8—Homework. Encourage client to practice Safe/Calm Place and word for cuing the safe and happy place.

Safe/Calm Place Protocol Instructions Form. Instructions for the Safe/Calm Place protocol follow. See Exhibit 4.1 for a Safe/Calm Place protocol worksheet.

Step 1: Describe image.
Step 2: Describe emotions and positive sensations (including location).
Step 3: Enhance imagery and affect with soothing tones.
Step 4: Introduce short sets of eye movements (four to six saccades).

If positive outcome, continue with several more short sets.
If minimal or neutral outcome, try alternative direction of eye movements.

If intrusions or negative response, explore solutions (i.e., containment of negative material, add more protective features to Safe/Calm Place) or switch to a different Safe/Calm Place or comforting resource image.

Step 5: Identify cue word(s). Guide child in holding cue word(s) and Safe/Calm Place together, as several sets of eye movements are added.
Step 6: Have child practice self-cuing, focusing on image and word(s) without eye movements.
Step 7: Have child bring up a minor disturbance. Therapist cues Safe/Calm Place.
Step 8: Have child bring up a minor disturbance. Child cues Safe/Calm Place.

Stop Signal

The Stop Signal is to empower the client to signal the therapist when the client wants to stop the desensitization process because the client needs a break or because the process is becoming too overwhelming.

Exhibit 4.1 Safe/Calm Place Protocol for Children Worksheet

Child: ______________________ **Date:** ________________

Image: ____
____
____
____
____

Positive emotions: ____
____
____

Physical sensations (location and description): ____________________
____
____
____

Cue word(s): ____
____
____

Minor disturbance for cuing/self-cuing practice: ___________________
____
____

Clinician's Signature: ____________________ Date: ____________

For children, this is a fairly straightforward process, but it is important to emphasize that the Stop Signal is for a purpose and not just for fun. The therapist may need to encourage the child to keep going even when processing becomes difficult.

What is more difficult with children is that a child may just leave and go play when the child wants to avoid the intensity of the processing. This can become very difficult if a child is unable to be redirected to finish the processing to come out on the other side of the stressful event. This is a point where more preparation may be needed for the child. We will discuss techniques for reengaging children in the process in the following paragraphs.

Instructions to the Therapist. Teaching the child a signal to stop or take a break from the processing/desensitization gives the child a sense of safety and control over the process.

Script. "Remember when we were talking about using _________ [BLS]? Well, I want you to know that you can raise your hand and tell me that you need to stop or take a break. Let's practice what you would do if you wanted to tell me to take a break." (Follow child's lead. Therapist may need to demonstrate raising his or her hand like a Stop Signal. After child has identified a Stop Signal, therapist will then repeat script.) "So I will know you want to take a break or stop if you do/say _________ [Stop Signal]."

Metaphor for EMDR

The purpose of the Metaphor is to give the client the sense of distance from the intensity of the affect the client may experience during desensitization with EMDR. In addition, the Metaphor is significant to processing because it conveys a sense of movement through the intense affect, which helps prevent the child from being overwhelmed by the potency of the emotion.

Children are typically motivated to avoid difficult situations, rather than confront the situation to overcome the negative impact of the experience. The Metaphor can also be used as a skill-building exercise to teach children how to manage intense affect by giving children a template to think about an unsettling or traumatic event.

Instructions to the Therapist. The Metaphor should be explained to the child before beginning desensitization to help support and encourage the child to continue to work through any intense affect that may arise.

Script. The therapist says to the child, "It's kind of good to have a way to help you feel like you can handle your thoughts and feelings so you can just notice it like stuff going by, like on a train, where you just watch stuff going by the window." The train Metaphor may not be in the child's realm of experience.

Other Metaphors that will work with children include the following:

1. "Imagine that you're in a plane and can change your seat or look out the window."
2. "Imagine that you are in a car or bus and you are just watching out the window at the bad thing passing by."
3. Even though there is some controversy about using the television or movie screen, we will use the Metaphor of watching the stressful event on a screen. If the client is having strong emotion and is unable to cope, the therapist can say, "Well, just put what's going on right now on a movie screen, and imagine that you're in the audience watching the movie." This allows the client to gain some distance from the process to prevent the client from avoiding the experience. This is referred to as a *decelerating technique* in the EMDR training. Techniques for decelerating and accelerating processing will be discussed in greater detail in chapter 6, on the Desensitization Phase.
4. A tunnel is another Metaphor for describing the therapeutic process to children. The therapist can ask the child, "Have you ever gone into a tunnel where it was dark, but then you could see the light at the other end, and after a while, you got out the other side of the tunnel?" The tunnel can be used as a Metaphor for explaining how the therapeutic process can feel difficult before the client feels better, like going into a dark tunnel and then coming out the other side.

Procedural Considerations

At this point, the therapist has taught the mechanics of the EMDR process and can decide that the next step in the therapeutic process is to begin the Assessment Phase. The clinical decision to proceed with the Assessment Phase is based on case conceptualization. The pace of therapy is based on the individual client and the treatment plan. The therapist needs to determine if the child has the necessary resources and skills to continue or if the child needs to be taught additional skills.

Some children can quickly move into the Assessment Phase because the child and the child's family are fairly stable. For other children, the therapist may need to spend a greater amount of time in the Preparation Phase. Some children will come to therapy with the skills to proceed, while others will need more scaffolding in place. Some children need emotional literacy, emotional regulation skills, containers, and the ability to titrate intense affect. If the therapist assesses the child to need additional skills, it is at this point in the therapeutic process that the therapist teaches and offers the opportunity for the child to practice.

Emotional Literacy. Emotional literacy is the ability to recognize, understand, and appropriately express our emotions. Children also need to learn to understand their own internal experiences and to comprehend the oral, physical, and nonverbal expressions of others. There are several sites online where you can read more about emotional literacy—the emotional literacy process has partially originated from the book *Emotional Intelligence* by Goleman (1995). What is most important is the question, How do we teach children emotional literacy? Part of psychotherapy with children is teaching emotional literacy. Through play therapy, books, and instruction, the therapist can teach even very young children to identify feelings and use those feelings to improve expression and processing of feelings.

There are many techniques for teaching children emotional literacy, including the following:

1. Teach children to identify feelings and facial expressions by looking in a mirror.
2. The child can practice making faces with the therapist. The therapist and child can take turns making different facial expressions and then labeling the feeling associated with the facial expression.
3. There are pages with pictures of facial expressions that the child can use to label emotions.
4. The therapist can have the child identify feelings from pictures in a magazine and then make a collage of feelings using the pictures from the magazine.
5. The therapist can teach children classic body Metaphors (i.e., *weak in the knees, butterflies in the tummy, heartache,* etc.). The therapist can actually have the child act out different body poses that exemplify an emotion and body sensation.
6. If the child can read, the therapist can give the child a homework assignment to look up two feeling words in a dictionary and bring those words to the next session to teach the therapist. If the child cannot read, the therapist can ask the parent to help the child find two new feelings words before the next session.

Emotional Regulation. From the time the therapist first meets the child, the therapist is assessing how the child and family express emotions and how the child manages or does not manage intense affect. The therapist also needs to consider how the child's family responds to the child's intense affect. Is intense affect allowed in the family, or is intense affect dangerous? What has the child learned to do with intense affect?

Just like with adult clients, some children may need resources to decelerate the pace of the therapeutic process if the intensity of the experience becomes overwhelming. The therapist needs to learn about how the child regulates emotion. Emotional regulation is part of a healthy attachment process, as children learn how to express emotions by observing and interacting with caregivers. Children with a history of chronic abuse and, more often, children from the child welfare system will need to learn skills to appropriately express and manage intense affect. Children with a poor or traumatic attachment history have not had a relationship within which to learn how to experience and express intense affect and will likely need additional preparation to proceed with the next phases of EMDR.

Children need to feel competent in managing intense affect to continue to be engaged in the therapeutic process. If a child feels unable to manage the intense affect, the child is more likely to avoid the process or dissociate, rather than to participate in reprocessing traumatic memories. When children feel competent to manage intense affect, they are able to maintain the dual attention required for reprocessing memories and will be willing to continue in therapy.

Since children do not typically initiate their own therapy, convincing children that the therapeutic process will be beneficial to them is crucial. To engage children in the process, front loading during the Preparation Phase of EMDR is extremely important. Children who have experienced success with EMDR and feel competent and prepared for managing intense affect are much more likely to be willing participants. This certainly makes the treatment process much more positive for both children and therapists alike.

Therapists may have indications that the child needs emotional literacy and emotional regulation skills during the Preparation Phase, but sometimes the therapist does not realize the child's need for emotional regulation skills, until the client is in the midst of reprocessing in the Desensitization Phase and the reprocessing becomes stalled. The therapist will again need to consider the possibility that the therapeutic process will need to return to the Preparation Phase to provide the child with the skills to continue with reprocessing and manage the intense affect.

In the Preparation Phase the therapist is trying to give the client the resources and skills to proceed through the experiences that have been stored maladaptively and determine what prevented the client's healthy information processing from working. Case conceptualization includes determining when the child needs emotional literacy and emotional regulation skills. When does the child need containers? What does the child need from the therapeutic process to return to healthy functioning? It is important to remember that containers can stop the processing, but sometimes a child may need a container to contain one memory, while finishing another memory network. If a new target arises during reprocessing, the therapist may suggest, "That's another target; let's contain it, and then we'll come back to it." This is a pivotal piece of clinical judgment, where the therapist must decide which memory network to follow.

Techniques for Distancing and Titrating Intense Affect

Techniques for distancing and titrating the intensity of reprocessing can also be used as containers. Tools for decelerating, including distancing and titrating, need to be taught for clients to be able to manage the intense affect that might arise from the Desensitization Phase of EMDR.

Children are very creative in using containers for affect management, which is taught in EMDR training; however, children often struggle with the tools that are more adult oriented and abstract. Using techniques like using television channels as a Metaphor for distancing when the affect becomes overwhelming in EMDR processing gives the child a feeling of being in a position of power and competency. Using the television and remote or the movie Metaphor as interventions are different than using the train Metaphor that is taught in EMDR Part 1 training because the train Metaphor implies that the client is in one place and memories are moving by, while using the television or movie screen is a distancing technique that is used for the deceleration that the client needs to be able to tolerate intense affect. Children first need to learn about the observer self. Children need to learn to be able to stand outside the emotion and body sensation to observe from a distant place, which often is a place of wisdom. This gives children perspective on the process and really stems from the place of adaptive information processing for children. This helps decrease the flooding of affect or the overwhelming experience of body sensations.

CONTAINERS AND TYPES OF CONTAINERS

Containers can be used for incomplete sessions to store activated but unprocessed material that may be potentially potent for the client between sessions.

Containers can also be used for children who are experiencing a high level of disturbance for affect tolerance and emotional regulation. Using containers will hopefully lay the foundation to allow the therapist to have the child return to the memory to continue reprocessing. This process will also give the child a sense of mastery over intense affect and, ideally, the willingness to continue with reprocessing traumatic experiences.

Containers can also be used to store new skills a child has learned for use in the future when he or she encounters situations that have previously been problematic. We often use the term *toolbox* for a container for new skills and techniques that the child can draw from for coping with difficult situations.

What tools does the child need to be able to contain an intense affect and be able to benefit from EMDR both in session and between sessions? Children are incredibly creative with container exercises. If the therapist cannot find a Safe/Calm Place or container that is grounded in reality, the therapist can use an imaginary container. Some examples of containers include the following: (1) Children can draw pictures of containers (see Figure 4.1) or create containers in the sand tray; and (2) Children can create art projects such as making a box or drawing pictures of the things the child wants to contain. We have used boxes that we have purchased and allowed the child to decorate the box, and then had the child write the word and put the word on a "worry rock" that can be placed in the container.

Children can be taught to compartmentalize the entire memory and put it in one or multiple compartments in order that the memory is not overwhelming or disturbing outside of the session. Containers for affect management can include a see-through container, where the child can see the traumatic experience through glass or plastic but not experience any of the emotions or body sensations. This allows the visual stimulus without experiencing the entire impact of the memory.

Containers can also be used to teach children how to fractionate memories as a way of managing the intensity of the memory. By placing different pieces of the incident into different containers, it is possible to fractionate the incident in order for the client to more effectively manage the severity of the experience. Once each piece of the memory is processed, it is easier to complete the incident. Children can be taught to take one piece of the memory out of the container and reprocess the piece of the memory. As each piece is reprocessed, the intensity decreases, until the entire memory can be combined and completed.

There are many types of containers that can also be used as deceleration techniques for titrating intense affect.

Movie Screen. The therapist can use the Metaphor of a movie theater several different ways. First, the therapist can ask the child to imagine sitting in a movie theater and looking at the incident on the screen. The therapist uses BLS to help the child watch the movie, but if the movie is overwhelming, the child can have a part of himself or herself walk to the back of the theater and observe the child who is sitting in the theater and imagine himself or herself consoling the child who is upset. Or the child can watch from the back of the theater or from outside the doors of the theater and imagine looking through a window of the theater door to watch the movie.

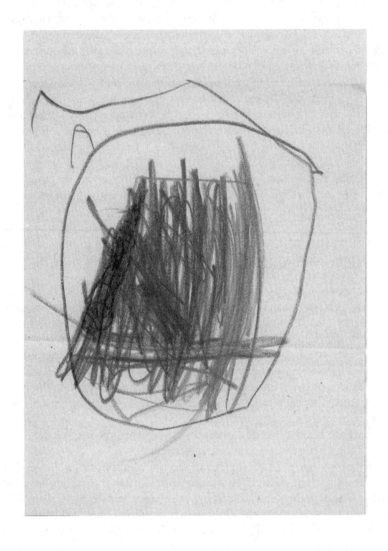

FIGURE 4.1 A picture of 3-year-old Sienna's container. She has drawn a makeup box to contain her worries.

Another way to use the movie screen is to again have the child imagine the memory on the movie screen and do BLS. If the movie is too difficult to watch, the child can be taught to pull the curtains over the movie, or make the movie black and white, or turn off the sound and just watch the movie. Another suggestion can be made for the child similar to a cognitive interweave by suggesting to the child that the child can bring a trusted adult or a superhero into the movie to protect the child. The therapist can also ask the child to describe the moral of the story or summarize what the movie is about.

Television and Remote. The therapist can teach the child to put traumatic memories on certain channels, while putting Safe/Calm Places on other channels and safe people on yet other channels. The child then imagines holding the remote and being able to move between channels for titrating the intense affect that may be stimulated by certain stations.

Instructions to the Therapist. It is helpful to teach children to use containers as a tool for intense affect and incomplete sessions; however, containers can also be used as a way to avoid dealing with painful issues. The therapist must use clinical judgment to determine if the child needs to learn to use containers or if the child has sufficient resources with which to proceed in therapy. I (R.T.) became so good at teaching children containers that many children did not want to return to the containers to process targets that were very well contained. What person in his right mind would want to take something out of a container if it was well contained and not causing problems?

Script. The therapist says, "Sometimes we have thoughts or feelings that get in our way at school or at home. Do you ever have thoughts or feeling like that? Well, I want you to know that if we need to, we can put those thoughts or feelings in a container like a box or something really strong that they can't get out of. What do you think we could use to hold those thoughts or feelings?" (Children may need to be taught examples.) "I want you to be able to put all of those thoughts or feelings, or what we worked on today, in that container. Sometimes we need different containers for different thoughts or feelings. Sometimes I like to draw pictures of my _________ [container] and make sure it's strong enough to hold everything that I need it to hold. Would you like to draw a picture with me?" After child identifies a container, proceed by asking the child, "OK, so we drew a picture [note how child identified container] of it, so now let's imagine that everything we worked on today is put in the container, and we lock it away until we get together again and can take it out to work on it again. If you start thinking about it or it seems to come out before our next session, you can just imagine putting it into the container and giving it to me or making sure that I have it."

ORGANIZING THE OFFICE FOR TREATING CHILDREN WITH EMDR

Any therapist working with children will need to have the office organized in a manner that is comfortable for the therapist and child. The office will need to have some basic supplies, including writing materials, drawing materials, and manipulatives. Some therapists have the luxury of playrooms with many toys and activities, while other therapists may not even have their own office and have to travel to different offices to see children. We would recommend that if you do not have your own office, you create a play basket or bag to carry the essentials you will need to conduct psychotherapy with children. One of the many advantages of using EMDR with children is that very few tools are necessary, besides a place to meet and the therapist's ability to move in a manner to create eye movements or some type of BLS. It is advantageous to also have a very simple play therapy bag that contains crayons or markers, paper, and a NeuroTek device. We agree that we can provide very effective psychotherapy with children with just those minimal tools.

RESOURCING AND MASTERY SKILLS

The Preparation Phase of EMDR includes establishing a healthy working relationship between the therapist and the client and providing the resources and skills necessary for the client to proceed to the Assessment Phase of EMDR.

Resourcing and mastery skills are also important tools for children to use for affect management and self-soothing. Children do not typically possess skills for managing intense affect. Specific techniques, including imagery, relaxation, self-soothing techniques, mastery techniques, and tangible tools for teaching children to effectively manage responses to EMDR, are taught in chapter 9.

SKILLS FOR DEALING WITH BETWEEN SESSIONS AND INCOMPLETE SESSIONS

Finally, the therapist must teach clients skills for dealing with incomplete sessions, including teaching clients the skill to use containers, along with relaxation and emotion management skills for clients to be empowered to deal with intense affect.

SUMMARY

The goal of the Preparation Phase is to prepare the child and the child's parent for the trauma processing that occurs through the remainder of the EMDR protocol. By the end of the Preparation Phase, the child and parent should have an understanding of EMDR, and the child should have skills for Safe/Calm Place, Metaphor, Stop Signal, and skills to cope with intense emotions.

PREPARATION PHASE SESSION PROTOCOL

Mechanics of EMDR include Stop Signal, Metaphor, Safe/Calm Place, and evaluation of the child's needs for additional skills and resources.

1. Therapist reviews first session and answers any questions from child and parent. Therapist assesses general functioning since initial session. Therapist reviews current status of any symptoms identified in initial session and explores any new symptoms: "Has anything changed since our last session?" Therapist reviews any symptoms identified on client monitoring system forms and notes changes.
2. Therapist presents the therapeutic rationale for EMDR.
3. Therapist teaches Stop Signal.
4. Therapist teaches Metaphor.
5. Therapist provides an explanation/rationale for the Safe/Calm Place exercise to child and parent. Therapist then completes the Safe/Calm Place exercise. Therapist completes Safe/Calm Place worksheet.
6. Therapist instructs parents to remind child to practice on a daily basis to connect with imaginary Safe/Calm Place.
7. For procedural considerations, therapist assesses the child's need for skills in emotional literacy, emotional regulation, and containers and makes a clinical decision on how to proceed.
8. Therapist reviews session with child and parent and answers questions as needed.
9. Therapist reminds child and parent to practice Safe/Calm Place for enhancement between sessions. Therapist schedules next session and escorts child and parent to waiting room.
10. The next therapy session may be a continuation of the Preparation Phase, with additional skill building, or the therapist may decide that the child is ready to proceed with the Assessment Phase.

CHAPTER 5

EMDR Phase 3: Assessment Phase

This chapter describes the procedural steps of the Assessment Phase of the EMDR protocol (Shapiro, 2001), with detailed explanations of the techniques and skills necessary for successfully steering a child through this phase.

As previously discussed, the therapist needs to be cognizant of the child's and parent's readiness for EMDR before proceeding with the Assessment Phase. The therapist also needs to take into account the previous evaluations of dissociation as well as the general assessment for cognitive functioning, expressive/receptive language issues, and sensory integration issues for the individual child.

With all the information gathered during the Client History and Treatment Planning Phase and the resources and skills developed during the Preparation Phase, the therapist moves to the Assessment Phase of EMDR. This chapter will explain in detail skills that the therapist needs for distilling the pieces of the EMDR protocol with children in the Assessment Phase.

During the Assessment Phase, it is also important to remind clients about the informed consent they signed when first starting therapy. We recommend therapists do this as a form of education about what the child and family can expect during the next stages of treatment.

We cannot emphasize too strongly that this psychotherapy process with children is not linear. The process is more like interwoven concentric circles that require flexibility from the therapist as the therapist follows the client's presentation. The therapist's role is one of teacher, guide, coach, cheerleader, artist, and follower, all in the moment. Therapists working with children must have some conceptualization of how psychotherapy with children requires a unique and fluid experience from the therapist to be attuned and dance with the child. The therapist needs to consider how theories and models of psychotherapy as well as clinical experience drive the implementation of psychotherapy, as we discussed in chapter 1. The therapist needs to continue to stay attuned to the client, continually observing and modifying the care conceptualization as the dynamic psychotherapy process unfolds.

PROCEDURAL STEPS OF THE ASSESSMENT PHASE OF EMDR

The Assessment Phase of EMDR includes specific procedural steps: guiding the client through identifying the target image, identifying negative (NC) and positive cognitions (PC), assessing the validity of cognition (VoC), identifying the associated emotion, determining the subjective units of disturbance (SUD) and associated emotion, and identifying the location of the body sensations. These are then tied together to start desensitization. This is the standard protocol for all clients.

The difference in working with children during the Assessment Phase of EMDR is that the therapist is interacting with the child and the parent. When interacting with the child, the therapist needs to adhere to the protocol, while changing the language to match the developmental level of the child. Tools for clinical solutions to eliciting the procedural steps of EMDR with children are included throughout this book.

With the procedural steps, it is important for the therapist to remember that typically children are present time and symptom oriented. For example, a child may say, "I can't get to sleep. There are monsters and shadows in the corner," or "Kids are mean to me," or "I'm afraid of robbers." Accessing the memory network with children less than 10 years of age requires that the therapist track the manifestations of the memory. The evidence of the memory is not always identified through cognitions and can be difficult for children to verbalize. Evidence of how children's traumatic memories are stored can be manifested in physical sensations, emotions, behaviors, odd beliefs, and unexpected symptoms. The stimuli for accessing specific memory networks with children often require unique interventions from the therapist. With AIP theory the therapist needs to find a way to assess how the memory is stored for the individual client.

Target Identification

The first procedural step of the Assessment Phase is to identify a target. Target identification begins during the Client History and Treatment Planning Phase and continues throughout the treatment process, with ongoing treatment planning and case conceptualization.

During Phase 1 of EMDR the therapist completed a comprehensive history and noted possible targets for reprocessing. The information collected during Phase 1 was elicited from both the parents and the child. During the Assessment Phase, the therapist explores in great detail the targets noted in the Client History and Treatment Planning Phase and also specifically looks for other targets that may not have been identified previously.

To identify a specific target for reprocessing, the therapist starts with the current symptom presentation that initially brought the client into therapy. These symptoms were explored during the Client History and Treatment Planning Phase of EMDR, while the therapist also noted possible targets that will now be explored. The therapist has the client return to these targets and themes to organize targets for reprocessing. If a client presents with a memory of child abuse but has no current symptoms, then the therapist needs to use clinical judgment in case conceptualization regarding what is happening for the client. If the client is not having any symptoms, then the therapist needs to consider that the memory of the abuse was already reprocessed through the client's own AIP system or that the client has dissociated from the impact of the abuse history. The most important issue to consider is why the client is seeking treatment now. Ultimately, it is not the memory that is the focus, but the current symptoms, and what is driving the symptoms that are the focus of therapy. The target memory is only as important as the symptom it is driving in the present. In other words, the symptom is the way to tap into the memory network that includes the memory that is stored maladaptively and thus provoking current symptoms. With children, the memory may not be as important as the symptom it has created that has brought the client into therapy. Some individuals have traumatic events occur in their lives that reprocess without intervention and leave no residual symptoms that would compel an individual to seek psychotherapy. This seems obvious, but is a critical point in EMDR therapy. The symptom is the focus of treatment. However, the therapist is searching for the maladaptively stored memory that continues to be aggravated by the current stimuli, thus causing symptom manifestation. For the purposes of clarification, stimuli are triggers in AIP theory. The client's reaction to the current stimuli needs to be changed; however, the current stimuli may be difficult to change in some cases.

Case Study: Sierra's Story

I (C.S.) had a young girl present for therapy with trichotillomania that started when the child entered kindergarten and had a teacher who yelled at the class. Initially, we targeted Sierra's response (symptoms consistent with trichotillomania; see chapter 11 for trichotillomania protocol) to the teacher's yelling (current stimuli) to decrease the symptom manifestation. We did not target the trichotillomania directly, but instead targeted the current stimuli or trigger, which was Sierra's experience of the teacher yelling. The maladaptively stored memory that kept getting triggered by the teacher yelling was actually an earlier experience in Sierra's life, when a coach had yelled at her and threatened to kill her. The symptom is the trichotillomania, and the current stimuli or triggers was the teacher's yelling, which was difficult for the child to cope with due to a previous threatening incident with a coach.

In case conceptualization, it is important for the therapist to recognize the relationship between current stimuli or triggers, symptom manifestation, and maladaptively stored memories to successfully identify targets for desensitization.

Clinical Implications

AIP theory focuses on state change versus trait change, with the goal of EMDR therapy being ultimately trait change. The client may have experienced state change to some degree during the first two phases of EMDR such that certain targets are no longer salient or new targets have arisen. Children may start to present as happy when they have experienced relief after reprocessing the initial event, yet the underlying traits can still be an issue. The client may present with additional or more expansive themes for treatment. Therefore we recommend that the therapist explore the child's targets again during the Assessment Phase to continue with effective treatment planning and reprocessing. Some children may experience state change and choose to suspend therapy because the initial symptoms have improved, yet underlying issues may need to be revisited in the future, when the child's new developmental issues tap into the target event. It is possible to have cleared the target but later have the target manifest in a different symptom presentation. This is not poor treatment, but the overlay of development. Targets change and mutate as the child develops new capacities for expression and understanding.

With this concept in mind, the purpose of target identification at this point in the protocol is to search for the touchstone event that may be driving the current symptoms to most efficaciously proceed with reprocessing during the Desensitization Phase. There are many ways to select targets, including simply asking the child and parent, using a floatback technique with the child, or conducting a formal target identification process.

Procedural Considerations. The therapist's clinical judgment is necessary at this point to determine if there is a salient target already identified. If so, the therapist may just "go with that," or the therapist may want to conduct a more detailed target identification procedure. This decision is guided by information the therapist has gathered about the particular client and by the therapist's clinical judgment. One critical question is whether the client presents with a single-incident trauma, multiple cascading traumatic experiences, or only symptoms with no specific target.

Single-Incident Trauma Target Identification. With a single-incident trauma, therapists need to consider that there are several options for addressing the traumatic event. The therapist can target the presenting event or use some form of a floatback technique to access an earlier image, emotion, or body sensation, or, if the child cannot remember, the therapist can explore the child's recollections of an event the parent presented.

First, if the child is brought to therapy because of an identified event, such as a dog bite, the therapist can decide to target the dog bite incident and continue with the procedurals steps without pursuing any additional targets.

Alternatively, the therapist can set up the procedural steps from the dog bite incident and then do a float back from the NC or emotion. For example, if the child selects the image of being bitten by the dog and then identifies the NC as "I'm not safe," the therapist can ask the child to float back to an earlier time when the child first remembered thinking "I'm not safe." At this point the child may identify an earlier incident and say, "I remember not feeling safe when my mom forgot to pick me up from school one time."

If the child identifies an earlier incident, then the therapist targets that earlier incident. If the child does not report remembering an earlier incident of not feeling safe, the therapist then continues with the dog bite as the target with the NC of "I'm not safe." This is still addressing the current target but tracing the channel to the past to see if there is an associated memory.

Children frequently stay with the current target, which is fine. Children will often say, "No, I don't remember another time," even if there was. If they have no previous associated memory, they target the current one. When you choose the target connected to the worst of the current active symptoms, you may also have a generalized desensitization effect on other traumas. A child's previous incident of molestation or physical abuse may get completely reprocessed by targeting the current trigger or trauma. The therapist should use drawing, clay, sand tray, and other techniques to elicit the trauma. This requires that the therapist have patience and become attuned to the child because the target may be expressed in nonverbal ways.

As a last resort, if the therapist determines that the child is unable to access the memory networks that are believed to be associated with the current symptoms, the therapist can request that the parent provide suggested targets. The therapist needs to take the time and invest the energy in the psychotherapy process to find procedures by which to elicit targets from the child because in doing so, the child is learning to express emotions and identify feelings and make the connections between how emotions affect the child and behavior. The energy invested in a thorough target identification process will lay the foundation for reprocessing as psychotherapy continues.

If the target is a single-incident trauma, then the therapist targets that event and proceeds with the protocol of the Assessment Phase by moving to distilling NCs and PCs. If the child's history is more complex and the therapist believes that there are most likely multiple cascading targets, then the therapist will need to conduct thorough target identification at this point in treatment.

Multiple, Complex Traumas and Target Identification. There are several issues for the therapist to consider when the child's history is more complex.

Length of Time and Number of Sessions Between Client History and Treatment Planning and Target Identification During Assessment Phase. One consideration for the therapist at this step in therapy is that it depends on how long ago the therapist conducted the Client History and Treatment Planning Phase of EMDR. If the initial contact with the child happened several weeks ago and the therapist was able to move through the Preparation Phase fairly quickly, the client probably has fewer targets and greater resources. If the client has a more extensive trauma history and fewer resources, the first two phases of EMDR probably took longer to address, and it may have been months since the therapist conducted Phase 1 of EMDR. The therapist will need to check the original symptom presentation and targets and ensure that those issues continue to be the targets that need to be addressed during the remaining therapy.

Client Resources for Coping With Target Identification. If the therapist decides to proceed with a more detailed target identification process, it is necessary to consider what resources the client may need to actively participate in the exploration of targets without decompensating. For example, is the child prepared to handle more in-depth exploration of the sexual abuse history at this time, and does the client have sufficient affect regulation skills to cope with this process? If the therapist determines that the child is struggling and needs more resources and coping skills, the therapist may decide to return to the Preparation Phase for additional resourcing before continuing.

Target Identification When Clients Present With Only Symptoms but No Specific Event. In some cases, the therapist may not be able to identify a specific event because there is no adult available to provide the child's history, and the child cannot report any events. There may be no obvious target because the parents and child do not report an event because there are no events that the parents consider to be relevant to the child's current symptoms. The therapist may then focus on a symptom and use the float back to explore potential events that are targets for desensitization. In case conceptualization, the therapist needs to consider that the child's and parent's inability to identify a specific event may be because the event was so early that it was the child's response to an unknown event, or the child cannot remember and the parent does not know.

Case Study: School Phobia

For example, I (R.T.) worked with an 8-year-old girl, Ellen, who initially was brought to therapy for treatment of school phobia. During Client History and Treatment Planning, neither the child nor her mother were able to identify any specific event that led to the school phobia. Both reported to me that the child had been able to attend school until second grade. During target identification, I asked the child's mother about her theory for why the child was refusing to go to school. The mother's theory was that the child had become phobic after returning from a trip where the child had shared a room with the mother. Mother also noted this was the first school year after the 9/11 attacks in New York. When I asked the child, she reported that she became anxious about going to school without her mother after throwing up in school. The child explained that the incident was even more traumatic because when the teacher called the child's mother, the mother was not available to come to the school, and the child was embarrassed. According to the child, the specific incident at school was the origin for the school phobia, which then escalated because the mother began staying at the school for progressively longer periods of time. Until therapy, the mother was unaware of Ellen's vomiting incident at school. During therapy, we targeted Ellen's image of throwing up at school first and then explored her feelings about the 9/11 attacks in New York City and processed those as well. After targeting both of Ellen's targets and the ones offered by the mother, the child returned to school and no longer needed her mother to stay.

The therapist can identify a target based on a single-incident trauma or on multiple traumatic events, or can assist the client in identifying targets by using a floatback technique.

If the therapist determines it is clinically indicated to further tease out targets during the Assessment Phase and the client handles the further exploration well, the therapist can proceed with the following target identification process with children.

TOOLS FOR TARGET IDENTIFICATION WITH CHILD CLIENTS

Touchstone Event

There are various techniques for target identification, as taught during EMDR training. This section will focus on techniques for target identification with children. The techniques range from basic clinical interviewing and focused questioning of the child and parents to various art and play therapy techniques. The therapist can use different clinical techniques to assist the client in identifying the first time the client can recall thinking that way, feeling that way, or having a similar body sensation. This is identifying a *touchstone event*. In AIP theory, the touchstone event is the original incident that has been maladaptively stored and is driving the current symptoms that brought the client into therapy. By probing for the touchstone event, the therapist is attempting to assist the client in processing through to healthy resolution, the foundational memory that is driving current problematic issues in the client's life.

To explore for a touchstone event, the therapist can use several tools, including a floatback technique or an affect bridge.

First, the therapist can simply ask questions to identify the touchstone event. The therapist can ask the child, "Do you ever remember feeling this way before?" or "Do you ever remember thinking this before?" Often, children are so current-focused that the therapist must consider possible touchstone events of which the child is unaware.

Case Study: Sara and the Wind

When my (C.S.) daughter Sara was 9 years old, she developed a wind phobia for no apparent reason. In Arizona, where we live, we have strong summer dust storms accompanied by lightning and thunder. Sara would stand at the door and shout to her friends, trying to still be involved with her friends playing but staying out of the wind. She would cry fearfully when the almost nightly monsoon would arrive.

I had Sara see a very good EMDR therapist, and after three sessions, the behavior had not changed. One night, when the wind was blowing hard, Sara had her arms around my waist crying and crying. I thought that I must do something. I asked if I could tap her shoulders. Normally, my children will not let me tap their shoulders or do any EMDR because I am their mother. But this time, Sara agreed. I was at a loss as to what the target was since she had already done the first, worst, and most recent times with her therapist.

I was trying to find out how the information was maladaptively stored when I asked Sara what the wind sounded like. She made an unusual sucking sound with her mouth that did not sound at all like the wind sounded to me. But I did recognize the sound—it resembled the oxygen being pumped into her incubator when she was born. Sara had been born 6 weeks premature and had been in the neonatal unit for 12 days.

I said to her, "Oh, that's the sound of the oxygen that they pumped into your incubator when you were born. That was a long time ago, and you are safe now." Then I tapped her shoulders. After a few repetitions, she relaxed her arms and looked up at me and said, "Really?" I said yes and did a few more repetitions. Sara's whole body relaxed; she hugged me and went off to play.

There is no perfect way to elicit the touchstone event. What the therapist and client first identify as a touchstone event may later change as the client reprocesses. The client will go wherever he or she needs to go to reprocess what is feeding the current symptoms.

Case Study: Allison

I (R.T.) worked with a 4-year-old child, Allison, who was brought to therapy because of specific fears. Allison's fears were so extensive that they were interfering with her willingness to attend preschool. Allison was almost 5 years old and was preparing to begin public kindergarten. Allison's history included extensive medical interventions due to being a micropremie. Allison's mother reported a traumatic incident at age 3, when Allison went into cardiac arrest and was flown to a nearby hospital. After conducting a thorough history and teaching Allison some emotional regulation and self-calming skills, we began reprocessing this memory. Allison's NC was "I'm all alone." During the Desensitization Phase, Allison began to reprocess body memories and feeling all alone in a "bubble thing." We processed Allison's memory through, and she came to "I'm with my family and I'm OK." Allison's mother reported she had never left Allison during the incident at age 3 but that she had left Allison in the neonatal intensive care unit, in an isolette, during the 3 months following birth. Allison's mother was surprised Allison appeared to have floated back to the touchstone event of being born and being in intensive care, even though Allison was just a newborn. After processing this event and several others, Allison was no longer afraid of the wind in the trees and was able to attend kindergarten. I cannot be sure that Allison understood what was happening to her, but she began to feel less anxious and not worry about getting sick. I have included this example as one of many experiences when the child's target identification and reprocessing is a surprise to both the parent and the therapist.

This is one example of how the original target thought to be the touchstone event was in fact being driven by even an earlier traumatic event that was the touchstone event.

Interviewing Children and Parents to Identify Targets

We recommend six steps to help more thoroughly explore target identification when interviewing children and parents. These six steps include (a) asking the child for targets; (b) asking the child what the child thinks the parent might identify as potential targets; (c) asking the parent about the parent's thoughts about possible targets; (d) asking the parent what the parent thinks the child might identify as possible targets; (e) asking the child about what the parent reported as possible targets; and (f) returning to share targets the child has identified with the parent because the parent is regularly unaware of some targets identified by the child. This information may have already come out during the Client History and Treatment Planning Phase; however, we include these steps here in order to help therapists create a template for organizing targets.

It is possible that new targets have arisen since the original sessions with the child and parent or as part of understanding the therapy process, children and parents may have recognized the need to address certain targets that were previously dismissed.

As part of the first contact with the family, previously discussed in chapter 3, the therapist makes a decision about when to interview the parents and the child. We recommend that with target identification, the therapist ask the child without the child having any influence from the parent.

Ask the Child. The first method of identifying targets with children is simply to ask the child. We emphasize this point because there is diversity in the EMDR community about how to do target identification with children. Some professionals have suggested that the therapist ask the parent, without ever asking the child. Best practice with any psychotherapy approach with children compels the therapist to ask both the parent and the child about potential targets for desensitization. Often, children's targets are more current. What the child identifies as the trauma may not be what the parent identifies as the trauma.

Case Study: Rottweiler Story

I (C.S.) treated a 9-year-old girl, named Brianna, who had been attacked by a Rottweiler dog 6 months earlier. She had previously been a happy, secure girl. She had developed clingy, whining behavior and was fearful around dogs, even the 8-year-old family dog.

Her mother thought we should target the emergency room where Brianna was getting stitches, but Brianna reported that the worst part of the incident was the actual attack, where the dog had viciously bitten Brianna's right foot in several places so badly that Brianna required numerous stitches.

I had her draw a picture on one half of a large piece of paper of the dog attack. The NC was "I'm in danger; I'm not safe," and the PC was "I'm safe now," and she drew a picture of herself walking the family dog (see Figure 5.1).

When they returned on their third visit, both mother and Brianna reported that the clinging behavior was gone and that Brianna had suggested going to a pet store across the street. They went to the pet store, and Brianna was fine around the dogs there. Most important, Brianna was able to enjoy the family's Scottish terrier again.

About 6 months later, the mother called wanting to bring Brianna back because her clinging behavior had returned. The

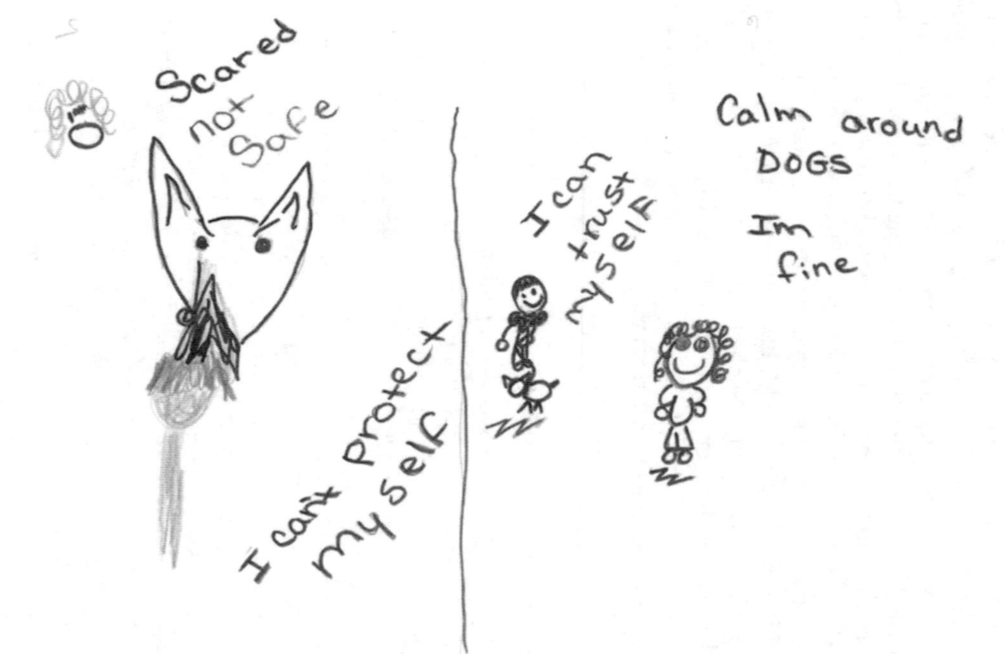
Scared
not
Safe
I can't protect
myself
I can
trust
myself
Calm around
DOGS
Im
fine

FIGURE 5.1 Nine-year-old Brianna's picture of the Rottweiler dog biting her foot shows how a child can draw the negative cognition and positive cognition on the same page to use for the desensitization process (chapter 6).

mother asked if EMDR wore off and needed a booster occasionally. I said no and inquired from both the mother and Brianna if something had happened or changed. The mother said no and that she had asked Brianna. When I was alone in the session with Brianna, I asked more specific questions regarding the return of her fearfulness. Brianna told me that they lived between two houses that both had Rottweilers, neither of which was the dog that had attacked her. She reported that within a span of a week, one Rottweiler had escaped the neighbor's house and stood viciously barking at her in the driveway, having to be restrained. The other dog, which is normally kept in a pen, was loose in the backyard and was ferociously barking at her when she jumped on the trampoline.

We targeted these incidents. The NC was "I'm not safe." The PC was "I can protect myself and have good caution around some dogs." In the follow-up session, Brianna again felt better and was back to her independent behavior.

By asking the child to identify targets and symptoms, the child will present what issues are bothering him or her, and then the therapist can consult with the parent to explore possible additional pieces of the child's memory experience. As we will emphasize throughout this book, it is important that the targets be identified primarily by the child, with ancillary input from parents and other caregivers.

Ask the Child What the Child Thinks the Parent Will Report. After asking the child to identify targets, we suggest that the therapist continue by asking the child to predict what the parent might report. For example, the therapist can say to the child, "*Why do you think your parents brought you here to me?*" Or, "*What did your parent tell you about why they were bringing you to my office?*" Sometimes children have discussed this with his or her parents and sometimes children will just know because he or she has figured out that his or her parent has been upset about something the child is doing. Other children may not have an idea. The child's responses give the therapist additional understanding into how the child and his or her parents interact.

Ask the Parent. The second method of identifying targets is to ask the parent. We ask the parent to further discuss and clarify what the child has identified. In this role, the parent provides additional evidence to assist the therapist in understanding what the child is processing. Even though it is not always necessary for the therapist to understand what the child has identified, at times, the parent can provide additional clarification.

Case Study: Sienna's X ray

I (C.S.) saw Sienna when she was 3 years old. She exhibited oppositional behavior with her mother, was very active, and had prolonged crying bouts, particularly around bedtime. During the history-taking process, I found that numerous traumas had occurred in Sienna's lifetime. Sienna had been born prematurely and had a serious medical condition at the age of 1 that required hospitalization. Her mother had gone through a miscarriage when Sienna was present, which was upsetting to her. Because her mother could not lift or hold Sienna during her pregnancy, Sienna felt sad and neglected. Her mother and I suspected that these traumas might be contributing to her behavior.

I explained EMDR to Sienna and her mother. The next session, Sienna knew I was planning to do the assessment and desensitization phases with her. She came into the session, grabbed the drawing paper and crayons, and began to draw what appeared to be a bunch of scribbles (see Figure 5.2).

Puzzled, I asked Sienna what she was drawing, and she said, "An X ray." "An X ray of what?" I asked. She replied, "An X ray of when I broke my arm." The mother was surprised and then said that Sienna had broken her arm last year and that this was the exact week a year later that it had happened.

Sienna's mother and I had speculated about the extent of the previous medical trauma. But Sienna chose her target as the X ray and knew what she wanted to work on. We targeted that initial target and reprocessed it successfully.

The parent presents his or her observation of what the child has demonstrated, observations which are filtered through the parent's own system. As we have discussed, the parent's own issues may impact what targets the parent identifies for the child.

Ask the Parent About What the Parent Believes the Child Will Report. Just as we ask the child to predict what the parent might report, we do the same with parents. We explore with parents what the parent believes the child will identify as potential targets for EMDR. For example, we might ask the parent "*What did you discuss with your son or daughter about bringing them to my office?*" Some parents will have discussed treatment with the child, while others may not. Again, this is valuable data for the therapist to use in treatment. Once we discuss the parents prediction of what the child might report, we can continue by discussing what the child actually identified.

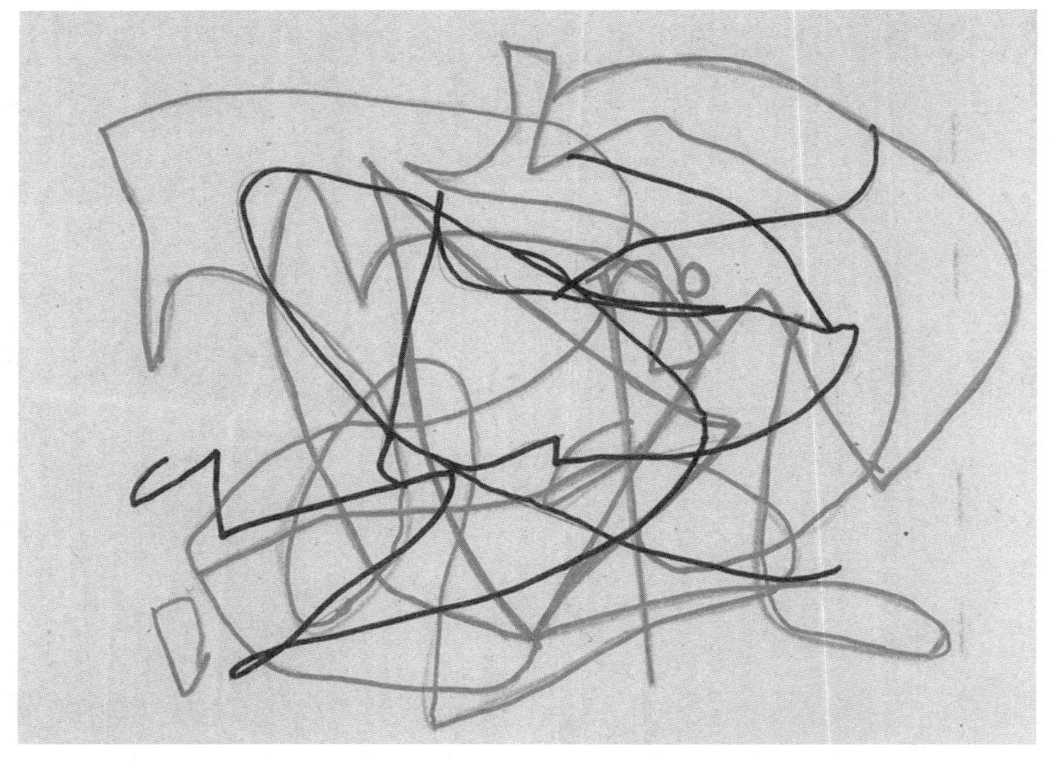

FIGURE 5.2 Sienna, 3 years old, chose to draw her target as the X ray of her broken arm.

Ask the Parent About What the Child Reported. Sometimes the parent is aware of the child's concerns, and sometimes the parent is surprised by what the child identifies as the target. Therefore another possibility is that the child may identify a target of which the parent is completely unaware. For example, a child may report an experience from school, and the parent is not aware of what happened to the child in school.

Case Study: Bethany and Selective Mutism

Several years ago, I (R.T.) was asked to try EMDR with a 7-year-old with selective mutism. Bethany taught me a great deal about children and EMDR. Let me begin with the end. When Bethany finally started talking after 8 months of working together, I asked her why she stopped talking, and she replied, "Because a boy on the playground said I talked funny." If only I had asked her first and targeted that memory with EMDR! Thank goodness Bethany was a very patient and tolerant little girl.

Initially, Bethany was referred to me by a child welfare agency for the treatment of trauma and the selective mutism. I was told that the last time anyone knew that Bethany had spoken was when she called 911 after she found her mother overdosed on the sofa in her home. I thought the target was fairly obvious. Bethany was in foster care by the time I met her, and she was transported each week by taxi, which often left her in my office for hours, and then a new driver came every time. This part was traumatic for both of us, but that is not the point of my case study. It was just Bethany and I were trying to work together regarding what she needed from therapy. Bethany and I had very little assistance from any other adults, with the exception of several telephone calls I had with Bethany's foster mother.

After building rapport and eating lunch each week, we began to write to each other on a clipboard. In the beginning, Bethany spelled everything phonetically, and then we also played charades to see if we could understand each other. At the time, Bethany was in first grade but presented as very bright and expressive. At this time, I was focused on the client history and treatment planning and preparation phases. We explored resources and installed mastery experiences about when she felt good about herself.

I then learned that this little one started answering the phone, even though she still did not talk anywhere else, so I put her on my phone in my office and then went to my waiting room phone and got on the same line. I ran back and forth from my office to the waiting room and did the entire EMDR protocol with the child talking on the phone, writing, or drawing. Finally, we targeted the 911 call and the police and emergency personnel coming to her home. I later learned that no one realized she was hiding in a closet in the home for many hours after she called 911, and they only took the other children out of the home, but not Bethany. I thought I was so smart and had a second target. So Bethany decided to reprocess this target by hiding in the closet in my office, while I sat outside the door with the tactile "buzzies" wires under the door for bilateral stimulation (BLS). She opened the door when I stopped the buzzies and then closed the door each time we continued with BLS. She would even slide notes under the door to respond when I asked her, "What happened now?"

Eventually, she came out smiling and did not close the closet door again. At the foster home, she started communicating more by ordering at restaurants and running to answer the phone, so we targeted ordering at a restaurant and then went to a restaurant for her to order lunch. I tried to use ordering in restaurants as a master experience and congratulated Bethany on her success. I made an agreement with Bethany that we could go to a nearby restaurant, and if she ordered, I would pay. The first time we went to the restaurant, she would not order, so we returned to the office. The second time, she ordered, and I bought her lunch. On our way back to the office, I asked her why she stopped talking in the first place—and she looked at me like I was so very dense. Once we targeted what the boy said on the playground, she did not stop talking.

I am not sure if targeting all the other events helped, but once we targeted the memory of the boy on the playground, Bethany did very well. She was held back in first grade, which made her angry, and rightfully so because it turned out that she was very bright but just had stopped talking, which later became another target.

I learned from this 7-year-old that I need to always ask the child for the target, at least initially. Since learning from this little one, I always ask the child for targets, no matter how old the child is—even tiny ones can draw, or set up the playroom, or use puppets or sand tray to communicate the image that bothers them or worries them or scares them, and the image can be real or imaginary. It does not matter what I think, but what the child knows to be true for him or her. I would encourage you to ask the child, look for the missing piece about why he or she stopped talking, and keep going with EMDR.

Ask the Child About What the Parent Reported. Finally, we check with the child about what the parent reported if the child is able to cope with what the parent reported. Sometimes the information provided by the parent may be overwhelming for the child and may not be part of the child's implicit memory, but by providing the child information from the parent, the therapist is offering information that can potentially assist the child in creating a narrative of the child's history. Once the therapist collects the information from the parent, the therapist can then explore what the parent reported with the child.

In addition to directly asking the child and the child's parents to identify possible targets, the therapist can use less direct techniques to elicit targets and to explore what touchstone event may be driving the current symptom presentation.

Floatback Technique

We suggest that the therapist consider what we call a *floatback cognitive interweave*. We created floatback cognitive interweaves both to assist in target identification and to jump-start blocked processing during the Desensitization Phase. During the target identification process, the therapist uses the floatback cognitive interweave to introduce information about the child's history and to introduce the concept of associative chaining to children. The therapist may be aware of information about the child's history of which the child is unaware or which the child is discounting because the child has not associated the event with current symptom presentation. With the floatback cognitive interweave, the therapist introduces a piece of information about the trauma to explore possible targets. The child may or may not make an association with this information. The therapist explores whether the link is not made because the child is developmentally unable to make the association or because the child is not aware of an association. The therapist's clinical judgment determines how to proceed. With the floatback cognitive interweave, the therapist suggests that the child consider an event of which the therapist is aware. The therapist can ask the child, "Do you remember that your mom told me you had this accident when you were 2 years old? Well, I was wondering if you think that the accident has anything to do with what you think about now when you feel scared or have that bad thought of 'I'm not safe.' Do you think those might be connected?"

Case Study: Jeremiah

Jeremiah was an 8-year-old boy, the youngest of three siblings, and lived with his parents in a middle-class neighborhood. He lost his left index finger in a bicycle accident a year ago. Before the accident, Jeremiah had been a happy, growing, hungry, adventuresome boy. I (C.S.) mention Jeremiah's hunger because in every session, despite having been recently fed, he would express being hungry. Even though he focused on eating, Jeremiah was a thin and active boy. Within the previous 6 months before coming to therapy, Jeremiah had developed clinging behavior; he would not play in the front yard, he slept in his brother's room, he would cry and have tantrums at the water park if his siblings were not nearby, and he checked the locks on the house at night.

When I took a history from the parents and Jeremiah, they reported that Jeremiah and his siblings were riding their bicycles down a hill and were going fast. There was a lot of construction in the neighborhood, and someone had removed a manhole cover and put it on the sidewalk. The oldest brother, who was first, quickly went around the manhole. The middle brother, who was second, also went around the manhole. Jeremiah, who was last, did not see the manhole cover in time and hit it. His hand was tangled up in the spokes, and he lost his index finger. His brothers were great and ran to get their parents. The parents responded quickly and rushed Jeremiah to the hospital. Jeremiah was surprisingly calm, and everything went as smoothly as could be expected.

In therapy, I had Jeremiah complete the mapping process (mapping is discussed in the next section of this chapter) during his second session. This was how I began to see how Jeremiah had maladaptively stored his trauma. He was afraid to be left home alone, was afraid of being kidnapped, was afraid of robbers, and was afraid of bad dreams. Jeremiah wrote this out phonetically on the piece of paper on which we were doing mapping. He then connected the items on his map that were related, such as his fear of being kidnapped and his fear his brothers would be kidnapped. His fear of robbers and gangsters gave him bad dreams. And watching the news made Jeremiah afraid of being alone for fear of being kidnapped. He rated that kidnapping did not bother him as much, but watching the news was his biggest worry. In the map, he did not put down the bicycle accident as a problem/worry, and when he was doing his map, I asked him specifically if that was a worry. He said no.

In Jeremiah's third session, he identified "the news" as his target. This new target required a great deal of time and patience for me to patiently tease out the NC. Then Jeremiah drew a picture of robbers shooting a policeman on the TV screen. Jeremiah's NC, which he asked me to write for him, was "Something bad might happen. I'm in danger." I then tried to identify Jeremiah's PC. At my suggestion, the good thought was "Bad things happen, good things happen, but I'm still OK." Jeremiah agreed to that, but his response was tepid. It did not resonate completely for him.

On his drawing, he had people happily walking together, and on the other part of the page, robbers shooting a policeman. And at the top, there was a picture of Jeremiah at a table eating chicken. He then spelled out phonetically, "Can I have some privacy? I'm eating," which surprised me. Jeremiah then responded with a statement that seemed to resonate for him. Jeremiah stated, "Bad and good things happen, and I'm just going about my life." See Figure 5.3 for Jeremiah's map.

In desensitization, children may process quickly or be very active, as Jeremiah was when he was getting BLS with the NeuroTek buzzies. He was very active as he imagined beating up the robbers. Jeremiah continued reprocessing his targets, and by the fourth session, 2 weeks later, we did a reevaluation of the target. Reevaluating the symptoms is the most reliable way of determining whether reprocessing has successfully occurred. You want to ask the parents and child together. Parents will often report external changes, while children will report internal shifts. Usually, they are surprised to hear each other's responses. And without both, the reevaluation is often incomplete. This is a very important part of the process.

In our session, Jeremiah reprocessed his fear of the news and the robbers he feared. On reevaluation, the majority of Jeremiah's symptoms were gone: The clinging was gone, he was sleeping in his own room, and so on. One small symptom that the parents reported on reevaluation was that Jeremiah was still checking the locks before bedtime. We continued reprocessing focused on Jeremiah checking the locks. His negative cognition was still "Bad things happen" and I told him to "Go with that." Then I used a cognitive interweave floatback and said to Jeremiah, "What about the bike accident?" Jeremiah replied, "Bad things happen." I said, "Go with that." And then Jeremiah spontaneously said, "Bad things happen. Good things happen. It's not my fault." Jeremiah then lightly threw the buzzies down.

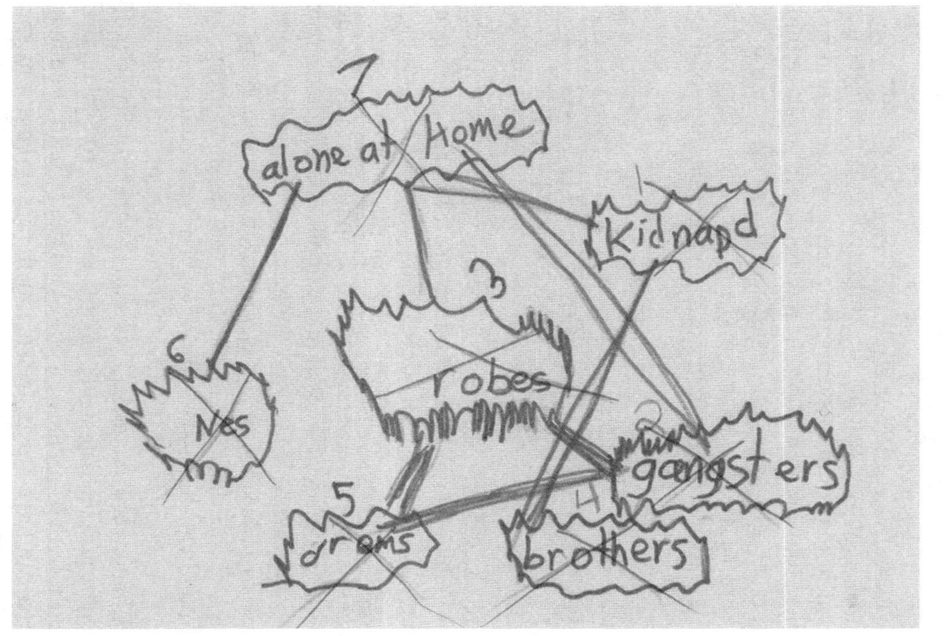

FIGURE 5.3 Here is an example of Jeremiah's map. You can see that he does not put the bicycle accident on the map of his worries. Instead, he puts his fears of being kidnapped, gangsters, robbers, his brothers being kidnapped, bad dreams, the television news, and being alone, in that order of importance. He then rates each worry with a subjective unit of disturbance level. Interestingly, at the next session, when we were at the beginning of our first desensitization session, he chose the bad news as his biggest worry. He then reported that the other worries no longer bothered him, and he crossed them out on the map.

I discovered that the missing piece to help in reprocessing was Jeremiah's sense of responsibility: "It's not my fault." When I talked with Jeremiah's parents privately, they were surprised. At no time had he indicated he thought that his accident was his fault. But it made sense—both of his brothers saw the manhole cover, but he did not. After this session, Jeremiah finished treatment and was reportedly fine at 6- and 9-month follow-ups.

A comprehensive target identification process includes some combination of all of the above. Asking the child to identify targets first, without the parent in the room, prevents the parent's presentation from contaminating the child's presentation. It may be helpful to have input from the parent, especially if the child is reticent to discuss issues or the child really is confused about why he or she was brought for counseling. Refer to the discussion of how parents are integrated into children's therapy in chapter 4.

CREATIVE TECHNIQUES FOR IDENTIFYING TARGETS FOR REPROCESSING WITH EMDR

The authors have created unique tools for identifying targets with children. These tools include Mapping and Graphing; art therapy techniques, including the sand tray, Play-Doh, and drawing on whiteboards or tablets; and the use of digital pictures to assist the therapist in identifying targets for reprocessing with children. Several of these techniques actually include one or more of the procedural steps. For example, the Mapping technique can actually be used to identify all the pieces of the protocol in the Assessment Phase to proceed with the Desensitization Phase. Mapping and Graphing assist the therapist in eliciting the steps of the protocol with children and can be integrated and used as case conceptualization for treatment planning in EMDR. Both techniques teach children to self-assess and enhance their metacognitive skills or their ability to think about their thoughts and feelings while having new tools to explain their experiences. Finally, both Mapping and Graphing can be used as containers where children can have any distressing memories or emotions stick to the paper until the disturbance can be resolved.

Mapping Targets for EMDR Processing

Mapping targets for EMDR (see Appendix V) is a technique utilized to organize the information collected when preparing for processing a client's issues with EMDR. Initially, I (R.T.) utilized this procedure to organize my child client's trauma history to identify targets for EMDR. However, as I utilized the process on a regular basis, I found that mapping targets is an effective tool for utilization when proceeding with the full EMDR protocol for clients of all ages.

Mapping targets begins with the initial phase of taking client history and treatment planning and proceeds through the entire protocol, including preparation, assessment, desensitization, installation, body scan, closure, and reevaluation. The following steps will outline the process of mapping targets as a process for organizing EMDR in psychotherapy. Even though I currently utilize this technique with adult clients as well, the following description of the mapping targets technique is focused on working with children.

When using mapping in EMDR with children, I once again begin by explaining EMDR to parents and children.

According to the standard EMDR protocol, when beginning EMDR with any client, the therapist screens for contraindications, including limited physical capacity for stress, emotional instability, and other risk factors. With children, this includes interviewing parents as well; however, I have regularly noted a discrepancy between what a parent identifies as targets for their child and what the child has identified as the target on his or her map. Therefore, after interviewing the parent, I will ask the child to assist me in completing a map of his or her worries that the child wants to "shrink, get rid of, or leave in the office with me." In addition, the parent's own issues may often distract from the child's issues, and based on the parent's issues and ability to tolerate the child's affective states, I may ask the parent to allow the child alone time with me (see Table 4.1 on decisions regarding including parents in sessions). It is important to assess the parent's emotional instability and risk factors in the child's home environment before proceeding with the EMDR protocol. Processing with EMDR will often be thwarted due to instability in a home where a child does not feel safe or in a home environment that is too stressful. If I note this to be true, I will often focus on a Safe/Calm Place, calming techniques, and resource development and installation, without pursuing trauma processing. If my assessment suggests that EMDR is appropriate at this time, I begin with the EMDR standard protocol using the mapping targets procedure (see Appendix V).

With every client, it is possible to begin EMDR with a Safe/Calm Place exercise that will empower the client and, with success, will also encourage the client to be more invested in the EMDR process, which at times can be very difficult. Once the client has been successful with using the Safe/Calm Place process, the therapist can then continue with the phases of EMDR.

As the therapist begins to explore the parameters of the problem based on parent input and discussion with the child, data regarding the client's trauma history will begin to arise; explain to the client that this is all important information that needs attention in order to help his or her brain fix the problem. The therapist can suggest to the child that talking about this information may bother the child a little; therefore, with the child's assistance, the therapist would like to create a map where he or she and the child can put all the important parts about the child's worries or fears. Suggest to the child that by putting his or her worries on the paper, the child might not have to worry as much. Show the child that he or she and the therapist are going to use a piece of paper and pen to begin to make a map of things that bother the child, and the child's help is needed to get the map correct. Suggest to the child that he or she can help with the map or do it entirely by himself or herself, if the child likes.

With the child's assistance, begin by drawing a large, odd-shaped figure (such as a cloud-shaped oval) in the center of the paper, and ask the child what the child thinks is his or her biggest worry. Depending on the child's description of the worry, put a single word or phrase in the center of the first shape. Then ask the child to continue with selecting more worries to add to the map. Then ask the child, "What do you think is your next biggest worry?" Continue to collect targets by asking the child to identify more things that bother him or her. Suggest things that the child's parent may have identified as well. For instance, "Your mom thinks you get in trouble a lot in school because you are mad about your daddy leaving. Do you think this is something we should put on your map?" Continue by asking the child if there are things that his or her mom does not understand or know about that should also be on the map. We continue with mapping all of the child's worries by adding to the drawing. Add additional pieces of paper, as needed, to identify all of the child's worries. Sometimes this process proceeds quickly, and we can move to the next phases of the EMDR protocol, while other times, this process takes an entire session. If the therapist notes that the child is becoming agitated while completing the mapping, offer cognitive interweaves, suggest that the child practice his Safe/Calm Place, or stop and conduct a resource installation in order for the child to cope with mapping targets (see chapter 10, on cognitive interweaves for children and resource installation for children). Throughout the remainder of this process, the therapist needs to try to become attuned to the child and use the child's language regarding how the child labels whatever problems or worries he or she has.

After completing the map, explain to the child that he or she can change the map at any time if we have forgotten something or if something changes. Encourage the child to make the map his or hers and know that he or she is in charge of what happens with the map.

After drawing the map, ask the child to rank the targets on the map. Say, "Could you help me understand which one of these targets is the biggest or bothers you the most?" Proceed with this ranking process from worst or most bothersome to littlest worry or "it doesn't bother me much at all." By doing so, we are basically creating a list of targets for processing with EMDR via the map.

After ranking the targets on the map, explain what SUD is to the child, and ask the child to rate the SUD level on each target on the map. With children, the SUD could be measured as "how big?" simply by using your hands and showing the child distance with your hands. Since we are working with a map Metaphor, ask the child to look at a map of the United States or the world and ask the child if his or her target worry is as big as Arizona (the state we live in), as big as the United States, as big as the whole world, or bigger than the whole world. One thing that is important to note is that sometimes what the child ranks as number one when ranking targets on the map will not be the target with the highest SUD. If this is true, first make sure that the child understands about ranking the targets from biggest to smallest and then review what a SUD means. After the therapist is sure that the child understands both ranking and SUD, check the SUD again for the targets. For example, "Maura, you told me that this target on your map was the second biggest of all your targets or worries. How much does it worry or bother you?" If the discrepancy between ranking the targets and SUD is still present, continue with the EMDR process and just note this discrepancy.

After collecting SUD for the child's targets, ask the child to draw lines between the targets to show what he or she might think about any targets being connected to other targets. Children frequently will make amazing and unexpected connections between targets.

Next ask the child how strong the connection between the targets may be on the map. This process teaches a child about how memories get linked into neuronetworks in the child's brain. Explain to the child that sometimes a thing might bother us more than we would expect because it is connected to something else that has bothered us before. For instance, if the child has identified anger as a target, ask the child if he or she thinks that his or her anger is connected to any other targets on the map—maybe part of the child's anger is from his or her dad and part of the child's anger is from getting in trouble at school, and another part of the child's anger is from the boy who picks on him or her at soccer practice. As the child diagrams the links between the targets on the map, suggest that everything that is happening to the child is related somehow and that by understanding how things that happen to the child make him or her feel a certain way, we can begin to understand how to make him or her feel better. Then ask the child if he or she would like help to find ways to make the child feel better or accomplish whatever goals the child has identified. This discussion leads to collection of the NC and PC.

Select a target on the map for reprocessing and proceed with collecting an NC and PC for the target. When attempting to identify NCs and PCs with children, explain to the child that we are looking for his or her bad thought about the target, and then we are looking for the good thought. Refer to the Kids' List of Cognitions (Table 5.1) for examples of NCs and PCs that are effective with children. With the child's permission, write the NC/PC on the map, and then ask the child to identify a VoC for the PC. The child and therapist will measure VoC based on the typical VoC scale process used with adults.

Next ask the child to tell you what feeling goes with the target. The therapist can utilize a child's list of feelings or suggest that he or she might feel bad, sad, mad, glad, or have other feelings that the child may have indicated during interaction with the therapist. Once the therapist has identified the child's feeling, combine this with the NC combination, and ask the child to demonstrate where he or she feels this in the body. Note all of this information on the map for the child and therapist to both see. Explain to the child that this map is important to help us get where we want to be, with the ultimate goal of the child feeling better and having the problems or worries go away.

Continue by explaining the different types of BLS available that will help shrink the target. Explain that the BLS is like putting laser beams on the target so we can shrink or blow up the target. Also suggest to the child that by putting his or her worries on the map and using the buzzies or whatever BLS was chosen, the child's symptoms will probably improve, or might even go away.

Resume the desensitization process per the standard EMDR protocol, including installation, body scan, closure, and reevaluation. As part of the reevaluation, ask the client to reevaluate the previous target, but also check on the other targets on the map to determine if anything has changed during the session.

Finally, ask the child if he or she would like a copy of his or her map, and ask if the therapist can keep a copy for the next time they work together. Offer the child a file or a tablet with his or her name on it to keep in a special drawer for each time the therapist and child see each other. The therapist can also offer the child an empty file, a tablet of his own, or an envelope for the child to keep copies of the work that he or she has completed. Suggest to the child that until the next time the therapist and child get together, if any targets, worries, or other things bother the child, he or she can use his or her container or draw a picture and put it in the file to show the therapist when they get together. Encourage the child to not let worries get too big without drawing or telling someone. Finish by reminding the child of his or her safe place and other tools the child has for self-calming and soothing.

Whether the parent is in the session or not, remind the parent that processing with EMDR most likely will continue between sessions, and if the parent is concerned or the child seems to be struggling, the parent should encourage the child to use the tools and self-calming techniques we have discussed, and if this is not successful, the parent should contact the office, as needed.

Instructions and Script for Mapping Targets

1. Per the protocol, start with Client History and Treatment Planning. Focus on attunement with the child and listening for negative cognitions and possible targets for EMDR processing. It is helpful for the therapist to make notes of the client's negative cognitions and potential targets.
2. In the Preparation Phase the therapist explains EMDR to parents *and* to children.
3. Then the therapist assesses the parent's current stability and ability to participate in EMDR process with child.
4. Teach Safe/Calm Place to child. During this process allow the child to experiment with the different types of bilateral stimulation from tapping, drumming, stomping, using the buzzies, and so on.
5. Teach the Stop Signal.
6. Interview the parent about identifying possible targets for EMDR.
7. Interview the child about identifying targets for EMDR and compare with parents' responses.
8. Explain mapping to the child. *"I would like you to help me create a map where we put all of your worries, owies, etc. Do you know what a map is?"* (If the child knows what a map is, continue with the Mapping process. If not, explain what a map is to the child.) *"Today we will start your map that shows where the things that bother you or the worries that you have are just like in your head"* (therapist can point to their own head and the child's head). *"Today we are starting with the map, but we can change it or add worries to it at any time. Remember it is your brain that will fix your worries and that I can teach you a way to help your brain shrink the worries and even make the worries go away."*
9. With large drawing paper and pen or pencil draw a large odd shape in the middle of the paper and ask the child to identify his or her biggest worry to start the map. *"On this paper, I want us to start drawing your map by picking the biggest worry that you have or the thing that is bothering you the most right now."* Help the child to write their biggest concern or symptom in the shape in order to begin the map. Have the child pick single words to put

in the figure on the map that will help to identify what worry is in each shape.

10. "*When we make the map, you might feel a little bit scared or worried, but remember you're safe here in my office and if you get too scared you can always practice using your safe place like we learned before. Do you remember how to use your safe place to feel better?*" If needed, review the Safe Place or continue identifying targets.
11. In addition to Safe/Calm Place, you can teach the child to use the figures on the map as Containers. "*Do you see this big worry here on your map? What do we need to do to keep that worry locked into that shape on the map so it won't bother you?*" Usually children are very creative and come up with many ideas, but you can assist as necessary. You might want to suggest to the child that the shape on the map can have steel walls with lasers to keep anything from escaping the shape. You can also add, "*When we put your worry onto the map, we're sealing it into the shape so it won't come off and bother you. It will stay stuck on the map until we take it off to shrink it. Is that OK with you?*" Continue to collect targets by asking the child to identify more things that bother them and suggest things that the child's parent may have identified as well. For instance, you may say to Johnny, "*Your mom thinks that you get in trouble a lot in school because you are mad about your daddy leaving. Do you think this is something we should put on your map?*" Continue by asking Johnny if there are things that his mom doesn't understand or know about that should also be on his map. Continue with mapping all of the child's worries by adding to the drawing. You can add additional pieces of paper as needed to identify all of the child's worries. Sometimes this process proceeds very quickly and you can move to the next phases of the EMDR protocol while other times this process takes an entire session. If you note that the child is becoming agitated in completing the mapping, you can offer cognitive interweaves, suggest that the child practice his Safe/Calm Place, or stop and conduct a resource installation in order for the child to cope with mapping targets. See chapters on cognitive interweaves for children and resource installation for children. Throughout the remainder of this process, try to become attuned with the child and use the child's language regarding how the child labels whatever problems or worries her or she has.
12. Continue to identify other worries to add to the map. Engage the child in helping you create the map or let the child create

the map as appropriate for the child's developmental level and understanding.

13. Explain to the child that you will also be writing notes because what she or he says is very important and you want to make sure you remember it correctly. *"I am writing down what you are telling me because it is very important and I'm old and I don't want to forget what you are telling me. Is that OK with you?"*
14. When the child has identified all the worries that he or she wants to put on the map for the day, remind the child that he or she can add to the map at any time. *"Remember we can change the map at anytime if we've forgotten something or something changes."*
15. Next ask the child to help rank the targets on the map. *"Now I want you to help me know which target is the biggest or bothers you the most. Would you show me which one is the biggest or worst?"* Proceed with the ranking process from worst or bothers me the most until littlest worry or *"It doesn't bother me hardly at all."*
16. After completing the ranking process, explain SUD to the child and ask the child to identify a SUD for each target on the map. *"I want us to be able to tell how much something bothers you so when I ask you to tell me how much something bothers you, we can use numbers or you can show me with your hands like this."* (The therapist demonstrates SUD based on distance between the therapist's hands.) The therapist then says *"Is it this big, this big, or this big?"* The therapist can also use other measurements for the SUD. SUD can be bigger than the whole world or universe or deeper than the ocean or the therapist can ask the child to tell what the biggest thing is that they can imagine. After that the therapist asks the child for the smallest thing they can imagine. Then the therapist asks the child to tell him how big each of the worry is for each target on the map and this is noted on the map. *"What's the biggest thing you can think of in the whole world?"* Whatever the child answers, the therapist explains, *"That tells me that your worry would bother you a lot if it's as big as* _______ (repeat child's answer)." The therapist then asks the child, *"What's the smallest thing you could image?"* Whatever the child answers, the therapist says, *"That tells me that your worry doesn't bother you at all if it's as small as* ________ (repeat child's answer). *That's how we will both know how much something bothers you."*
17. When I (R.T.) do this process because I'm already working with a map Metaphor, sometimes I will ask the child to show me how big the worry is on the map or globe. I will say things like *"Is it as big as Arizona or bigger?"* (We live in Arizona.) If it's bigger than

Arizona, I say, *"Maybe it's as big as the whole United States or bigger?"* If it's bigger than the whole United States, we continue with "as big as the whole world, the whole universe or infinity and beyond." Be creative and help the child feel validated in how big the worry is for them.

18. After completing the SUD, review the SUD compared to the ranking. The therapist notes if the SUD and ranking do not match as a way to assure that the child is understanding the concept of assessing how distressful the target is for them.
19. After completing SUD, the therapist also uses the map as a way to explain how worries or memories get connected in our brains. *"In our brains sometimes memories or worries get connected. Like you told me that when you think about your dad you are sad and when you think about your dog dying you get sad. On your map let's show how strong you think the connection is between the worries."* The therapist demonstrates to the child how to draw lines between the worries and then can make the line very thick or thin depending on how big the child thinks the connection is between the two targets. This serves to help the child understand how his or her brain works and why when feeling sad the child thinks of their dad and their dog. In addition to being educational for the child, we are also creating links that will ideally assist in linking the two memories when we proceed with desensitization.
20. After the SUD, ask the child to help the therapist understand what the bad thought is that goes with the memory. *"When you think about that worry, what's the bad thought that goes with that worry?"* If necessary I offer suggestions or use the "Kids List of Cognitions." Then ask the child what he would like to think instead or "What's the good thought?"
21. After identifying NC and PC, assess for a VoC. The therapist can use the example of the VoC bridge by saying, *"If we put your bad thought here* (put bad thought on the left side of the paper) *and your good thought here* (write the good thought on the right side of the paper) *and we make a bridge with seven steps from your bad thought to your good thought* (therapist draws seven steps on an imaginary bridge between the bad thought and the good thought), *where do you think you are right now?"*
22. After the VoC, ask the child to tell the therapist what the feeling is that goes with the target. Sometimes the therapist may need to offer feeling words to the child. *"When you think of that thing that bothers you and the bad thought, what feelings do you have about that?"*

23. Once we've identified feelings for the particular memory, look for links between targets for the child. Explain to the child that sometimes things bother us more than we expect because the feeling is connected to something else that bothered us before. For example, if Johnny has identified anger as a feeling associated with one of his targets, ask Johnny to identify other targets where he also might have felt angry and ask if he thinks those are connected to each other. Finally, this may also assist in identifying other feeder memories that are associated with feeling sad, mad, or other feelings.
24. After identifying the feeling, ask the child where he feels that feeling in his body. Sometimes the child can point and tell you where he feels the worry, while other times we need to take a break and teach mindfulness. "*When you think about that thing that bothers you and the ________ feeling, where do you feel that in your body? Some people feel it in their heads, some people feel it in their hearts, some people feel it in their tummies, and some people feel it in their legs and feet.*" (The therapist can point to different parts of their body to demonstrate where the child might feel the disturbance.)
25. Once the child has identified the body sensation, the therapist can then explain, "*This map helps to tell us what we need to work on to help you with* ______ (repeat child's concerns, symptoms or behavioral problems). *Each time we work together we will chose something on your map to work on until we can cross all of these off of your map. Do you have any questions? Let's pick the first thing we want to work on today or next week*" depending on the amount of time remaining in the session.

Each session the therapist can check in with the child to ask if any changes have occurred that would suggest something should be added or removed from the map.

Graphing EMDR Mastery Experiences, Targets, and Symptoms

Graphing is a multifaceted technique for elucidating various steps in the EMDR protocol. Graphing involves the therapist teaching the child to use a simple bar graph for identifying and assessing mastery experiences, targets, or symptoms; or evaluating progress in treatment; and/or as a container. The purpose for graphing is to help the child develop the observer self and to have a concrete technique for understanding and documenting the pieces of the EMDR treatment protocol.

Graphing for mastery experiences is used for the purpose of identifying resources, activities, abilities, and experiences that have created a positive experience for the child. For example, Riley feels good about how far he hit the ball in his baseball game. Riley would then note hitting the baseball as a mastery experience on his graph. The use of identifying and graphing mastery experiences provides the child with positive associations to the EMDR process, as well as developing a positive internal scaffolding in preparation for the Desensitization Phase.

For target and symptom identification, graphing helps the child create a list of his problems, worries, or "bothers" through drawing them in a concrete, visual manner. The purpose of graphing targets assists both the therapist and the child in selecting which targets should be reprocessed first.

As an evaluation tool, graphing can be used at the end of the session or for reevaluation in the following session. After the child has identified either resources or targets, the child and therapist can measure the strength of the resource or the level of competency over the target and then reevaluate progress. Graphing is not used as a SUD scale.

Graphing can also be used as a container during or at the end of the session if the child is flooded by disturbing emotions. The therapist can instruct the child to have worries or bothers stay on the paper like a container.

The therapist can have the child make different graphs for each type of graphing technique, or some of the graphs can be combined. Graphing is a fluid and ongoing part of the treatment protocol in EMDR.

See Figure 5.4 for a sample child's graph.

Instructions and Script for Graphing

1. First I (C.S.) explore whether the child understands the concept of a graph. Often children as young as 6 years old have already learned about simple bar graphs in school. Many times, even a 4 year old can draw a rudimentary graph with a therapist's help. If the child has not heard of a graph, educate him or her to the idea by saying something like, *"I'm going to show you how to draw a graph. A graph is a way to measure things. Today we are going to measure things that you feel good about and things that you think are problems or worries or bothers."*
2. The therapist demonstrates what a graph is by drawing a large *L* with a crayon on a piece of drawing paper. The therapist divides the vertical line with 10 small, evenly spaced lines to indicate

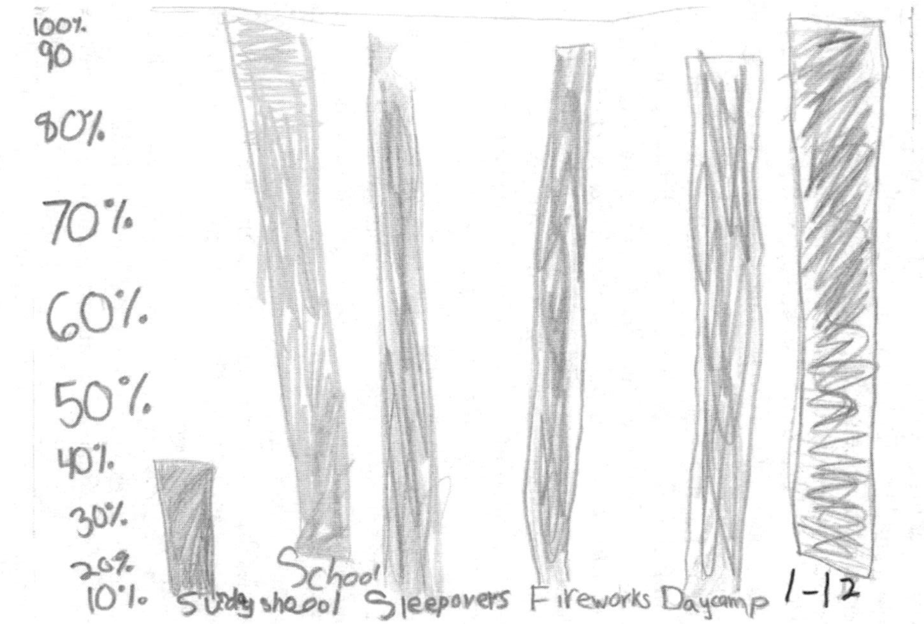

FIGURE 5.4 Polly was 9 years old when she listed her worries on the bottom of the graph. She worried about not being picked up by her parents after Sunday school, her mother forgetting to pick her up at the school bus, sleepovers, fireworks, day camp, and the scariest time of the day for her, between 1:00 P.M. and midnight. She originally drew each line to show how bad she felt about each worry. The goal was to feel better about the worry at 100%. Reaching 100% meant she no longer felt bad about that target.

percentages. At the bottom of the vertical line the therapist puts a 0 and in increments of 10, at each line, writes 10%, 20%, and so on, with the top of the line showing 100%. "*This line is how we can measure things with numbers where 0 is we don't feel good about them at all and 100 is where we feel really good about something.*"

3. On the bottom horizontal line the therapist can write or draw examples of either mastery experiences/activities or problems and worries that a child might identify for the graph.
4. For mastery the therapist says, "*We are going to make a list of the things that you feel good about on the bottom so we can measure them. Can you tell me something you feel really good about?*" The Mastery (or Good Things) Graph can be used in every session. To make a Mastery Graph you ask the child to tell you something that they feel like they do well, or something that makes them feel good about themselves, and list those items at the bottom of the horizontal line in one- or two-word descriptions. "*Can you tell me something else that makes you feel good?*" After collecting mastery experiences, the therapist then asks the child to draw and color in a line vertically that goes up to or as close to 100% as possible. "*Can you draw a line that shows how good you feel about that thing? Ten percent is you feel a little bit good and 50% is you feel pretty good, and 100% is you feel the best about that thing.*" The 100% represents how good they feel about the experience or activity. For instance, if Phoebe feels good about her drawing and art, we draw a line from the bottom of the horizontal line all the way up to 100%, meaning she feels as good as she can about her drawing. Then we identify several other activities that she feels positive about and she draws the line somewhere from 0% to 100%, demonstrating how good Phoebe feels about those positive experiences.
5. Then we install the mastery experience by having the child choose one of these positive experiences and enhance the good feelings in his or her body with bilateral stimulation, similar to the abbreviated RDI protocol. The therapist says to the child, "*So I want you to think about how good that* (mastery experience) *feels in your body and hold on to the buzzies for a second.*" The therapist can use whatever type of BLS the child had chosen to install the mastery experience.
6. When completing a Targeting (or Worries and Problems) Graph, use a separate piece of paper and again have them make an L-shaped graph with percentages on the vertical axis, and list on the bottom the child's reported problems, worries, or bothers.

The child then draws a bar or line that represents how much better or more competent the child feels regarding that target, with 100% demonstrating that the problem is resolved and/or the child feels competent to handle the problem or issue. Zero means that the child feels unable to handle the problem at all. *"Now we're going to make a worries or problems graph and we're gonna put all your worries or things that bother you on the bottom and this is how we're going to measure how good you feel about that problem. When it gets to the top or 100% you know you can handle the problem. It's kind of like a report card where we know you can handle that thing and it doesn't bother you or worry you any more."*

7. The therapist can then refer back to targets on the graph at the end of a session, to assess the target. *"OK, so we've worked on this problem, and where do you feel you are with handling that problem now?"* The child can draw the bar upward toward 100%, showing how much better he or she feels regarding the target. Often when one target is resolved, the child will spontaneously report that other targets are resolved. The child can then draw lines on the graph representing how much better he feels about each target.
8. The graph is also very useful to use in the next session to reevaluate the targets. The therapist says, *"Well, do you remember what we worked on last time? Let's take out our graph and look at it now. So with that problem we worked on, where are you now?"* The child may have increased feelings of competency with handling the problem and the percentage goes up, or occasionally the child is more worried about the problem, so the therapist can give the child a black crayon or marker to show that his or her feelings of competency over the problem actually went down. Children often feel empowered by the process of graphing because they can see their progress.
9. The Targeting Graph can also be used as a container at the end of sessions to assist the child in not having strong emotions or acting out behaviors between sessions. The therapist can simply say, *"This is your worry or bother graph and we're leaving them here on this paper in my office today. If for any reason these problems bother you when you go home, then you can imagine putting them back on the graph in my office and leaving them here."*

There are variations on graphing and we encourage you to use your own ideas to adapt the graph to your own client's needs after you have practiced the basic concept.

Additional Techniques for Target Identification of Children

Body Pictures. Children can be assisted in identifying targets that are associated with body sensations by drawing pictures of a person's body and marking on the picture where that person feels uncomfortable on the inside. It is also possible to have the child lay on a piece of butcher block paper and have the parent trace the child's body with a marker. We then have the child stand up and identify where he or she feels the distress, discomfort, or whatever word the child uses to describe feeling yucky. I (R.T.) have boxes of Band-Aids and have the child put Band-Aids on the picture where he or she feels hurt or feels the yucky feelings in his or her body. I explain to children that when we get hurt, sometimes we bleed, and sometimes we get bruises or black and blue marks, but sometimes we hurt and you cannot see it on the outside. I ask children to identify any place that they feel hurt that cannot be seen on the outside. We then use the drawings as targets or as potential floatbacks to memories when the child first felt that way.

Target Container. There can be confusion between a target container and a containment exercise. For the purposes of this book, a target container is used for target identification. We recommend that therapists not teach containers as a containment exercise during this phase of treatment. Instead, we suggest that the therapist only introduce a containment exercise if the child is overwhelmed by the target identification process or needs a container exercise as a tool for closing an incomplete session.

A target container is used during target identification as a technique for exploring targets with children. A child is asked to choose or make a container in therapy that can be used to hold targets in for later reprocessing. One example is using small stones as worry rocks, on which a child labels a specific target or worry. I (R.T.) use small glass decorative stones that I have in a basket. Children choose as many stones as they need on which to label worries. I use small stickers for the child to write a word or a picture to label the worry rock. The child then places the sticker on the worry rock, and worry rocks are then deposited in the child's container. Children leave the target container in the office and can make deposits into the container any time that a new target or worry arises. Some children come in each week and make deposits to the container. In therapy, we can then make withdrawals or pick a worry rock to work on in the session.

While conducting a formal target identification process, do not try to contain other memories unless you are out of time—let whatever happens happen; let it go wherever it goes. As the child begins to make associative links during target identification, the therapist needs to just note the child's responses for later processing. There is a progression that occurs where the therapist follows the client wherever those memory networks go, including the possibility that new substantial targets will arise that were not previously identified. At the end of the session, contain only what continues to be disturbing. The use of containers as a containment exercise for incomplete sessions will be discussed in chapter 6.

The next step in the protocol is to identify an image that represents the worst part of the image related to the specific target.

Selecting the Image/Picture. Starting with the list of traumatic experiences and targets established during client history and treatment planning and further expanded or clarified during this target identification step, the therapist decides, in collaboration with the child and parent, what to target first. When choosing a target to reprocess, the therapist should select the target most associated with the current active symptoms the child is experiencing. After the therapist and child select the target, the therapist asks the child to identify the picture or image that represents the worst part of the memory. We have included specific wording for the therapist to use with a child client.

Script to Elicit the Image or Picture. The therapist inquires about the most disturbing image or picture: "*When you think about what happened, what do you see? What's the worst/yuckiest part of the picture?*" If there is no picture, ask, "*When you think about that thing, what happens now?*"

If the child cannot verbally identify an image, there are other techniques that can assist the therapist and client in identifying the image for reprocessing.

Techniques for Setting Up the Image With Children. There are many techniques that assist children in communicating the image of the target. This is an excellent place to integrate play therapy techniques. Children can communicate through artwork, including drawings and collages, digital pictures, and through play in the sand tray or with puppets, toys, or a dollhouse.

Drawing. This is the simplest manner for eliciting a target image from children. Give the child choices of paper and drawing tools. Provide paper and crayons, markers, or colored pencils of various colors from which the child can choose to draw the picture. Once the child has selected the art tools, then repeat the script, "*When you think about what happened, what do you see?*" and have the child draw the picture. Once the child has completed the picture, continue with distilling an NC and PC.

I (C.S.) use Post-It notes and have children draw on them in between sets of BLS if they have difficulty communicating verbally. They draw on the Post-Its in between the BLS and then stick them on the wall in sequence of their processing, somewhat like being on a train. I do not have them revisit the previous pictures they have drawn, but this helps to titrate the information as the children move through reprocessing. This is especially helpful for children who obsess about their drawing because they have a smaller area to draw on, and I can take the Post-It note and have the children move to the next drawing to help the children focus and stay on the train.

With other children, I (C.S.) might take a large piece of paper, draw a line down the middle, and, on the left side, have the child draw the worst part of the image and have the child write the bad thought. If the child is unable to write, I write what the child says. Then I ask the child what the child is feeling and write that on the same side, and I also rate and write the SUD on that side of the picture. On the right side of the paper, I have the child draw what the child would like to believe—the good picture with the good thought and the VoC rating of how true it feels. Right before the start of BLS, I have the child look at the bad picture as a starting place and turn the picture over as the child is processing. When I think the child has reached the end of a channel, I have the child draw a new picture and ask him or her what the child gets now. If the picture is neutral or positive, I take a SUD. That is when I know the target has been reprocessed, and we check the VoC on the good picture. For an example of this drawing technique, see Figure 5.5.

Collaging. With various magazines (often old magazines from my waiting room), I (R.T.) ask the child to cut out a picture that represents the worst part of the target memory. Once the child has cut out the picture, we can either paste the picture on another piece of blank paper or just use the picture from the magazine. It is important to provide the child with various appropriate magazines to cut out pictures from for making collages.

Digital Pictures. Our colleague, Dr. Kim Johnson, has used digital pictures to assist the child in connecting with the image of the event. Dr. Johnson takes pictures of specific things that seem to be triggering for children and then let the child determine if there was a picture that represented the worst part of the image.

Case Study: Elijah and the Dumpster

Four-year-old Elijah was referred by Child Protective Services and his foster parents for treatment of trauma associated with a significant abuse history. One of Elijah's current symptoms was his terror of garbage dumpsters. Whenever Elijah saw a

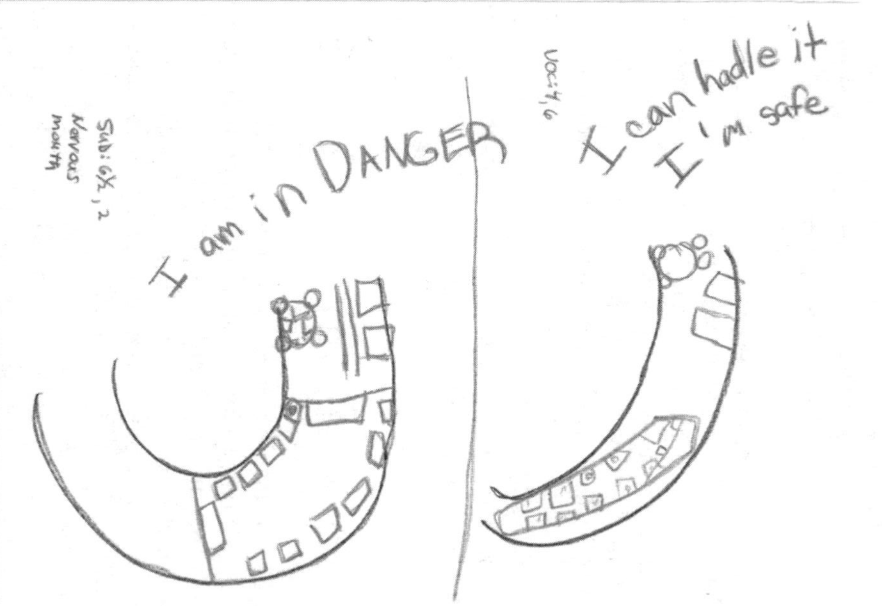

FIGURE 5.5 Polly's picture depicting her worry that her mother will not pick her up at the bus stop. The left side of Polly's picture shows her in the school bus parked on the street and her mother's car farther down the road. Polly is afraid and upset. Her negative cognition is, "I'm in danger." The right side of the picture shows the school bus is there; her mother's car is still not there, but Polly is feeling OK and handling it. Her positive cognition is, "I can handle it, I'm safe."

dumpster or his foster mother parked next to a dumpster, Elijah would have a meltdown; however, Elijah's verbal skills were significantly limited, and he was unable to draw what scared him. The therapist took pictures of several types of garbage dumpsters and had Elijah pick the digital picture that was the picture that bothered him the most. At the sight of one of the pictures, Elijah became extremely distressed. After targeting the picture, Elijah reported, "That bad man put me in the dumpster and I got all yucky." After this, Elijah no longer noticed garbage dumpsters, and his speech improved dramatically.

Play Techniques. This is an ideal place to incorporate play therapy techniques. The therapist can allow the child to create an image in the sand tray or in the playroom. Some children will choose toys from the playroom to reenact the image. Some children will set up the image in the dollhouse. Other children might set up the image with the puppets. Providing the child with various play tools from which to choose will allow the child to express the worst part of the image in a manner that is most expressive for the child.

Once the child has identified an image that represents the worst part of the incident, the therapist continues with the next step of the Assessment Phase.

NEGATIVE (NC) AND POSITIVE COGNITIONS (PC)

Training in EMDR explains that an NC is a presently held, irrational belief expressed as a self-referencing statement that is able to be generalized. Given that children may be in earlier stages of cognitive development, as discussed in chapter 1, NCs may look slightly different with children. For examples of possible negative and positive cognitions for children, see Table 5.1.

One of the most confusing things about identifying an NC for both the therapist and client alike is perspective. The NC is what the client believes as the client is sitting in your office looking back at the image. Clients of all ages will ask, "Do you mean what I thought about it then or what I'm thinking about it now?" The therapist needs to take the time to help the client understand that the NC is what the client believes as he or she is sitting in your office now, looking back on that experience that was identified as the image. This may take some time to process, but it is important not to skip over this part of the EMDR protocol. With children, this process may be different because children are so present-oriented, yet it is important to retain the essence of

TABLE 5.1 Kids' List of Cognitions

Bad Thoughts (NC)	Good Thoughts (PC)
I'm bad	I'm good
I'm in a fog	I'm in a clear place/I'm in sunshine
I'm going to blow	I'm calm
I'm going to explode	I'm calm
I'm hot	I'm cool (as a cucumber)
I don't belong	I do belong
I am stupid	I'm smart
I am dumb	I'm smart
I'm sick	I'm all better
I can't do it	I can do it
I'm hurt	I'm better
I don't understand	I do understand
I can't get help	I can get help
I messed up	I did the best I could
I don't know nothing	I do know
I'm dying	I'm alive
I'm hungry	I'm satisfied
I'm not lovable	I'm lovable
I'm fat	I'm just right
I'm lost	I found my way
I almost drowned and I got very scared and that made me hold my breath.	I tell myself, you should be glad you could hold your breath that long.
I couldn't come out from under the water.	I'm glad I can swim.
I didn't get to go the hospital with dad.	I get to go to the hospital with dad.
I'm not comfortable	I am comfortable
I am uncomfortable in my skin	I fit in my skin
Basic/Common Cognitions:	
I'm not safe	I'm safe now
I can't protect myself	I can protect myself
I don't have control	I do have control
I can't trust	I can trust

Therapists can choose to organize NCs and PCs into categories of Safety, Responsibility, and Choice; however often times kids cognitions are so concrete that it is difficult to determine the specific category in which the NC or PC falls. (See also Appendix IX.)

this part of the protocol as the therapist makes adjustments for child development.

It is very important that the NC and PC match. Typically, they are polar opposites. If the NC and PC are different, the therapist needs to take the time to find NCs and PCs that match. For example, if the NC is "I'm not good enough" and the PC is "I'm safe now," the cognitions are significantly different, and the therapist needs to ask the client which resonates more for the specific image. If the PC resonates more, it is appropriate to then change the NC to match the PC.

Also, it is important to ensure that the NC makes sense with the specific target. For example, if the client's target is the memory of a rape and the client's NC is "I'm not good enough," the therapist may want to explore whether or not that NC truly fits for the client or if the client is confused about the EMDR process.

Identifying NCs and PCs With Children

Identifying NCs and PCs is a critical part of the protocol for EMDR, and some therapists often find this step to be especially difficult with young children because of the child's level of cognitive development. Therapists may consider omitting this critical step in the EMDR process because the therapist is struggling to elicit cognitions from the child; however, this section will provide clinical tools and case examples to assist therapists in identifying cognitions with young children.

If the therapist simply asks the child, "When you think about the thing that happened to you [the target], what's the bad thought about you now?" the therapist can then continue by asking, "What is the good thought about you now?"

Children can present NCs in many different ways. Children can present their cognitions in concrete statements like "I want my hand back."

Case Study: Michelle and Reddy

I (C.S.) first saw Michelle when she was 3 years old. This was 3 months after she had lost her hand in an accident. The father, who is a minister, wanted her to try EMDR so that the incident did not affect her later years. I first did EMDR on the father and mother. I later did EMDR on the older sisters who were present when the accident happened. Because Michelle had a speech impediment, I kept the mother in the session to help me understand Michelle. She was a very active child, so I used the NeuroTek buzzies in her shoes. First I had her draw the incident of losing her hand, which turned out to be a black scribble. I asked her the bad thought, and it was "I want my hand back." Now, *this is a trauma-specific NC, but I thought this represented her helplessness. Her PC was "This is the way God supposed to make me," which I believed represented acceptance since she came from a religious family. Her feeling was sad, and she used her hands to show she was sad at a SUD of 10. In between each repetition, she scribbled more, and with each successive picture, she had more and more color, until it had rainbow colors. I had a hand-drawn VoC scale that was similar to the Humanitarian Assistance Programs (HAP) scale. She started drawing a frowning picture and continued drawing faces in between until there was a smile. We did EMDR for 15 minutes and then played. She said she felt "way good," with outstretched arms: "This is the way God supposed to make me" (see Figure 5.6).*

Her urinating outside of the toilet, tantrums, and nightmares stopped. She was able to sleep through the night again. We did two more sessions that covered upsetting parts of the memories. Michelle reprocessed quickly and was happy at the end of each session. She named her stump Reddy and began adapting. I did not see her again for a year, after she had been retraumatized by a new girl in the choir who saw her stump and started screaming. We targeted that in EMDR, and again, she quickly improved.

For some children, the cognition may be described in a fantasy such as "I'm a witch" or "I'm a princess." This can convey the child's experience and feelings of self-esteem. If the child says "I'm a witch," the therapist can choose to probe further by asking the child, "If you believe 'I'm a witch,' what does that say about you?" Younger children especially will tend to identify the NC as a monster or dragon or vampire or some disturbing creation from current children's literature: "I'm Draco" or "I'm Harry"—an example of a child who uses the Harry Potter books as a means to describe experiences and feelings.

A child may demonstrate the NC in pictures and/or play activities. For example, the therapist can ask the child to split the sand tray in half and create the bad thought on one side and the good through on the other side, with a bridge between the two sides of the sand tray. The bridge then leads to a Metaphor for identifying the VoC, which will be discussed in the next section.

Children will label a cognition as a feeling because the NCs and PCs may be single emotional words like *sad* versus *glad.* If the child has verbalized an emotion, that can be considered a cognition because

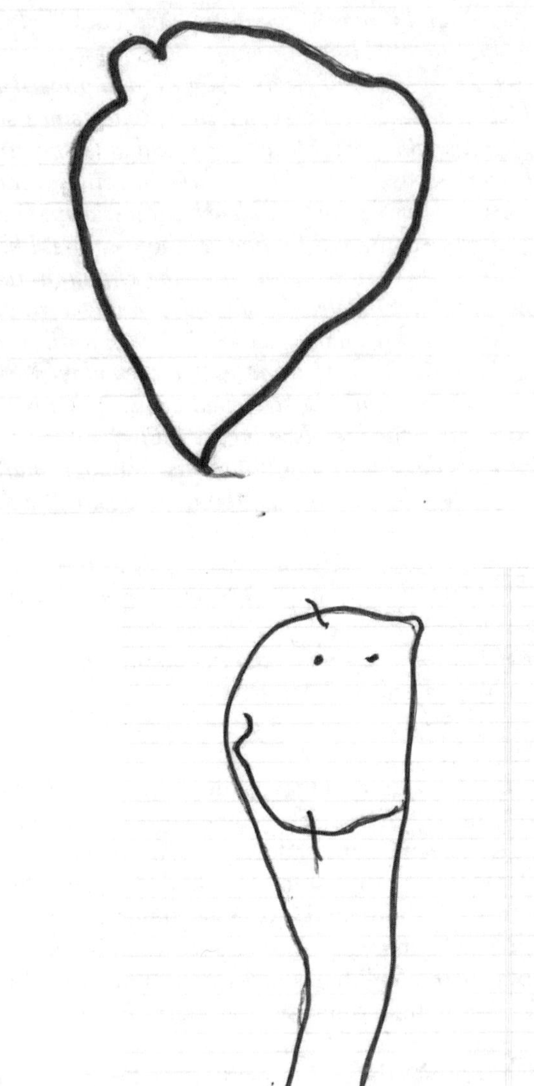

FIGURE 5.6 A series of pictures that 3-year-old Michelle drew based on her negative cognition "I want my hand back." As you can see, each successive picture adds a detail, from just a circle to a face to appendages, and the final picture shows Michelle with her whole arm and her stump with a big smile. Her positive cognition was "God supposed to make me this way," which is her expression of acceptance.

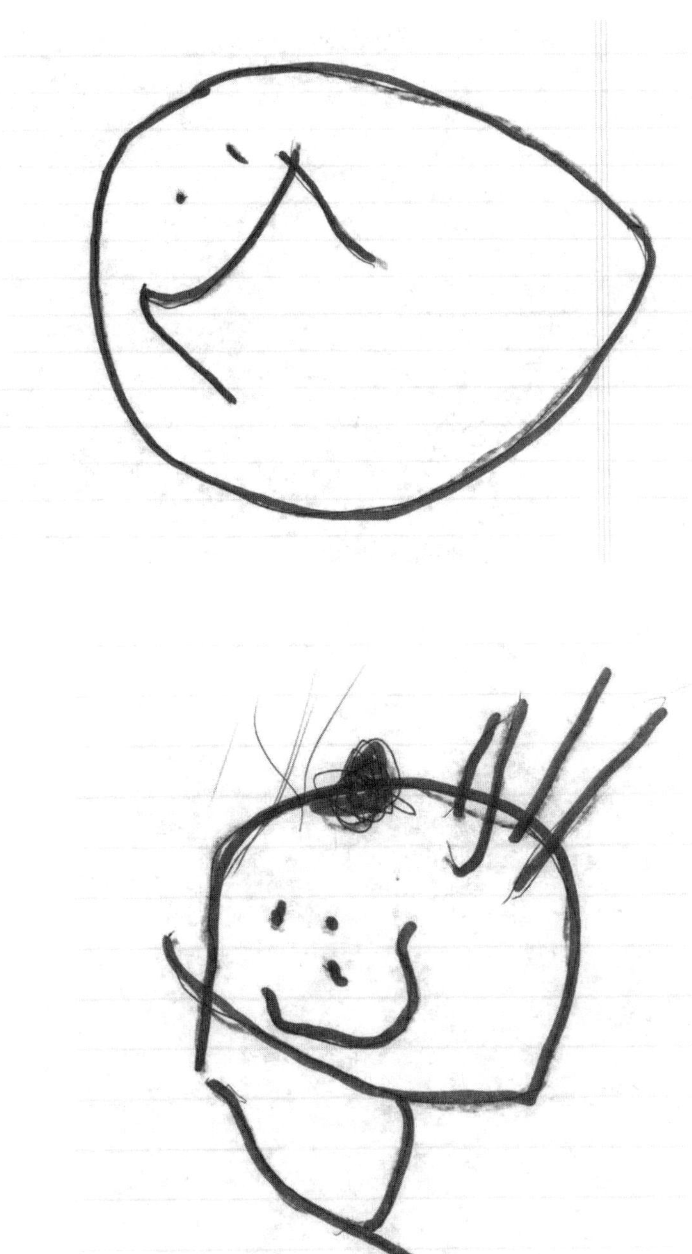

FIGURE 5.6 (continued)

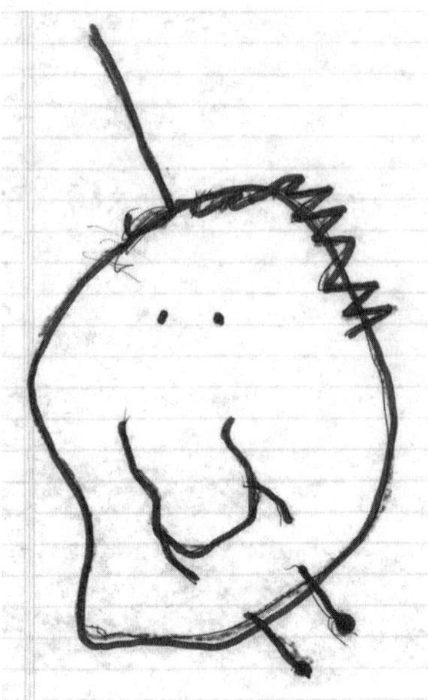

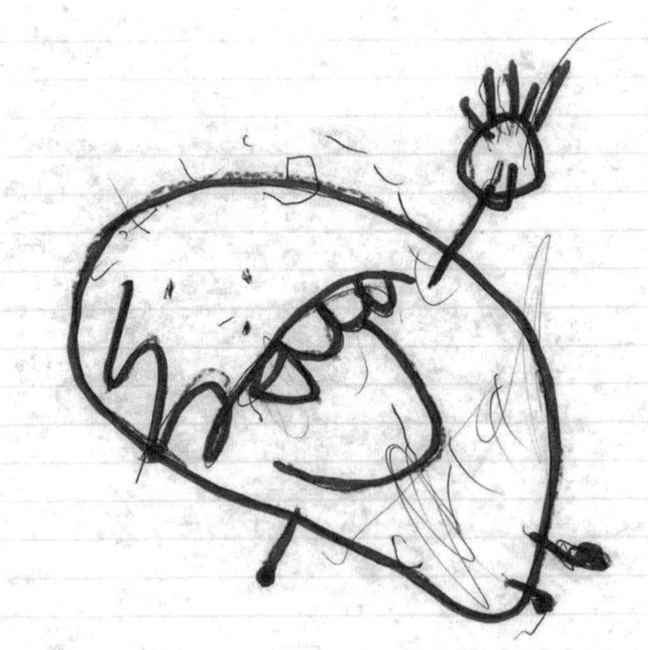

FIGURE 5.6 A series of pictures that 3-year-old Michelle drew (continued)

developmentally, the ability to verbalize a feeling indicates the child has moved beyond just experiencing the feeling into a cognitive process of verbalizing the feeling.

Children often express an NC in the third person to protect themselves from the full impact of the cognition. In addition, younger children tend to use speech that is telegraphic such as "David hurt," with a PC of "David feel better." The therapist can assist the child by eliciting NCs and PCs utilizing knowledge of the child's current live stressors. For instance, if we know that Katie has to go to the doctor, the therapist might say, "doctor scary" and then suggest that "doctor fix Katie's owie."

In addition, children may provide very concrete NCs and PCs, like "Jeff bad" versus "Jeff good." These concrete cognitions are often related to the child's current level of cognitive development and language acquisition level. While some children present NCs and PCs in very concrete terms, other children may utilize fantasy to express their thoughts about themselves. For instance, 6-year-old Mollie may say, "I'm a witch" versus "I'm a princess." The child's current media exposure can contribute to the child's expressions related to what he or she thinks about himself or herself.

Children also tend to be more trauma-specific when identifying their NCs and PCs such as "I was scared of the dog" versus "The dog can't get me anymore." For Melissa, being scared of the dog is related to having been unable to protect herself, while she may also be feeling unsafe in the environment in which she currently lives.

Children who struggle with verbalizing NCs and PCs may often find greater ability to express themselves through drawings, sand tray, or other expressive techniques. For instance, asking the child to create his or her worst world in one area of the sand tray, while creating his or her best world on the other side, may lead to identifying cognitions. This is true for drawing, creating with clay, and other expressive opportunities that provide greater opportunity for expression than verbal expression alone.

Ultimately, it is important to take the time to elicit NCs and PCs from children to be most effective with EMDR. As with adults, the NCs and PCs should resonate for the child. Children will oftentimes make eye contact, give verbal feedback, or change direction in their play behavior when the NC or PC fits. When the most appropriate NC and PC are identified for the child, the next phases of EMDR tends to be more valuable.

Sometimes children cannot come up with an NC but have a PC, so the therapist can work backward by getting the positive thought first, and then the therapist can ask the child for the NC. See Figure 5.7.

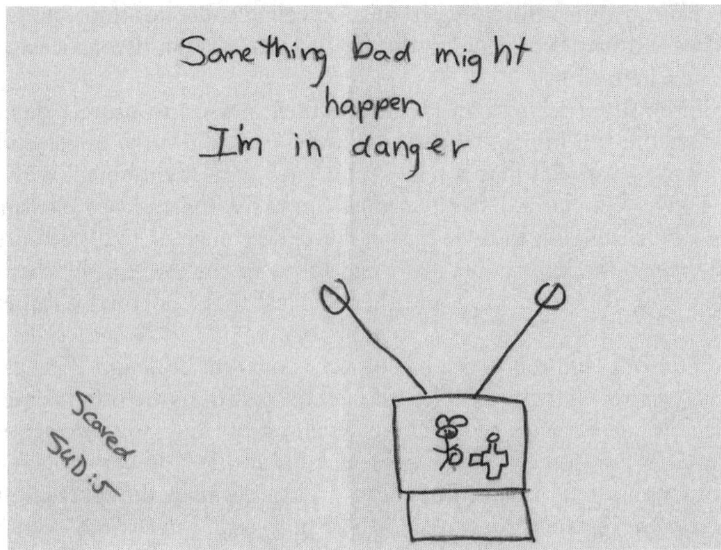

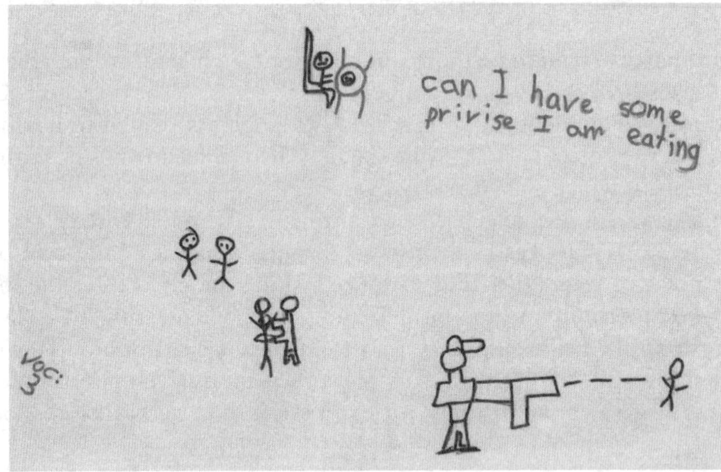

FIGURE 5.7 Jeremiah's negative and positive cognitions. If you remember Jeremiah's story about his fear of the news, his negative cognition was "Something bad might happen, I'm in danger." This picture shows the television with a robber shooting someone, which demonstrates his negative cognition. His positive cognition is drawn on the page showing him eating chicken at a table; the news is on, and somebody is shooting someone, and other people are just walking by holding hands. His positive cognition was "Can I have some privacy? I'm eating my chicken," which exemplifies his positive cognition, "Good things happen, bad things happen, but I'm OK."

Cognitive Themes: Responsibility/Safety/Choices

NCs are theoretically organized around three primary themes: responsibility, safety, and choices. People in general, when they have trauma, seem to typically assume a sense of responsibility for the traumatic event. This is especially true with children, who are developmentally egocentric.

Responsibility. When working with children, it is important to process NCs and beliefs that are associated with misattributions of responsibility, for example, a child exposed to domestic violence who says, "It's my fault. My mommy and daddy were fighting because I didn't get good grades in school." This child is assuming responsibility for events to feel powerful. In other words, "If I get good grades, my mommy and daddy won't fight anymore." By targeting the client's misattributions of responsibility, the therapist can assist the child in moving toward appropriate attributions of responsibility. Once the child is appropriately attributing responsibility, the child can then release the self-blame and internal critique. This allows the child to feel angry and turn the emotion toward the appropriate target, rather than internalizing the anger.

Case Study: The Twins

I (R.T.) worked with 8-year-old identical twin girls who had been molested by a nanny. Even though the twins had always been together when they were molested, the girls had completely different reactions to the abuse. One of the girls, Taylre, struggled with feeling responsible for the abuse. The nanny had told the girls to take down their pants, and the unsuspecting children had complied, and then the nanny told them to pull up their pants, but before the girls could pull up their pants, the nanny touched them inappropriately. Taylre reported that the nanny told her that it was Taylre's fault she was abused because she did not pull up her pants fast enough. Taylre had to work on reprocessing the responsibility that Taylre felt because the nanny had convinced Taylre it was her fault and that if Taylre told anyone about the abuse, Taylre would be arrested.

It is important to ask sexually abused children about what the perpetrator said as perpetrators often groom children to believe it is the child's responsibility. This is often a target that goes missed and must be reprocessed to help the child with misattributions of responsibility.

Safety. Once the child has come to the appropriate attribution of responsibility, this allows the child to feel safer on several levels. First, it is safer for the child to experience his or her own intense emotions and in the present, and it allows the child to explore issues related to current safety. Examples of NCs and PCs related to themes of safety include the following: I'm not safe now/I'm as safe as I can be now and I'm in danger/I'm no longer in danger. If you consider Jeremiah's case, the last missing piece of his reprocessing was his realization that it was not his fault. And when he got clear on the appropriate attribution of responsibility, he felt safe and quit checking the locks at night.

Choices/New Choices. The issue of choices for children revolves around issues of power and helplessness because many times, children do not have choices, and especially not the same choices as adults.

In overall case conceptualization, misattribution of responsibility tends to be a past orientation, while safety is a more present orientation, with choices/new choices being a current and future orientation. This is a gross overgeneralization, but in case conceptualization with NCs with an overlay of past/present/future targets, it is important to consider the interplay between the two concepts.

NCs and PCs and Cognitive Interweaves

The relationship between NCs and PCs and cognitive interweaves is that the cognitions offer insight into possible cognitive interweaves to be used during reprocessing. It is important for the therapist to be considering what cognitive interweaves the client might need, if stuck processing occurs during desensitization. We will discuss cognitive interweaves in greater detail in chapter 10.

We have suggested a Kids' List of Cognitions in Table 5.1. After trying to elicit NCs and PCs directly from the child, the therapist can offer suggestions or allow a child that can read to look at the table.

Assessing the Validity of Cognition (VoC)

Once the therapist has identified a target and distilled the NC/PC, the therapist then assesses the validity of the cognition by asking the client to hold together the image and the PC and determine how valid the cognition currently feels. With adults, the therapist will ask the client, "When you bring up that incident and those words [repeat the PC], on a scale of 1 to 7, where 1 is completely false and 7 is completely true, how true do those words feel to you now?" The therapist then notes the client's response and continues. We suggest that the therapist first attempt the VoC by asking, and if the child struggles, then we have several additional techniques for eliciting a VoC from a child.

Procedural Considerations for Measurements in EMDR

To measure the VoC and subjective units of disturbance, the therapist can attempt to use the same instructions as with adults, but some children may struggle with the explanation because the explanation of how the VoC is assessed is lengthy and abstract. If the child struggles to comprehend the adult explanation for the VoC, the therapist can refer to the image that the child created and repeat the PC and ask the child, "How true does it feel right now?" It is important for the therapist to demonstrate a measurement tool that the child can understand, without confusing the child about the differences between the VoC and the SUD. Because the VoC measures how true the PC feels and the SUD measures how disturbing the incident feels, sometimes children get confused because the stronger feeling of the VoC is positive, while the stronger feeling from the SUD is negative.

Measuring the VoC

The therapist can use any of the following child-friendly measurement tools for establishing the VoC.

How True? The therapist can demonstrate the measurement of the VoC by showing the distance between the therapist's hands. The therapist can move his or her hands apart and ask, "Is this true? This true? This true?" The child will either mimic the therapist or tell the therapist where to stop his or her hands.

VoC Bridge. The VoC bridge is a very simple way to measure the VoC with even very young children. I (R.T.) have the child identify the bad thought (NC) and the good thought (PC) either on sheets of paper or the whiteboard. I then create a bridge from the bad thought to the good thought, with seven steps on the bridge. This can be done by drawing the bridge on a piece of paper, or I have whiteboards that are magnetic and use one for the bad thought and one for the good thought, and then I put the whiteboards on either side of seven metal bars that I purchased at IKEA. I then have the child take a magnet to put on the bridge to demonstrate how he or she feels about the bad thought and the good thought. Most children will start with putting the magnet on the bad thought and then spontaneously move the magnet to the good thought during the installation phase of EMDR. See Figure 5.8 for an example of a VoC bridge.

HAP Sheet. The therapist can purchase a laminated sheet from EMDR HAP (http://www.emdrhap.org) that has cognitions on one side and faces on the other side, with measurements for the VoC and the SUD.

Movement. The therapist can have the child hold a symbol for the NC while the therapist holds a symbol of the PC, and the therapist moves

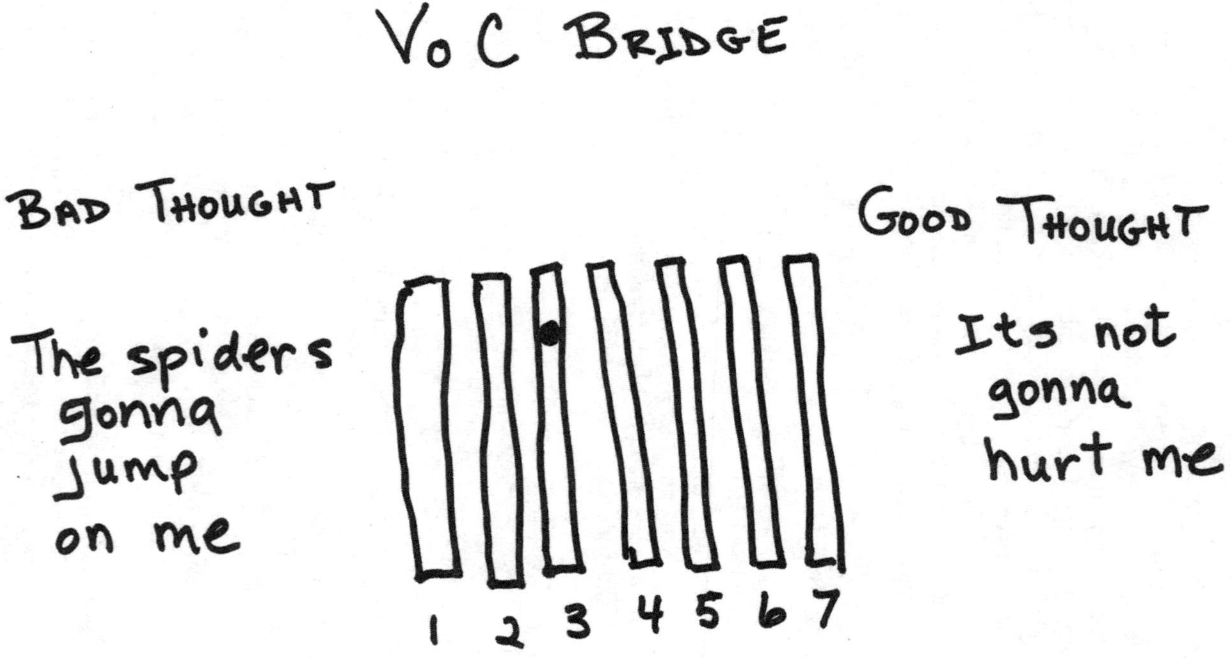

FIGURE 5.8 Validity of cognition bridge.

away from the child and asks, "From where you stand to me, how true does that feel now?"

Once the therapist has taken a measurement of how true the VoC feels, the therapist continues with the procedural steps by asking, "When you bring up what happened and those words [NC], what do you feel now?"

Identifying Emotions or Feelings and Body Sensations

Identifying feelings and body sensations are steps of the EMDR protocol that are often omitted by therapists because therapists struggle to teach children how to actively participate in this process. Teaching children emotional literacy (http://www.lionheart.org) and mindfulness are significant in successfully applying EMDR in therapy with children. The therapist's role can be of translator and teacher for feeling identification, mindfulness, and body sensations. One way of teaching kids emotional literacy is reviewing emotions on a feelings chart, with pictures starting with basic emotions like happy, sad, or mad. Another way therapists can teach emotional literacy is by having the child label expressions the therapist makes with his or her face and body or by having the child look in a mirror and practice the different expressions. This also helps the therapist to become attuned to the child as the child explains how he or she feels when making a certain expression. Teaching emotional literacy can be done throughout the EMDR process as children learn about feelings and how feelings affect their lives. For more information on emotional literacy, there is an online course available from http://emotionalliteracyeducation.com/index.shtml. There is also valuable information on emotional literacy provided by Steiner (2002).

Children may have difficulty understanding the difference between feelings and body sensations. This is especially true with children who are more dissociative. If a child reports that he or she does not feel anything or does not notice anything, it is important to explore the degree of dissociation. We discussed assessing for dissociation in chapter 3 and explore using EMDR with children who are dissociative in chapter 11. Once the emotion has been identified, the therapist then asks the child to remember the incident and the NC and then establish the amount of the disturbance the child is experiencing. This is how the SUD is determined. Our experience is that establishing the SUD is a fairly simple process, even for children.

Measuring the Subjective Units of Disturbance

Measuring the SUD can be a very simple process, especially with children. We have included several ways therapists can teach children to evaluate the level of disturbance they are experiencing.

How Much Does It Bother You? It is important to be attuned to the child's language and choose a question to establish the SUD that is consistent with the child's language. For example, if the child frequently talks about things that bother him or her, then the therapist should ask the child to tell how much it bothers him or her now. Or if the child uses the word *yucky,* ask the child, "*How yucky does it feel to you now?*"

Evaluating the subjective units of disturbance with children needs to be as simple as possible in order that the therapist stays focused on the procedural steps.

Identifying Body Sensations. The child may have previously described a body sensation, and the therapist needs to check if the body sensation remained the same or ask where the child notices he or she feels the disturbance in his or her body now.

We have noticed that children as well as adults, when asked where they feel something, will report feeling the emotion in their head. If the child identifies the feeling in his or her head, the therapist may need to teach mindfulness in order that the child learns to notice and associate body sensations with feelings and memories.

Children may need instruction on body sensations that can be taught by the therapist demonstrating that "sometimes people feel weak in the knees or feel butterflies in their tummies or feel heartbroken," while the therapist points at the associated body part. In teaching mindfulness, the therapist may say to a child that "butterflies in your tummy can sometimes mean that people feel nervous." Or a therapist can explain that an expression like *heartbroken* is where the child's heart is broken because of being hurt. Another example is the saying "I'm weak in the knees," which is what people might say when they are scared or excited or anxious. The purpose of this intervention is that the therapist is linking up body sensations with possible associated emotions to teach the child emotional literacy.

Therapists can use pictures from books or magazines, posters that contain facial expressions that suggest emotion, drawings, or activities that teach children about body sensations.

The purpose is for the therapist to become attuned to the individual client and learn how the client processes in his or her body. We have worked with children who only express feelings in their legs or in their stomachs, but have no images or memories. This happens quite often with children, and we just have the child notice what happens with the feeling. It is also possible to have the child float back to an earlier time, when he or she first noticed that feeling in his or her leg or stomach or hands.

Procedural Considerations for Body Sensations

Clients who experience a great deal of anxiety often live in their head and do not notice emotions in their body sensations. Children will say, "I feel it in my head." That is often an indicator that this is an anxious child who probably struggles with anxiety and is out of touch with his or her own body. It is helpful to explore other possible body sensations with the child to teach the child mindfulness and to check to make sure the child is reprocessing in his or her body. In our experience, anxious children report feelings in their head, and again, we can do a floatback or just have the child notice the feeling in his or her head and see what happens. These children will also be more likely to experience anticipatory anxiety, which can be addressed with a future template.

Body language is how others might interpret how we are holding our body. So the therapist can explain to the child that when the child crosses his or her arms across the chest, the therapist will notice and wonder about how the child is feeling when the child does that. We often will use this opportunity for the therapist to teach the child about how others may interpret nonverbal behaviors as a means of communication. We use body language as a way to teach children to again be mindful of their body and how their reactions and emotions are expressed both verbally and nonverbally during therapy. This further explores the body scan to children as the therapist may initially have to teach the child to make the links between nonverbal expression and emotions.

After completing the setup for the Assessment Phase of EMDR by identifying the image, NC/PC, VoC, emotion, SUD, and body sensations, the therapist proceeds immediately to the desensitization process, which is detailed in chapter 6.

SUMMARY

This chapter has described the procedural steps of the Assessment Phase of EMDR, with particular focus on eliciting the pieces of the protocol with young children. To further explicate this process, we have included the following script for the Assessment Phase of EMDR with children.

PROCEDURAL STEPS OF THE ASSESSMENT PHASE

The procedural steps of the Assessment Phase are included in one connected script for ease of use during a session with the child.

Review stop signal: *"If at any time you feel you want to stop, remember that you told me that you would do* ______________ (stop signal previously identified)*."*

Review and check Safe/Calm Place and resource images: Briefly review the Safe/Calm Place and resource images established in earlier sessions. *"Remember that safe place that we talked about before?"* The therapist names the Safe/Calm Place and offers descriptive cues. *"We can use that safe place when we are talking about what you remember, if you need to. I also want to make sure you remember what you told me about* __________*."* The therapist describes the resource images and associated feelings, qualities, or capacities if needed. Optional: *"Do any of these* ______________ (resources) *feel like they could really help us right now? Do you think there are any people, pets, or objects that you would want sitting with you who could help you feel better when we talk about that thing that happened?"*

Target identification: *"We have talked about things that worry or bother you before and, remember, we picked this one from your map, so how about we start with that one today?"*

Picture: Image: *"What's the worst/yuckiest part of the picture?"* If no picture: *"When you think about that thing, what happens now?"*

Cognitions: Negative cognitions: *"When you think about that thing/picture, what words go with that?"* Or, you can say, *"What's the bad thought that goes with that,"* especially with younger children who may need education.

Positive cognition: *"When you think about that thing/picture, what words would you rather say to yourself instead?"* Or you can say, *"What's the good thought that you want to tell yourself instead?"*

Validity of Cognition (VoC): *"When you say those words*__________ (repeat PC), *how true do those words feel right now, from 1, that means it's not true at all, to 7, that means it's really true?"* The therapist can use distance between the hands or other types of measures to which the child relates that are developmentally appropriate to demonstrate the validity of the cognition.

Emotions/Feelings: *"When you bring up that picture* (or incident) *and words*____ (negative cognition), *what do you feel now?"* If the child needs further explanation, the therapist can use the feelings chart or some other type of educational tool to help the child identify emotion. Explore the emotion(s) that the child feels in the present.

SUD: *"From 0–10, where 0 is it doesn't bother you at all to 10 it bothers you a lot, how much does that thing bother you right now?"* Therapist can use distance between the hands or another type of measure to which the child relates.

Body sensation: "*Where do you feel it in your body?*" If the child is not initially able to answer, the therapist teaches the child mindfulness of body sensations by pointing to body parts as the therapist says, "*Sometimes people feel it in their head, or their tummy, or their feet. Where do you feel it in your body?*"

Instructions to the child before beginning desensitization: "*What we're going to do is we're going to do the* ____ (BLS) *on that thing* ____ (target) *and I'm gonna do it for awhile and then I'm gonna stop and tell you to blank it out and take a breath and then we'll talk a little about it. Sometimes things will change and sometimes they won't. There is no right or wrong answer. What you think or feel is exactly what I want to know and you can tell me anything.*"

CHAPTER 6

EMDR Phase 4: Desensitization

The Desensitization Phase of EMDR begins once the therapist has identified all the pieces of the procedural steps of the Assessment Phase and is ready to begin bilateral stimulation (BLS). The therapist instructs the child to hold the image together with the negative cognition and determines where the child feels it in his or her body, then explains to the client what to expect and begins BLS. This is the starting place for reprocessing the target.

In this chapter, we have attempted to capture the phenomenon called *reprocessing,* which is at the core of EMDR and subsequent healing from trauma. With Adaptive Information Processing (AIP) theory, the Desensitization Phase is where the work takes place for the client.

THE GOAL OF THE DESENSITIZATION PHASE

The goal is for the therapist to provide the initial instruction to the client to fully access the experience. Once this occurs, there is typically overt evidence that the client has linked to the maladaptively stored information that is driving current symptomatology. Clients may display affect or behaviors that indicate to the therapist that the target resonates for the client. Clients may demonstrate a wide range of indicators that the target resonates. Some clients may show strong emotions, while others may show some physical indicator of recognition that the target is accurate. The therapist just observes the client's breathing, activity level, pallor, affect, facial expression, and overall nonverbal presentation, in addition to what the client reports. It is our experience that there is obvious evidence that the target resonates for the client.

With children, evidence that the target resonates may be more subdued or understated but still evident. This is where the therapist's observation skills and attunement to the child are invaluable. As the therapist, it is important to ask yourself, "How will I know or how can I tell with this child?"

Procedural Considerations

Once the desensitization process is launched, the image usually changes and is rarely the same again. However, occasionally there is the client who becomes stuck, and the image does not change, which is an indicator of blocked processing. Blocked processing will be discussed later in this chapter.

As reprocessing occurs, some clients will report pieces of the original incident, while other clients will follow a stream of memories that are somehow linked for the client. Sometimes what the client reports will sound like a logical course or chronology of the event, while for other clients, the information flow will appear to be a flood. Yet for other clients, there may be many tributaries that are sometimes logical and sometimes confusing for both the client and the therapist alike. The responses the client reports during the Desensitization Phase suggest the connections the client is making as things shift in ways that can be surprising and unusual, but that is AIP. This is all reprocessing in EMDR.

EVIDENCE OF REPROCESSING DURING DESENSITIZATION WITH CHILDREN

The therapist needs to learn what movement looks like with children when reprocessing a target. Normal reprocessing covers a broad spectrum of responses from children. During desensitization, the image, cognitions, emotions, body sensations, and beliefs may change in subtle ways. Any change is evidence that the memory is reprocessing and indicates that the therapist should continue without intruding on the client's process.

For example, one adolescent client I (R.T.) worked with presented with a severe trauma history and an inhibited type of reactive attachment disorder. Once she identified all the pieces of the Assessment Phase, we began the process of desensitization with tactile BLS. Each time the therapist would check in and say, "Take a deep breath. Tell me what you got." The adolescent would respond, "It's in my stomach." Even though the adolescent was verbally reporting the same information, physically, she was moving and eventually was lying on the office sofa and yawning. After several sets, the therapist asked the adolescent to describe any changes in what was happening in her stomach, and the client reported, "It went from feeling hungry to feeling full." Even though the client was reporting each time that it was in her stomach, the body sensation was actually changing with each set of BLS. The therapist must be cognizant of what reprocessing looks like with each client.

Children Process Quickly

Initially, the therapist may be surprised at how quickly the child has processed the memory and will need to check in with the child. Following the associative chaining process is much simpler with children because children's memory networks have fewer channels and associations because children are younger (see Figure 6.1).

Even though some children may have experienced extensive traumas and distress in a short period of time, not as many years have gone by since the child had the experience.

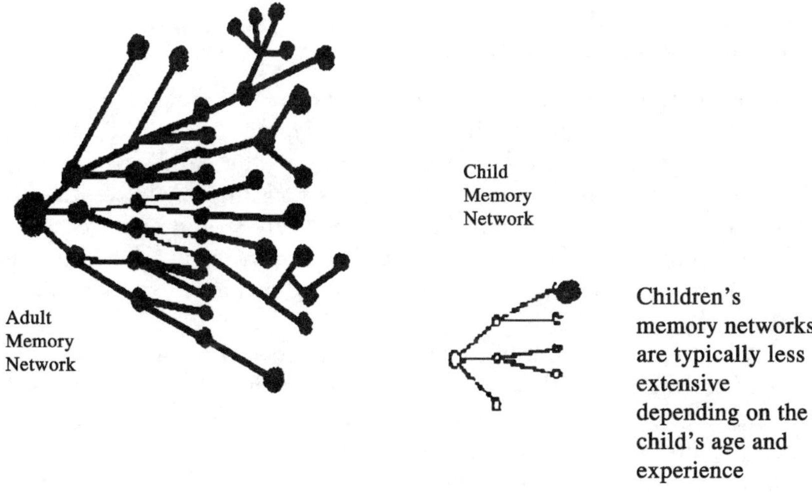
Adult
Memory
Network
Child
Memory
Network
Children's memory networks are typically less extensive depending on the child's age and experience

FIGURE 6.1 Neuronetworks.

Affective and Behavioral Indicators of Reprocessing With Children

How children process memories is as unique as the individual child. Some children are very restless and need to stop and play for a while. Then they may be able to come back and continue processing. Other children may be annoyed at the process or frustrated and need to move to a different activity or change modality of BLS. Yet other children may get very quiet, and it looks like nothing is happening, and then the child reports or demonstrates a significant shift that can surprise even the therapist.

The same child may process each target differently as well. Following the client and establishing a synchronicity with the individual client promotes reprocessing and the relationship between the therapist and client. Therapists' fluidity and flexibility in working with child clients enhances the efficacy of EMDR. Therapists' awareness of the individual child and the child's current development must be interwoven in reprocessing. Using the child's language and life experiences to translate the process assists in engaging the child in treatment.

In the case of Jeremiah discussed in chapter 5, as he reprocessed his fear of robbers, he actively kicked and punched the air, making fighting sounds as he held the "buzzies" for BLS. Jeremiah's reprocessing was very active, while other children may be quiet and still.

Implication of Developmental Milestones on Reprocessing

Because children are still working through developmental tasks and the child's personality is also still developing, the child's trauma history has not been as deeply ingrained into the child's personality. This is one of the most important reasons for using EMDR with children. By processing through the maladaptively stored experiences at a very young age, therapy can change the trajectory for the child and prevent those experiences from manifesting in more extensive adult pathology.

Children are constantly changing even between sessions, indicating a need for the therapist to be ever aware of the individual child's learning and developmental gains. As the child learns from participating in therapy and in life, the therapeutic process also changes. This dance of awareness continues throughout psychotherapy with children. The various stages of psychosocial development are an ever present overlay for the therapeutic process.

USE OF BILATERAL STIMULATION (BLS) WITH CHILDREN DURING REPROCESSING

The types of BLS were explored in chapter 4 and will not be repeated here, but instead, we will discuss the nuances of how BLS is actually used during the Desensitization Phase.

Sets of BLS

Children may not need a full 24 saccades or number of sets to process a memory. In general, children process more quickly than adults and may make links that they do not even notice. Again, the therapist needs to monitor the child's verbal and nonverbal responses. As we notice the child beginning to give indicators of an affect shift or overt recognition that he or she has made a connection, we will stop the BLS and ask the child, "What happened?" or "What did you notice now?"

Sometimes the therapist may need to go longer with the BLS when children are distracted or playing with the NeuroTek device. It is our experience that most children will play with the buzzies by putting them on their face and ears and experimenting with the buzzies to see what they feel like or put them together to notice the noise that the buzzies make when they connect. Whether with tactile stimulation or eye movements, it is important to assess that the child is engaged and focused. This may mean that the therapist needs to work harder to engage the child by wiggling his or her fingers or moving around the room to stay connected with the child.

Need to Change Type of BLS or Play or Focus

With children, therapists may also need to change the type of BLS more frequently to sustain the child's attention. Again, in an effort to stay in sync with the child, the therapist may need to notice when the child is distracted or habituated on the type of BLS. The therapist can change the speed, intensity, or volume of the BLS to keep the child engaged in desensitization.

Eye Movements

With their eyes, children process more quickly than adults and may not be aware they are really done. Children as young as 4 years of age are able to do the BLS with their eyes and are able to cross the midline. Often, a therapist does not even need props like puppets. Some children actually prefer eye movements.

ISSUES UNIQUE TO DESENSITIZATION WITH CHILDREN

In our experience in working with children, we have noticed interesting and unique responses to desensitization.

Children May Display Hesitancy and Avoidance Behavior

Therapists may notice that a child is hesitant or avoids reprocessing the target. This is not an oppositional child, but rather a child who has not bought into the purpose and efficacy of the therapeutic process. The therapist must consider what the individual child needs to become engaged.

Children may also be avoidant, which is a symptom category for posttraumatic stress disorder. In case conceptualization, it is important for the therapist to consider what the child might need, both internally and externally, to proceed. We have discussed using resourcing and mastery skills for the child to feel more competent with emotional regulation and emotional literacy. Teaching these skills to children is detailed in chapter 9. The circular process of EMDR with children includes returning to the Preparation Phase to improve the client's skill set at any time in order for the child to be able to continue with desensitization. Teaching children distancing and titrating techniques, including containers, is detailed throughout this book.

Young children typically have not initiated the therapy process but are brought to therapy by caregivers. Discussing the child's feelings about therapy is important, and asking the child to invest in treatment validates the child's opinion and gives the child a sense of empowerment. We are not suggesting that the child be given an option to not participate in therapy, but rather that the therapeutic process include the child's opinion about how to proceed. We both will admit that we have at times made deals with children, including allowing the child to choose a play activity for ending the therapy session. This is about setting the template for therapy and teaching the child what to expect. For example, we might say to the child, "We need to work for 25 minutes, and then you can choose an activity for 15 minutes, and then we will talk with your parents."

I (R.T.) may even suggest that the child can check the clock in the office, which gives the child some sense of power over the therapeutic process and builds a sense of predictability and even trust in my commitment to respect the child's opinion.

Some children have participated in previous psychotherapy that was uncomfortable and/or overwhelming for the child. If the child has previously participated in psychotherapy that was difficult for the child, the therapist may need to begin with previous therapy as a target. As with any target, I (R.T.) ask the child to begin with the worst part about the previous therapy, identify a negative cognition or bad thought about the previous therapy, and then continue with the procedural steps of the Assessment Phase.

We strongly encourage therapists to explore with child clients any previous therapy experiences and responses to the therapy. The previous therapy experience may be the root of the child's or even adult client's resistance to the therapeutic process or avoidance of a specific target.

Fluctuations in SUD Ratings

With all clients, it is not unusual for the subjective units of disturbance (SUD) to increase initially. This is a predictable part of reprocessing, as the client accesses the potency of the memory network. It is important to predict and normalize this for the client, and especially for children. Reminding children of the Stop Signal and Metaphor, along with other resources that the therapist has established for the child, is helpful at this point.

Yet it is often the therapist's discomfort that is more prominent when the child displays an increase in affect or disturbance. Therapists must explore their own countertransference issues and ability to tolerate the pain of a child for the therapist to be beneficial to the child. It is the therapist's responsibility to hold the space for the child and convey to the child that the therapist can tolerate the child's intense affect or behavioral responses and that the therapist can assist the child with reprocessing the traumatic event. This is where the dance between demonstrating care and concern, while guiding the child along and responding to the child's activity level in a gentle and solid relationship, becomes the foundation for reprocessing. The therapist needs to be able to stay out of the way because in doing so, the therapist is letting the child know that intense affect is OK and that the therapist has confidence in the child's ability to get through the target. The timing of the interactions with the child is in and of itself an art, especially during reprocessing. Being attuned to the client's need for the therapist to stop and start BLS, offer a tissue, change the type of BLS, or offer simple encouragement of "that's it" must be based on the child's needs, not on the therapist's needs. The nuance of observing the client's nonverbal responses and having a toolbox of clinical choices from which the therapist can select as the client's needs indicate is the art of reprocessing. The fluidity and flexibility of the therapeutic relationship requires steadfastness and creativity, especially with children. Sometimes the therapist needs to follow the thread until the child processes through the experience. The tenacity to hang in there and not panic is a hallmark of a good EMDR therapist.

Therapists also need to be resolute in the process and not be driven by their own feelings or need to interpret the child's responses. The therapist must have confidence in the client's own wisdom and allow for the surprise and true discovery that arise during reprocessing with EMDR. Believing in the client's own AIP ability is often tested during the Desensitization Phase. It is not uncommon to be confused by what a child is reporting or for a child to report disconnected pieces that at times have a connection with reality, while at other times are obviously fantasy, yet are the child's own process. Children will at times use imagination and fantasy woven together with pieces of reality to create a coherent narrative of the target. It is not necessary for the therapist to understand everything that the child is experiencing or reporting to know that movement is occurring and that the target is being reprocessed.

Children May Process in Fantasy Before Processing in Reality

Confronting a specific traumatic event may feel overwhelming to a child, and the child may need to initially approach the target from a distance.

Case Study: Andrea and the Teddy Bear

I (R.T.) worked with a 7-year-old girl who had been with her mother when her mother had overdosed. In therapy, Andrea wanted to use EMDR to work on her worries about her friends at school. Even though I knew about Andrea's past traumas with her mother, Andrea was so avoidant that we decided to first work on the issues Andrea chose to target. Andrea targeted her friend issues and gained confidence in the usefulness of EMDR. Andrea then decided that my teddy bear needed help to deal with his problems with his mother. While I was her assistant, Andrea led the teddy bear through the Assessment and Desensitization Phases of the EMDR protocol by putting the buzzies on the paws of the teddy bear until the teddy bear felt better. Andrea was also experiencing the bilateral stimulation as she held the buzzies on the teddy bear's paws allowing her to reprocess the target to adaptive resolution.

The child may describe or create the narrative of the event in third person perspective or through fantasy. The child's experience of the event and current stage of development impact how the child will present the maladaptively stored information. This is not a memory test, but a representation of the individual's unique experience. What the child expresses represents how the memory is stored and nothing more. Some children will process through play, art, sand tray, or in drawings. Whatever medium the child chooses to use to process and convey the experience is only as important as what matters to the child. Even if the original target appears to be grounded in reality, the child may process partially or totally in fantasy.

At the end of this chapter, we have provided a detailed case with transcript of a desensitization session, in which a 3-year-old reprocesses monsters that are keeping him from sleeping in his own bed.

THERAPIST'S ROLE

One of the most difficult parts for therapists is staying out of the way of the client's experience and understanding the flow of reprocessing that uniquely unfolds with each client. Therapists need to understand the underlying theory of AIP and what associative chaining looks like as the client's maladaptively stored memory connects with greater insight and understanding and reveals what has been driving the symptomatology with which the client originally presented for therapy. The connection originates from the client's internal processing as the therapist takes a more passive role than during the first three phases of EMDR.

The therapist's role is to follow the client wherever the associate chaining takes the process. The reprocessing continues by having the therapist use BLS to desensitize the original incident and any associated memories to link up with more adaptive information.

The therapist's role is to stop the BLS to check in with a client to see if things are changing and to insure that the client is straddling the past and the present as well as the internal and external experience.

Therapists' Skills, Tools, and Use of Self in Therapy With Children

Therapists need to use all their clinical skills to stay in sync with the child during reprocessing of a target. The therapist's role continues to be a very active role in a client-centered process. As with any therapy, it is helpful to listen to body language, stay attuned to the child, and be aware of what processing looks like and what is truly blocked processing or looping. The therapist's natural instinctive and intuitive response adds to the art of being with the child during the desensitization of a target. This is where we struggled with capturing the essence of what we do in therapy to convey it to the reader. This has been a struggle for words that truly articulate what happens, especially with children. As the child is reprocessing the memory with the aid of BLS, we are constantly considering how the client has stored the information, determining what piece might be missing, and creating options to choose from should the child need more assistance than the therapist just saying "what do you get now?" and then "go with that."

Desensitization is so much more than BLS. It is an unfolding of the reprocessing of maladaptively stored information that has been interwoven in the child's life and development, while simultaneously trying to follow the client's expression of the experience in the therapeutic environment.

It is also the therapist's role to be aware of when the client is struggling and needs assistance to either slow the process that is unfolding or to connect with the experience when it is difficult.

STRATEGIES FOR REGULATING THE SPEED OF REPROCESSING

Reprocessing needs to proceed at a speed that the client can tolerate, while also adequately accessing the target memory. Too much information or too little can impede the Desensitization Phase.

Flooding

Just like with adult clients, children need resources to decelerate reprocessing when the intensity of the experience becomes overwhelming. *Flooding* occurs when the client becomes overwhelmed with the intensity of the experience and needs assistance to continue. Flooding can present as multiple and rapid images, racing thoughts, intense affect or emotion, and confusing or intolerable body sensations. Flooding is a unique experience for each client with each target. Theoretically, the client has tapped an encapsulated memory that has been maladaptively stored because at the time of the incident, the client was unable to tolerate the event. The memory then is accessed for reprocessing during EMDR. Flooding cannot be measured simply by the display of emotion or affect but is instead the client's ability to tolerate the desensitization and stay with the reprocessing. Clients who cannot continue processing because they are unable to tolerate the process need assistance from the therapist.

During the initial phases of treatment, the therapist has attempted to evaluate the client's ability to manage intense affect and taught the client skills during the Preparation Phase of EMDR; however, sometimes neither the therapist nor the client have been able to accurately predict how the client will respond during the Desensitization Phase. If the client becomes flooded and cannot proceed, the therapist may need to teach the client skills for distancing and titrating affect.

Evidence of flooding with children may resemble what happens with adult clients, but may also occur when a child throws the buzzies and walks away, refuses to participate, appears very blank, or starts to yawn and appears to be getting sleepy. Children who appear to be getting sleepy may still be processing; however, it is important for the therapist to stay attuned and aware of what is happening with the child.

The word *abreaction* has been used with various definitions; however, the psychoanalytic term *abreaction* refers to connecting with a traumatic memory to discharge the affect associated with the memory. By using this definition, abreaction can be a product of reprocessing a memory that is beneficial to the client; however, abreaction is not necessary to desensitize a traumatic event. If a child begins to abreact and can tolerate the intense experience and proceed with reprocessing the memory, it is the therapist's responsibility to modulate and guide the process in order that reprocessing the memory is not another traumatic event, but instead a release or catharsis. To achieve the cathartic effect of adaptively reprocessing a traumatic event, children may need techniques for distancing and titrating the intensity of the experience.

Techniques for Distancing and Titrating Intensity of Memory Reprocessing With Children

Techniques for distancing and titrating the intensity of reprocessing can also be used as containers. Tools for decelerating, including distancing and titrating, need to be taught for clients to be able to manage the intense affect that might arise from the Desensitization Phase of EMDR. This is important for several reasons.

Children need to feel competent in managing intense affect to continue to be engaged in the therapeutic process. If a child feels unable to manage the intense affect, the child is more likely to avoid the process or dissociate, rather than to participate in reprocessing traumatic memories. When children feel competent to manage intense affect, they are able to maintain the dual attention required for reprocessing memories and will be willing to continue in therapy. Since children do not typically initiate their own therapy, convincing children that the therapeutic process will be beneficial to them is crucial. To engage children in the process, front loading during the Preparation Phase of EMDR is extremely important (see chapter 4). Children who have experienced success with EMDR and feel competent and prepared for managing intense affect are much more likely to be willing participants. This certainly makes the treatment process much more positive for both children and therapists alike.

Children are very creative in using containers for affect management, which is taught in EMDR training; however, children often struggle with the tools that are more adult oriented and abstract. Using techniques like the television channels as a Metaphor for distancing when the affect becomes overwhelming in EMDR processing gives the child a feeling of being in a position of power and competency. Using the television and remote or the movie Metaphor as interventions are different than using the train Metaphor that is taught in EMDR Part 1 training because the train Metaphor implies that the client is in one place and memories are moving by, while using the television or movie screen is a distancing technique that is used for the deceleration that the client needs to be able to tolerate intense affect. Children first need to learn about the observer self. Children need to learn to be able to stand outside the emotion and body sensation to observe from a distant place, which often is a place of wisdom. This gives children perspective on the process and really stems from the place of AIP for children. This helps decrease the flooding of affect or overwhelming experience of body sensations.

Containers

Containers can be used for incomplete sessions to store activated but unprocessed material that may be potentially potent for the client between sessions (see chapter 4 for teaching containers).

Containers can also be used for children who are experiencing a high level of disturbance for affect tolerance and emotional regulation. Using containers will hopefully lay the foundation to allow the therapist to have the child return to the memory to continue reprocessing. This process will also give the child a sense of mastery over intense affect and, ideally, the willingness to continue with reprocessing traumatic experiences.

Children can be taught to compartmentalize the entire memory and put it in one or multiple compartments in order that the memory is not overwhelming or disturbing outside of the session. Containers for affect management can include a see-through container, where the child can see the traumatic experience through glass or plastic but not experience any of the emotions or body sensations. This allows the visual stimulus without experiencing the entire impact of the memory.

Containers can also be used to teach children how to fractionate memories as a way of managing the intensity of the memory. By placing different pieces of the incident into different containers, it is possible to fractionate the incident in order for the client to more effectively manage the severity of the experience. Once each piece of the memory is processed, it is easier to complete the incident. Children can be taught to take one piece of the memory out of the container and reprocess the piece of the memory. As each piece is reprocessed, the intensity decreases, until the entire memory can be combined and completed.

There are many types of containers that can also be used as deceleration techniques for titrating intense affect.

Movie Screen. This is discussed in detail in chapter 4.

Television and Remote. As previously discussed in chapter 4, the therapist can teach the child to put traumatic memories on certain channels, while putting safe places on other channels, and safe people on yet other channels. The child then imagines holding the remote and being able to move between channels for titrating the intense affect that may be stimulated by certain stations.

The child can also be taught to turn down the volume or change the channel to black and white.

The therapist can offer the child a blanket or stuffed animal to hold, or some children may choose to sit in the parent's lap or sit beside the parent to more effectively cope with the intense affect and feel more secure.

On the other end of the continuum, clients may struggle with not being able to access the memory network and need assistance to begin or stay with reprocessing.

Incomplete Accessing

Incomplete accessing occurs for several reasons. Sometimes the client is distracted and not focusing. Other times, the client is avoiding the process. Some clients may experience alexythymia and not be in touch with their emotions or body sensations and may need to be taught additional skills. Yet other clients are confused and need additional instruction about the process. Finally, some clients are dissociative and need additional support and skills, as will be discussed in chapter 11. In our experience, it is more likely for clients to display incomplete accessing at the beginning of the Desensitization Phase.

Cognitive Interweaves

Cognitive interweaves are another tool used during the Desensitization Phase of EMDR to jump-start blocked processing; however, using cognitive interweaves with children creates unique challenges for therapists. Even though cognitive interweaves are typically used during reprocessing, cognitive interweaves will be discussed in detail in chapter 10. It is important for the therapist to always be thinking about what cognitive interweaves may be most helpful to the unique characteristics of the client.

Procedural Considerations

The therapist needs to be able to differentiate between incomplete accessing versus actual reprocessing. A client may no longer be able to access the target because the target has reprocessed. This is especially true of children, who process very quickly. To determine if the client is experiencing incomplete accessing or if the client has already reprocessed the memory, the therapist should return to the original target and ask the client, "What do you get now?" Whatever the client reports, add a set of BLS. As the therapist, if you still are not sure if the client is having difficulty accessing or has already reprocessed the memory, take a SUD measurement.

Clients Who Struggle With Focusing. Clients may begin the Desensitization Phase struggling to be able to completely access the target and can require assistance to focus and reorient to the original components of the procedural steps. This is when the therapist may have to repeat the image, negative cognition, emotion, and body sensation to assist the client in accessing the target to start reprocessing. Other clients may access the target initially but then become avoidant or lose focus.

Clients Who Appear to Be Avoiding Reprocessing. If the therapist concludes that the client is avoiding reprocessing the target event, the therapist needs to evaluate what is driving the avoidance response and when this is occurring. It is also important to consider if it is conscious or unconscious avoidance. No matter what the etiology of the avoidance, it is the therapist's responsibility to assist the client in being able to access and tolerate reprocessing. The therapist needs to ask himself or herself, What does this client need to participate in successfully reprocessing a target event? Does the client need additional resources or affect tolerance, or is the client not convinced of the efficacy of the process? Is the child tired or hungry, or does the child just need a break for the day?

Children will often change the subject or distract themselves simply because it is more fun to talk about cartoons than about a car accident. Helping children understand why targeting a memory can be helpful is the role of the therapist. We use stories from books and Metaphors to engage children in the process. We will discuss using mastery experiences and installing resources in chapter 9.

Modulating the flow of information at a pace that the client can tolerate can also be controlled by BLS.

Using the Speed of BLS and Number of Saccades to Adjust Reprocessing. The use of BLS to regulate the speed of reprocessing is the art of EMDR. Using the speed of BLS to slow the flow of information or increase the flow of information can be very productive. If a client is flooding, titrating the amount of information by using shorter sets of BLS can help the client to artificially space the information into manageable portions.

If the client is struggling to access the entire target event, longer sets of BLS allow the time for the client to access the event. It is often difficult for clients who are very analytical and who tend to stay in their heads to sustain the analytical stance with longer sets of BLS. For some clients, this may mean 80–100 saccades. This is especially true for gifted children and anxious children who may tend to stay in their heads. Longer sets of BLS can be helpful for children who are struggling to focus and are fidgety. It may take longer sets for the child to play with the buzzies and settle into the experience of reprocessing the memory. Being attuned to how the individual child responds is pivotal to decision making. Some children may be overstimulated by longer sets. It is the dance between the therapist and the child that is the key.

Changing the type of BLS is also beneficial in modulating the flow of information from the target. If a child is having difficulty with body sensations and mindfulness, it may be beneficial for the therapist to use tactile stimulation.

THEMES FOR COGNITIVE INTERWEAVES: RESPONSIBILITY/SAFETY/CHOICES

Themes for cognitive interweaves are significantly impacted by human development and the child's mastery of specific stages of development, including cognitive and moral development and the ability to mentalize. How children organize their beliefs about themselves and the world within which they live impacts their interpretation and reaction to traumatic events.

In AIP theory, cognitions are organized around three themes: responsibility, safety, and choices. In exploring the child's bad thought about the traumatic event during the procedural steps of the Assessment Phase, the therapist tapped the cognitive part of the memory network that was maladaptively stored.

We discussed the cognitive themes of responsibility, safety, and new choices in chapter 5. During the Desensitization Phase, the therapist is ever aware of the three cognitive themes to be prepared with an appropriate cognitive interweave at the point where the child becomes stuck or loops. The cognitive themes provide a clue to possible cognitive interweaves if the child becomes stuck or begins looping.

Because both children and adults struggle with misattributions of responsibility regarding traumatic events, the therapist may need a cognitive interweave that suggests jump-starting the process of resolving misattributions of responsibility. Cognitions that revolve around the theme of safety involve the client's ability to feel safe in the present moment. Sometimes this has to do with the current environment, while other times, this is related to the client's feelings about life and the universe. If the child becomes stuck on a cognition of safety, this suggests that the cognitive interweave would contain information to assist in jump-starting the resolution of cognitions involving safety. Once the child has resolved the appropriate attribution of responsibility and has achieved the ability to feel safe in the present moment, the child now has the opportunity to process cognitive themes of choices that include a sense of empowerment. Of course, children do not have power over their entire lives, but children often come to the belief that "I can walk away when other kids are misbehaving." Other children might conclude, "I can sleep in my own bed and call for my mom and dad if I need help." For children especially, there is something energizing and healing about having choices for new behaviors, thoughts, and feelings. Again, if the child's reprocessing becomes stuck around negative cognitions that suggest the child is unable to identify new choices, cognitive interweaves would focus on helping the child link up with resources providing new choices in the present.

There can be a circular process that occurs with cognitions: Once a client feels empowered to make new choices, then the client often experiences a greater sense of release of responsibility for being victimized and acquires new choices for safety. At any point in the child's reprocessing, the child may need the associated cognitive interweave to continue. Cognitive interweaves are discussed in detail in chapter 10.

The Desensitization Phase continues until the therapist believes the child is at the end of a channel and the therapist needs to return to check the target, or the therapist is confused about where the client is in the process, or time is running out at the end of a session and the therapist needs to close down reprocessing.

End of a Channel

If the therapist believes the child is at the end of a channel, the therapist needs to return to the original target and check in with the child. The therapist might suspect the child is at the end of a channel because what the child is reporting is either neutral or positive and staying positive. We would suggest the rule of threes. If the child is saying the same positive response three times, this suggests the child is at the end of a channel and that the therapist should return to check the target.

A client may report positive connections that suggest that the client is generalizing and making positive associations to adaptive resolutions, but this is not necessarily an indication that the client is at the end of a channel. The client may be linking to positive memories and even make spiritual connections. Even children make spiritual connections. I (C.S.) worked with a little girl whose sister was run over by a bus and killed. During reprocessing, the little girl saw her sister waving good-bye to her and telling her she was going to be with God. It is important for the therapist to be cognizant of when the client needs to continue with reprocessing because the memory is becoming more adaptive, versus when the client has actually reached the end of a channel and it is time to return to check the original target.

Checking the Target

If the therapist assesses that the client is at the end of a channel, the therapist returns to the original target and asks the client what he or she gets now and does a set of BLS. If the client reports new information, the therapist continues with BLS. If the client continues to report positive information, then the therapist can take the SUD. If the SUD is greater than 0, continue reprocessing. If the SUD is 0, then the therapist checks the validity of cognition (VoC) and proceeds to the installation phase, which is explained in the next chapter. We have included the entire script for desensitization and checking the target at the end of this chapter.

Incomplete Sessions

An incomplete session occurs when the session is over and the client has not reprocessed the memory. If the client has continued to report disturbing information, the therapist stops BLS and then follows the directions for an incomplete session by helping the client close down the disturbance and prepare for in between sessions.

Procedure for Closing Incomplete Sessions

An incomplete session is one in which a child's material is still unresolved; that is, the child is still obviously upset, or the SUD is above 1 and the VoC is less than 6. The following is a suggested procedure for closing down an incomplete session. The purpose is to acknowledge the child for what he or she has accomplished and to leave the child well grounded before he or she leaves the office. Tools for closing an incomplete session may also be necessary during desensitization, installation, or body scan. (The reader is referred to chapter 7 for additional application of procedures for closing incomplete sessions during other phases of EMDR.)

1. Explain the reason for stopping and check on the child's state: "We need to stop and clean up now because it's time to go. How're you doing after the thing we talked about today?"
2. Give encouragement and support for the effort made: "We worked hard today, and you're awesome. How are you doing right now?"
3. The therapist can use a process to access containers and safe place for the child to close the desensitization process: "Let's stop and do our container and our safe place one more time before we go. Remember your safe place? I want you to think about that place. What do you see? What do you smell? What does it feel like to be there? Where do you notice it in your body?"

SUMMARY

The Desensitization Phase of EMDR requires patience and consistency from the therapist using skills for reprocessing events with children. The therapist needs to stay attuned to the child and the child's body language and be aware of demand characteristics. Demand characteristics can arise when children realize that telling the therapist that a SUD is 0 means the child can go and play. The therapist must use clinical judgment and reports from adults in the child's life to assess the efficacy of the desensitization process. Once the child processes the associated memory networks, the therapist may need to bring the child back to the original incident several times before completing one target. When the target is reprocessed as evidenced by a 0 SUD, the therapist then continues into the Installation Phase of EMDR.

INSTRUCTIONS TO THE CLIENT AND THERAPIST'S SCRIPT FOR DESENSITIZATION PHASE

1. "I'd like you to bring up that picture [label and describe using client's word] and the words [repeat the negative cognition in client's words], the __________ feeling, and notice where you are feeling it in your body and __________ [therapist uses whatever BLS was previously identified]."
2. Begin the BLS. (You established the BLS method and speed during the introduction to EMDR.)
3. At least once or twice during each set of BLS, or when there is an apparent change, comment to the client, "That's it. Good. That's

it." With children, the type of BLS may need to be changed often to assist the child in sustaining attention.

4. If the child appears to be too upset to continue reprocessing, it is helpful to reassure the child and to remind the child of the Metaphor identified with the child prior to processing. "It's normal for you to feel more as we start to work on this. Remember, we said it's like _________ [Metaphor], so just notice it. It's old stuff." (Only if needed, if child is upset.)
5. After a set of BLS, instruct the child by saying, "Take a deep breath." (It is often helpful if the therapist takes an exaggerated breath to model for the child, as the therapist makes the statements to the child.)
6. Ask something like, "What did you get *now*?" or "Tell me what you got." Or if the child needs coaching, say, "What are you thinking and feeling? How does your body feel, or what pictures are you seeing in your head?"
7. After the child recounts his or her experience, say, "Go with that," and do another set of BLS. (Do not repeat the child's words or statements.) As an optional phrasing, you can say, "Think about that."
8. Again, ask, "What do you get now?" If new negative material presents itself, continue down that channel with further sets of BLS.
9. Continue with sets of BLS until the child's report indicates that the child is at the end of a memory channel. At that point, the child may appear significantly calmer. No new disturbing material is emerging. Then, return to the target. Ask, "When you think about that thing we first talked about today, what happens now?" (Remember that children may not show affect and may often process very quickly. So there may be no more disturbing material for the child to access or describe about the target memory.) After the child recounts his or her experience (children may verbalize or draw or otherwise demonstrate through play therapy what they have experienced), add a set of BLS.
10. If positive material is reported, add one or two sets of BLS to increase the strength of the positive associations before returning to the target. If you believe the child is at the end of a channel, that is, the material reported is neutral or positive, then ask, "When you go back to that first thing we talked about today [therapist references the picture, sand tray, or whatever was used by the child to identify the original target], what do you get now?" Whatever the child reports, add a set of BLS.
11. If no change occurs, check the SUD. Ask the child, "When you think about that thing, from 0 to 10, where 0 is 'doesn't bother

you at all' and 10 is 'bothers you a lot,' how much does that thing bother you right now?" (The therapist can use one of the alternate ways of checking the SUD described in the Assessment Phase.)

12. If the SUD is greater than 0, continue with further sets of BLS, time permitting. If the SUD is 0, do another set of BLS to verify that no new material opens up. Then proceed to the installation of the positive cognition. (Remember: only proceed to installation after you have returned to target, added a set of BLS, no new material has emerged, and the SUD is 0.)

CASE PRESENTATION: EMDR SESSION WITH A 3-YEAR-OLD CHILD

The following is a transcript of a session with a 3-year-old that includes all the pieces of the protocol during the Assessment Phase and continues with desensitization, installation, and body scan.

Case Study: Michael

This is a brief overview of a child named Michael and a summary of Michael's history. When I (R.T.) met Michael, he was 16 months old, and his case manager had received a call that his foster mother could no longer care for Michael because 2 days earlier, Michael's foster dad had fallen over dead from a massive heart attack. We still are not sure what Michael witnessed, but we do know that the man who had cared for Michael for 7 months was gone and that Michael saw the emergency personnel in his foster home. This foster home was Michael's sixth foster placement. Michael was born heroin exposed and was removed from his mother's care at birth. After meeting with the foster family, the case manager put this child in a car seat in the back of her van, and I sat next to Michael as we left his foster home, where he has never returned. Michael had been giggling and chasing his other foster siblings prior to leaving the home, but now Michael was blank, with no affect. I sat in the back of the van talking to Michael, telling him that he would be safe even if he was scared right now. I spoke softly and tried to reassure Michael.

When she got the call to remove Michael, the case manager could not tolerate putting Michael in a shelter, so we called a certified adoptive home with whom we had worked. We asked them to take Michael, and they agreed. Michael was placed with his new family within 4 hours of my call to the adoptive home. For the next 2 years, Michael had visits in my office with a biological grandmother and his now adoptive family. The family repeatedly reported that Michael's sleep was disturbed by terrible nightmares that increased after visits. Michael was evaluated by a psychologist, who reported that developmentally, Michael was on target or advanced in many areas, but she suggested that his sleep disturbance was due to anxiety and trauma. Michael has a poor immune system and has had frequent infections. The pediatrician also suggested that Michael's anxiety needed to be addressed.

After many months of visits with various family members, a wise judge decided that Michael needed to stay in his foster home and be adopted.

Since the waiting list for mental health services for toddlers is very long, and very few mental health professionals in Arizona are trained to use EMDR with children, the family asked me if I would try EMDR with Michael. They knew the impact of EMDR because their 14-year-old daughter Nina sees me, and we have used EMDR with her with great success.

Michael calls me "Tapia Tapia." On many occasions, Michael has been in my office playing with me, and I have frequently discussed Michael's functioning with his parents. One day, Michael and I talked about the monsters and if he would like to try something to make the monsters go away. I showed Michael the buzzies, and we played with them for a while. I asked Michael if he would come back to play with me and make a movie about his monsters. He agreed, and the following transcript is of this session.

Michael is now 43 months of age and has been adopted for 9 months. The family signed the appropriate documentation for me to share this transcript with the reader.

I had an extensive client history with 2 years of observations of Michael. The treatment plan was limited to processing Michael's nightmares to improve his sleeping. The only preparation I chose to do was to explain the buzzies and how Michael could tell me to stop. My playroom is a safe place for Michael.

Transcript of a Therapy Session

The following is a transcript of an EMDR desensitization session with Michael and Dr. Adler-Tapia. The session is in no way perfect, and the astute therapist will note that initially, I (R.T.) missed evaluating the body sensation. Michael's sister Nina is present in the transcript and videotaped the session.

ROBBIE ADLER-TAPIA (R): Yeah, are you gonna help me make a movie?

MICHAEL (M): Yeah.

R: Cool, Michael.

NINA (N): Say hi again.

M: Hi.

N: How old are you?

M: [*laughs*] Three.

R: Wow.

N: Three. When's your birthday?

M: Ummmm . . .

M: November. November.

R: Do you remember that? Then we need these little things that buzzed on the floor?

N: He's turning it on already?

R: You know we've got to plug it in. If we don't plug it in, it won't work. Do you want to plug it in? Oh, you've got it turned on already. Good job. Do you want to plug in these things that go right here? Put this in there.

M: This one?

R: Good job! Wow! Now do you want turn it on? Do you remember how you turn it on?

M: Yeah.

R: All right. Do you remember that?

M: Yeah.

R: Yeah. Do you know what these are for?

M: What?

R: **Image.** Do you remember when you told me about the monsters when you tried to sleep? These are to help with the monsters. Remember when we said we were gonna do that? Can you help me to draw pictures of the monsters? So we can squish them like you said? How big did you say they were? . . . Here, let's go over here so you can draw some pictures of what the monsters look like. OK? **Negative Cognition.** Can you show me what the bad thought about the monsters? What's gonna happen with the monsters?

M: Squish them.

R: You're gonna squish them? Do they make you scared?

M: Yeah.

R: How come?

M: 'Cause.

R: What are they gonna do?

M: Eat me.

R: They're gonna eat you? OK. Can you draw a picture of that? What they look like? Do they have big teeth, or what?

M: Big teeth like this.

R: Big teeth like that. OK.

M: And they look like this.

R: Wow. Those are big teeth, Michael. That's a great picture. You know what?

M: They look like that.

R: What's the scariest part about the monster? Are you in bed, or where are you? What's the scariest part?

M: They're in my bed.

R: In your bed? In your new room?

M: In my room.

R: Are you in your big room in your new house? Where are you?

M: In my room.

R: Yeah.

M: Yeah.

R: Do you have a Spider Man room?

M: Not yet.

R: Not yet, but that's how you're gonna make your room? So the worst part is they're gonna eat you. OK. What would you rather have happen instead?

M: Stomp 'em.

R: So you wanna stomp them? Instead of the monsters eating Michael, you'd stomp the monsters? Would that make you feel not so scared anymore?

M: Yeah.

R: So how about over here? Look at this thing. Can I show you? Will you help me? We need special markers to write on here. Do you have the markers that write on the board?

M: What markers?

R: We need the special markers to write on the boards.

M: These ones?

R: Can you draw a picture of the bad thought that they're gonna eat me?

M: This one doesn't work.

R: It's not working. OK.

M: There it is.

R: That worked. What's that? That's what it looks like with the monster's teeth that they're gonna eat you?

M: Yeah.

R: **Positive Cognition.** OK, and then the good thought, the happy thought. What do you want to draw on this picture?

M: This is the happy thought.

R: What is the happy thought?

M: Stomp 'em.

R: You're gonna stomp the monsters instead. OK, let's pretend we're gonna put them on the bridge, the monster's teeth and then the happy thought when you stomp the monsters. Let's pretend, remember these things you like to play with, that this is a bridge. OK. Remember those sticky things that you had on the board over there? Can you get one of those?

M: Yeah.

R: Yeah.

M: One?

R: Yeah. Do you want just want one?

M: I got one.

R: **VoC.** Can you show me from the scary thought, the monster's teeth and if Michael goes across the bridge to the happy thought, where are you on the bridge?

M: Here.

R: Can you put your sticker right there for now? When you're right there and the feeling where the monsters are gonna eat you? **Emotion.** Is it a scared or sad or a different one? What's the feeling? What's the feeling when the monster's gonna eat me? Is it your scared feeling?

M: Yeah.

R: Is it your scared feeling or a different feeling?

M: A different one scary . . .

R: What is it?

M: Where does this stone go?

R: Is that the basket of stones over there? Over there, honey. See, right there. Is it behind there? Is that where the basket of stones is?

M: Yeah.

R: Thank you so much. **Emotion.** So on your scary thought, is there a scary feeling? Michael, can you show me how big the feeling is? Is it this big, or this big, or this big?

M: It's this big.

R: So it's a really big scary thought, huh?

M: Yeah.

R: OK, so can we turn on the buzzies now? **Desensitization.** What you think about when you're in your bed and you see the monster's teeth and the monsters are gonna eat you . . .

M: What are these for? Where do these go?

R: Remember that's the Lite Brite.

M: Where do these go?

R: The Lite Brite thing? I don't see it. What happened to it? It might be in the playroom. Can we put it on the table and take it in there after we're done, when you go play? Would that be OK?

M: Yeah.

R: Thank you.

M: Now can we make the movie?

R: Yeah, well, Nina's making the movie. Look. Can you tell her about this picture of the monster's big teeth that scare you when you're in your bed? Look at it. Here's the buzzy things. Remember? Do you remember what we said they're for? OK.

M: Oh, it's not in.

R: Oh, these got unplugged. Can you help me? Where should we put them?

M: They go in here.

R: OK, remember these buzzy things, do you want to put them in your hands or in your socks or in your shoes? Where should we put them?

M: In my shoes.

R: Do you want to do it or do you want me to help you? Is that working? Oh, look, you're doing it. Do you want to stand up or sit down?

M: I want to stand up.

R: OK, can we turn this on? Oh, are you OK?

M: Yeah.

R: Can you bring up that scary picture of that scary picture monster with the big teeth and "he's gonna eat me," and can you close your eyes and see the monster, and I'm gonna turn the buzzies on? They're in your shoes. Are you ready? Are they working?

M: Yeah . . .

[44 SACCADES]

R: OK, can you take a deep breath? Go like this. Wipe it out? Wipe your face like this? Can you wipe it out like this? Do you want to tell me what happened or do you want to draw a picture?

M: Draw.

R: Yeah. You can leave them in your shoes for when we do it again. [Michael takes out buzzies] Do you want to stand up or sit down to draw your picture?

M: Ummm . . .

R: You can sit down if you want to. There you go. You can take them out and then we can put them back in later. OK, so can you draw me a picture on the paper? What happened when the buzzies were in your socks?

M: This page can't work.

R: Do you want a new page?

M: Yeah.

R: OK, we've got lots of pages. What happened when the buzzies were in your socks?

M: Like that.

R: What is that?

M: Buzzing.

R: Buzzing, OK, and what happened with the monsters?

M: Like that.

R: Like that. Can you tell me a story about this?

M: I can't read it.

R: You can't read it?

M: No.

R: That's OK. It's a picture. It's a picture that you can tell me a story about.

M: From that page to this page.

R: OK. It's the same as this picture?

M: No. It's this.

R: Did this picture change?

M: Yeah.

R: What happened?

M: I don't know.

R: You don't know. OK, so do you want to put the buzzies back in your socks? Or in your hands? What do you wanna do?

M: In my hands.

R: OK, do you want to turn it on? Are you ready?

M: Um, yeah.

R: So that picture that you just drew?

M: Which one?

R: OK, so that picture that you just wiped out.

M: Which one?

R: That one that you just drew me. Can you close your eyes and bring up that picture and see what happens?

M: Sure.

[44 saccades]

R: What happened? Take a deep breath. And, wipe it out. And, what happened? Is it a new picture? Can you draw it for me or tell me about it?

M: This one doesn't work.

R: OK.

M: I want another one. I just did that one.

R: You just did that one so you want to change. [Michael picks up an orange marker] Does it smell like oranges?

M: Yeah.

R: Do you want to use that one to draw your new picture?

M: But it's the same color.

R: Yeah, what color is that?

M: Orange.

R: Yeah, do you like that color?

M: Not really.

R: You need red.

M: Where's the red one? Where's the red one like this one?

R: Do you want to use this one?

M: Oh, yeah.

R: Oh, yeah, OK.

M: That's his head and that's his mouth.

R: That's his head and that's his mouth. He has a really big mouth. **Body Sensations.** And Michael, when you get scared from that big mouth like that with those big teeth, where do you feel that scary feeling in your body? Is it in your head, in your ear, in your heart, in your tummy . . .

M: In my head.

R: In your head. It makes your head hurt?

M: Yeah.

R: OK, so let's put the buzzies, do you want to hold them in your hands and put them on the monster's teeth and see what happens?

M: Yeah.

R: Yeah.

M: Right there?

R: Yeah. Can you hold both of them with both of them, with both hands and put them on there? Can you do that?

M: Yeah.

R: Just like that. Hold them down there just like that. There you go.

M: Why's this buzzing?

R: Hum. [BLS commences; Michael giggles because of the sound of the buzzies] What are you doing to that monster's teeth?

M: I'm using this to make them go away.

R: You're making his monster teeth go away?

M: Maybe this will make it go away.

R: Hum?

M: Maybe this noise on the monster can make him go away.

R: It's making it go away. Is it helping?

M: Not really!

R: Not really. What if we try a different way?

M: Yeah.

R: What if we pick a different marker. Pick the black marker in there. Do you want to try the black one? Can we use that marker to make the monster's teeth go away?

M: Yeah.

R: Let's put the buzzies in your socks. And make them go away like this. Can you do that with that marker?

M: Like this?

R: Put them in your feet.

M: Yeah.

R: Or, let me see if I can find my special markers to make it go away. You put them in your feet and I'll look for those special markers.

N: Put it in your other shoe, Michael.

R: Is that working? OK, do you see this special one?

M: Yeah.

R: This is the one that you can use to make his teeth go away. I'm gonna put your name on it so we know it's Michael's special crayon. Is that OK? Do you think this will work?

M: Yeah.

R: How can we make those teeth go away? Can I turn the buzzies on? What's that? Can you try like this? Back and forth and back and forth and back and forth. The other way to make that monster go away. [Michael colors across the picture.] Make that monster go away . . . is it working?

M: Yeah.

R: Keep going. Can I put it closer or put it on your lap? Will that work?

M: Yeah . . . it's all gone.

R: It's all gone. Keep going. Can you see it or is it all gone?

M: All gone.

R: It's all gone.

M: It is all gone.

R: All gone. Monster's teeth are all gone. OK, can you draw me a new picture?

M: With this?

R: Whichever one you want. Do you want to use that one?

M: That's not the scary part. This is.

R: That's not the scary part. What's the scary part?

M: That one.

R: What is that?

M: The monsters, the monsters, the head.

R: The monster's head. OK.

M: And his mouth.

R: And his mouth.

M: And that's his mouth and that's his head.

R: OK, can you close your eyes, and the buzzies are in your socks and can you see the monster's head and his mouth? And see what happens? Can you close your eyes? Are the buzzies going? What do you think? [BLS commences] Are you done? [Michael shakes his head no] OK, can you take a deep breath and wipe it out? OK, do you want to draw another picture?

M: Nah.

R: No more pictures. What happened to this picture?

M: It's scary.

R: It's still a scary picture. What do you need to help with the monster? You're turning it off. Huh?

M: Does this go in there?

R: The other one. There you go. OK, do you need to put the buzzies on the monster picture? That scary picture?

M: What buzzies?

R: These buzzies? Do you want to put them on this picture? Do you want to do that?

M: Yeah, I need this.

R: Yeah, what are you gonna do with it?

M: Make it go away.

R: Make it go away. OK. All right.

M: Yeah. I'll fix it. This goes on there.

R: I told you the wrong way. You were right. There we go. Are you gonna put them on the scary picture? Can you hold them? There you go.

M: I think these didn't work.

R: You don't think they're working?

M: No.

R: No. What do you need to make that go away?

M: Can't do it.

R: Can't do what?

M: Make these go away.

R: What if we used your magic crayon? What if we do that? Do you want this? Can you do a whole bunch really fast? Really fast. Make it go away so we can't see it. Make that monster go away faster, faster, faster. There you go. Get all of it. What's this part? Do you want to make it go away, too?

M: It's all gone.

R: It's all gone? Wow. Let's draw a new picture. That one's all gone. Now what?

M: Now it's like this.

R: OK, do you want a different color than your magic crayon to make it go away?

M: I don't want to do any more pictures.

R: You don't. OK, you're done with your pictures?

M: Yeah.

R: OK, Michael, remember what we were drawing pictures of? Do you want to put that in your pocket? That's good, in case you need it at home.

M: All right.

R: All right. Keep it at home in case you need. OK, Michael, remember when I asked you about that picture and how scary it was? Is it this big, this big, or this big? How big is it now?

M: This big.

R: It's still really big. Oh my goodness, what are we gonna do?

M: I don't know.

R: What do you need, do you need Spider Man to help you?

M: I could do it.

R: You can do it. How can you do it?

M: I can.

R: You can make it not be so scary.

M: No.

R: No. I'm confused. Can you make that part not so scary anymore? Do you need Spider Man to come with you?

M: Uh huh.

R: Maybe you could unzip him and get inside of him and have Spider Man there to help you.

M: I can do that.

R: You could do that?

M: Yeah.

R: What would Spider Man do?

M: Push him out of my room.

R: Push him out of my room. Can you do that? Who else do you need to help you push him out of your room?

M: I could do it.

R: Wow, you could do it? All by yourself? Wow, let's put these buzzies on and see if you can push him outside of your room all by yourself. Can you do that for me? Can you put this on and see if you can push him out of your room all by yourself?

M: Yeah, I could.

R: You could. Good job.

M: I'm gonna hold them.

R: You're gonna hold them.

M: Yeah.

R: You could take your shoes off if it would make it easier to put them in your socks. What do you think?

M: Hey, a bug!

R: Hey, a bug. Oh, you're right. What should we do? [A bug walked across the office floor.]

M: What?

R: Just let him go or what should we do? Squish him?

M: Yeah, Squish him.

R: Well, hey, maybe you could put the buzzies in your pockets because I think your pockets usually work pretty good. Oh, you got him.

M: I just got him [referring to the poor bug].

R: I'll put him in the trash can, OK? Do you want to put the buzzies in your pocket?

M: Yeah.

R: Do you want to try that? Oh, there you go. Now what are you gonna do to him? Are you gonna push him out of your room?

M: Yeah.

R: OK, are you ready? Do you have your muscles? Have you got everything you need? Are you ready? OK, let's close your eyes. You ready, got your muscles? Let's go. [BLS commences] Take a deep breath. What happened?

M: I pushed him out?

R: You did? The whole way out? Can he come back in?

M: Nope.

R: Never? Never, ever, ever? OK, what do you need? What are you gonna do to him so he can never come back in?

M: I'll push him out.

R: Push him out. OK, Michael, OK, remember we said about that thing and how much it was scaring you . . . how much it was bothering you. How big is it now? Is it this big, or this big, or this big?

M: This big.

R: It's this little for real? OK, can we do the buzzies one more time so you can get really strong? What do you think, back in your socks or your ears?

M: My ears.

R: You wanna try them on your ears. We'll make sure we've got all of you with the buzzies your socks, your feet, tummy, head, and now ears. Do you want them on your ears? Are you ready?

M: Yeah.

R: OK. [BLS commences] Take a breath. What happened?

M: I pushed him out!

R: You pushed him out. Uh oh. Hey, Michael, now that you pushed him out all gone, do you remember these pictures that you drew when you were over here at this scary, the bad thought, where Michael is now on the bridge from the sad thought to the happy thought? Where's Michael now?

M: The happy thought?

R: Where does it go now? [Michael moved his magnet and placed it on the PC.] Wow, the whole way over there? How about where that feeling was in your head? How does your head feel now?

M: Good.

R: What did you find back there? Are there more bugs back there?

M: No.

R: OK, Michael, so can I ask you tonight when you go home and you're in your bed and if that monster comes, what are you gonna do?

M: Push him out of my room.

R: And how about tomorrow night? What are you gonna do tomorrow night?

M: Stay in my bed.

R: But what are you gonna do to the monster?

M: Push him out!

R: Push him out. Hey, can we do buzzies one more time? Because we forgot part, we forgot your knees. OK, and we've gotta make all your body really strong to push him out. OK, do you wanna do your knees? Do you wanna hold them on your knees?

M: I don't wanna do my knees.

R: Can we do your knees and then we'll go play? To make you big and strong with the monsters. Where are your knees at?

M: Right there.

R: Do your knees so tomorrow night you become your biggest strongest, you can push him out of your room.

M: Yeah.

R: Take a deep breath and you're really strong. Are you super strong?

M: Yeah.

R: So are you ready to go play?

M: Yeah.

R: Are you all done?

M: Yeah.

R: Thank you for helping me make a movie.

CHAPTER 7

EMDR Phases 5, 6, and 7: Installation, Body Scan, and Closure

This chapter is a detailed description of how to integrate the Installation, Body Scan, and Closure phases of the EMDR protocol. The chapter includes procedural considerations for clinical decision making in EMDR psychotherapy with children through these three phases of the EMDR protocol. Because these three phases can occur very quickly with children, we decided to include all three phases in one chapter.

PHASE 5: INSTALLATION PHASE

After completing the Desensitization Phase, with the child reporting a Subjective Units of Disturbance (SUD) of 0, the therapist then will coach the child through installation of the positive cognition. The goal of the Installation Phase is to strengthen the validity of the Positive Cognition until it becomes a 7.

During the Installation Phase, the therapist links together the initial incident and the positive cognition and then checks the Validity of Cognition (VoC) with the child. When the therapist proceeds with the installation of the Positive Cognition, the therapist first checks to make sure the positive cognition initially chosen still fits or if another positive cognition now fits better for the child. Specific instructions for wording to use with young children is included later in this chapter.

After the client reports the VoC, the therapist proceeds with bilateral stimulation (BLS) and each time checks the VoC. This can be very annoying to clients, especially if the VoC gets stuck at less than a 7. If the VoC stays at a rating less than a 7 for several sets of BLS, the therapist then can ask the child, "What would it take for it to be a 7?" or "What would it take for the positive thought to be stronger?" Children typically will express what is preventing the positive cognition from strengthening. For example, some children may be very practical and say things that are very present oriented like, "It will get stronger once I get to eat" or "It will get stronger after I get to play." I (R.T.) asked a child what would help the VoC get stronger, and she simply reported, "Time." Some children will say fun things like, "It will get stronger when I kick that monster's butt." Children are dynamic and unpredictable. Again, it is the therapist's attunement to the child that will assist in clinical decision making about the child's progression with strengthening the VoC.

The installation process proceeds fairly quickly with children, to the degree that therapists may question the success of the process. With the installation process, children will just be done, and this can happen quickly. If the therapist used the VoC bridge when initially identifying the negative and positive cognition, some children will spontaneously get up and go to the VoC bridge and move the marker to show that the child is at the good thought on the VoC bridge. Sometimes the therapist can ask the child to report where the child is on the VoC bridge. This can be conducted with any technique the therapist used to initially identify the negative and positive cognitions and measure the VoC. Children will frequently move from a VoC of 1 to a VoC of 7 with occasional steps on the bridge. If the child reports a VoC of 4, use BLS to strengthen the positive cognition.

The speed and rate of the BLS should replicate what was used with the child during the Desensitization Phase. If the therapist was using 24 repetitions during desensitization, then continue with 24 repetitions during the Installation Phase.

Installation of the positive cognition is different than the procedure for safe place. When installing the positive cognition, the therapist wants any new and unprocessed material to come up. If the child reports new disturbing material, the therapist simply says, "Go with that." If new material arises during installation of the positive cognition, the EMDR process is actually once again in the Desensitization Phase, and the therapist continues with BLS. This continues until the channel has cleared or the time is over for the session, and the therapist needs to close down an incomplete session, as described in chapter 6.

Children do not typically report new material, but it is important to complete this step of the process. Once the child reports the VoC as a 7, it is helpful to continue installation of the positive cognition (PC) beyond a 7 to see if the child can make even more positive associations because that is when the child gets generalizable effects. Children may struggle with generalizable effects because children tend to be more concrete and present oriented, but a child may make associations to other situations or events in his or her life.

For example, I (R.T.) worked with a child who was reprocessing an incident with a friend at school, and during the Installation Phase, the child began to connect the positive cognition with relationships with other friends. The child reported, "You know, I know how to be friends with David. But you know, I have more new friends like Andrew and Max, too." The child had generalized his ability to be a friend to other children and was noting how his new beliefs about himself had impacted all his friendships.

Sometimes children will make additional associations, and sometimes the child will not report further associations, but reports from parents and the school may indicate that the child's behavior has changed in several areas, suggesting that the positive cognition has actually generalized and the child is feeling better about himself or herself. Children may start reporting more positive memories or even more positive current experiences. Some children may come to sessions even with a more positive outlook on life. Installing a positive cognition with a child seems to have a greater impact in that children feel more competent and capable of tackling difficult experiences in their lives. It is almost as if installing the positive cognition and the child's experience of thinking one thing positive about himself or herself gives the child a template for future experiences both in therapy and in his or her life. Children seem to experience a sense of accomplishment and belief that things can get better and that therapy can help.

Once you get to installation, it can go very quickly and naturally. Children move easily to more positive thoughts and adaptive solutions.

Script for Installation of Positive Cognition (PC)

Installing the PC is about linking the desired PC with the original memory/incident or picture:

1. "Do the words _________ [repeat the PC] still seem right, or are there other positive words that would be better now?"
2. "When you think about that thing we talked about at the beginning and you say those words _________ [repeat PC], how true

do those words feel right now, from 1, 'it's not true at all,' to 7, 'it's really true'?"

3. Say, "Now think about that event and say those words, _________ [repeat PC], and follow," then do a set of BLS.
4. Then check the VoC again. "When you think about that thing we talked about at the beginning and you say those words _________ [repeat PC], how true do those words feel right now from 1, 'it's not true at all,' to 7, 'it's really true'?"
5. Continue doing sets of BLS as in Step 2, as long as the material is becoming more adaptive. If the child reports a 7, repeat Step 3 again to strengthen, and continue until it no longer strengthens. Then go on to the body scan.
6. If, after several sets of BLS, the child still reports a 6 or less, check the appropriateness of the PC, and address any blocking belief (if necessary) with additional reprocessing.

Challenges to Installing the PC With Children

Because some children feel so much better after installing the PC, it may be difficult to get the child to continue with the body scan. With young children, the cognitions, emotions, and body sensations are so closely related that there is a simultaneous improvement in all areas. The positive cognition, emotion, and body sensation improve almost as if the pieces are all one unit, rather than separate processes. The therapist's awareness of the child's developmental mastery and previous interactions in therapy should cue the therapist to this possibility. For example, if the negative cognition is an emotion, installation of the positive cognition may concurrently alleviate the disturbance of the emotion that is integrally related to the body sensation. For younger children, the differentiation between thoughts, emotions, and body sensations appears to be less than with older children and adolescents. We are not suggesting that the therapist omit these steps of the protocol, but instead, this is a way for the therapist to conceptualize the child's responses during the Installation and Body Scan Phases of EMDR. We still recommend that the therapist check the SUD and the body sensations.

Children often feel good at this point and may even refuse to do the body scan or may report what the child thinks the therapist wants to hear in order that the child can go play. Because emotions and body sensations are so closely linked in young children, or because emotions and body sensations may even be the same thing for young children, children report that they feel good and do not require a body scan to complete the process. However, if at all possible, it is important to ask the child to scan his or her body for any additional disturbance.

Procedural Considerations

As with each step of the EMDR protocol, the therapist needs to focus on managing clinical time in a session. Once the VoC is installed, the therapist must determine if there is sufficient time to complete the body scan. It is important not to stop a session during body scan, if at all possible. With children, body scan is typically a very quick process. The best predictor of how the child will process the body scan is based on the therapist's previous experience working with the child. The therapist will have had experience with the child and have some insight into how the child functions from teaching skills to the child during the Preparation Phase. It is not always possible to predict what will happen with a child during the body scan process, but if the therapist is attuned to the child, this should be a fairly predictable phase of the EMDR protocol.

If there is not sufficient time in the session, the therapist should continue with the steps to close an incomplete session. If there is time in the session and the therapist feels pretty comfortable proceeding, then the next phase is body scan.

PHASE 6: BODY SCAN

Once the positive cognition has strengthened and holds at a VoC of 7 or greater, the next phase of EMDR is the Body Scan Phase. The goal of the Body Scan Phase is to clear any physical disturbance associated with the target memory. If the child is reticent to complete the body scan, the therapist can ask the child to participate in a different type of BLS such as changing from taps to butterfly hugs. Or, if using the "buzzies," the therapist can ask the child to put the buzzies on his or her head and then move to the child's ears and then arms, and continue until the child holds the buzzies on his or her toes to make sure everything is "cleaned out." This is where the therapist needs to be creative to keep the child in the process until it can be completed. However, we would not suggest that the therapist prolong the body scan any longer than necessary. By observing the child's body language and affect, the therapist will have indications as to how the child is feeling.

Children may need to be taught how to do a body scan. Initially, the therapist can simply follow the script. Some children relate easily to the body scan, while others may need encouragement to continue because the child has lost interest in the therapy process or because the child has lost focus and needs help to return to the body scan. This is where the child may need to be reminded of the skills the child learned during the Preparation Phase regarding mindfulness and body sensations. The therapist may have to remind the child by saying, "Some people feel it in their heads. Some people feel things in their heart, or tummy, or legs." The therapist can demonstrate a body scan. There can be a great deal of overlap between installing the positive cognition and the body scan with children, especially when the child moves through these phases very quickly.

Body scan goes along with emotional education; children will often say, if you ask them to scan their body, "I have a Band-Aid here" or "I cut my knee." Through coaching children to notice where their body is relaxed or tense, strong or weak, with butterflies or other disturbances, the child learns mindfulness and awareness of body sensations.

Script for Body Scan

We have found that the body scan procedure can require more active direction and demonstration from the therapist. We will use our hands to demonstrate to the child that the child is to scan from the top of his or her head to the tip of his or her toes.

"Close your eyes; concentrate on that thing you told me about and the words _________ [repeat the final PC], and notice your whole body, from the top of your head to the bottom of your feet, and tell me where you feel anything." If any sensation is reported, do a set of BLS. If a discomfort is reported, reprocess until discomfort fully subsides. Then do the body scan again to see if there are still any negative sensations. If a positive or comfortable sensation is reported, do BLS to strengthen the positive feeling. If discomfort is noticed, have the child focus on the discomfort and use BLS to address the negative feeling until the child reports a clear body scan.

Procedural Considerations

If the child reports a clear body scan, and there is time in the session, the therapist can process through current symptoms and possibly even move forward to a future template. With children, reprocessing a target from past to future can go very quickly and be accomplished in one session.

As with adults, children with more complex trauma may require several sessions to process a target from the past. We have found that with children, you cannot predict how long it will take to process a target. Some children with what would seem to be small *t* traumas may take some time to reprocess, while other children with big *T* traumas may process very quickly. We can only encourage therapists to stay attuned to the individual child and be tenacious.

If you, as the therapist, get confused, ask the child to confirm that the positive cognition is installed and the body scan is clear, and that there is nothing currently bothering them. Again, if the current belief is positive and the child reports no disturbance, the therapist then does several BLS to help the child assimilate the information and develop a positive template for future action. This is the three-pronged approach of EMDR.

Future Template, Closure of an Incomplete Session, or Closure? At this point, the therapist will need to use clinical judgment to determine whether to continue with present triggers and future template, proceed with closing an incomplete session, or determine that the session is complete and that it is appropriate to continue with closure. Sometimes a therapist will not have enough time to complete this future template process all in one session. If time is limited, the therapist should omit future template at this point and proceed with closure of an incomplete session to end the current session. If future template is omitted, the therapist should return to the future template process in the next session immediately after completing reevaluation. With EMDR, this is the three-pronged approach of past–present–future, where past events, present or current stimuli, and then future template are implemented.

If there is time in the session and the past event is reprocessed, and the client is reporting that in the moment, the symptoms related to the target are cleared, then the therapist assists the child in developing a future template.

FUTURE TEMPLATE

The future template of EMDR is like rehearsal for the future. With the therapist's help in imagining any challenges that would prevent the client from being successful in a future endeavor. The future template can be conducted either imaginarily/in vivo or, if appropriate, as live practice for the future. We help clients practice in the safety of our offices with our support and guidance so when the client goes out in the world, he or she feels prepared and competent.

Future template can be confusing because the future template is not about the incident or event, but about the symptoms and the positive cognition. If a child comes to therapy because of anxiety about riding in a car, and the Touchstone Event is a car accident, the future event is not the child imaging being in another car accident. The future template is about the child imagining riding in the car and becoming anxious and practicing the positive cognition, such as "I can handle riding in the car," and new skills, such as "if I get nervous, I can practice deep breathing and listen to my music so I can relax." This would be a future template about a specific skill the child wants to develop. See Figure 7.1 for an example.

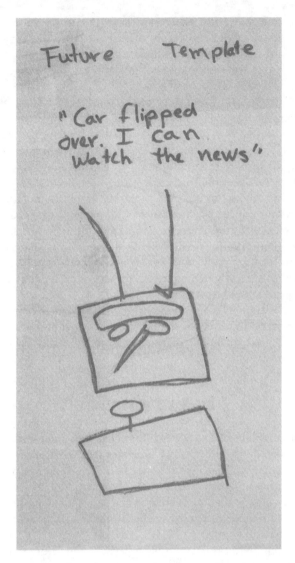

FIGURE 7.1 This is a picture of Jeremiah's future template showing his desire to be able to watch the news. The picture he has drawn is of a television depicting a car accident with the car flipped upside down on a TV news story. He tells me (C.S.) to write, "Car flipped over. I can watch the news."

The future template can be set up in general terms or as a specific rehearsal for future events: "When you think about the work we've done since we've been together, you've done a great job working on all the things that were bothering you. So let's see how that might help you with now and tomorrow. What is something you would like to be able to do?" Sometimes you get "I want to get ice cream." OK, so the therapist may have to offer some guidance. For example, when you started therapy with the child, you noted that one of the child's symptoms was that she has not been able to sleep over at a friend's house because she gets scared. So the therapist might say, "Before you told me that you wanted to be able to go to sleepovers, but you get too scared. Would that be something we could imagine you doing in the future?" Then you proceed with the client imaging sleeping at a friend's house and associated adaptive responses.

With the future template, the therapist identifies the desired response and the negative and positive cognitions, along with the remainder of the procedural steps, and then desensitizes the future template. While processing the future template, the therapist needs to do the same number of BLS saccades as during desensitization because the therapist wants negative material to come up. The number of saccades for future template can be confusing because the purpose of longer sets is to reprocess the target. Future template is a target, not a mastery installation. Future template is to focus on anticipatory anxiety or a missing skill set. If the child is missing a specific skill, the therapist may need to stop and teach a new skill, such as relaxation or deep breathing, or just remind the child of a skill that can be used in the future. Some children may need to be taught assertiveness or how to speak up. The therapist may need to use a cognitive interweave to make a link for the child with the future desired behavior and a skill that the child may need to successfully enact the desired behavior. For example, the child may be processing a future trip the family is taking in the car, but the child is continuing to be anxious or fearful of taking the trip. The therapist can then offer, "Well, you told me that you can help yourself relax if you listen to Hanna Montana's music and take deep breaths. I'm wondering if that would be something you can try while riding in the car?" We are not suggesting that the therapist stop processing the future template to teach deep breathing, but instead use a cognitive interweave to help the child link up with a skill that the child has already learned and has reported to work in other situations and that they might be able to use in the future situation.

If new negative material emerges during future template, then that is the next target. How do you determine if it is the same target or a new target? Clinical judgment: If it is a new target, the therapist can instruct the client to contain the new target for reprocessing later.

We recommend that future template with children be more immediate. Instead of processing all past events and present symptoms before moving to the future, we suggest that after a child has processed a past event and current symptoms, that the therapist take that process to the future. Because children are more present oriented, children need current positive behavioral actions to practice, which can be empowering to them. By learning new skills and feeling more competent both in therapy and in their lives, children often experience a positive association to the therapy process. Therefore we suggest that with children, once earlier memories and present triggers and symptoms are adequately resolved regarding the specific target, the therapist explore how the child would rather feel and act in the future. The therapist may have to teach the skills to the child (e.g., social skills, assertiveness, anger management), but the process is adjusted for children in that the three-pronged approach is applied in a more immediate fashion with children.

Future Template Script

Target. "What would you like to be able to do?" (positive behavior like "sleep in my own bed").

NC/PC/VoC. "When you think about that thing you'd like to be able to do, what's the bad thought?" (Therapist identifies new negative cognition [NC] for future action.) Therapist then asks the child, "What would you rather tell yourself instead?" or therapist explains, "What's the good thought?" Then therapist elicits VoC for new PC by asking, "When you think about that thing you want to be able to do and those words __________ [therapist repeats PC], how true does that seem to you right now, from 1, being completely false or not true, to 7, being completely true?"

Emotion. Therapist continues by identifying emotion by saying to the child, "When you think about that thing you want to be able to do, what's the feeling that goes with that?"

Subjective Units of Disturbance. Therapist continues by identifying SUD by saying to child, "How disturbing does that feel?"

Body Sensation. Therapist then identifies body sensation by asking, "Where do you feel that in your body?" (Therapist can use examples of body sensations, as discussed previously.)

Once the therapist has elicited a future target, NC/PC, VoC, emotion, SUD, and body sensation for future desired behaviors/actions/feelings, therapist continues by saying, "Sometime in the next day or so, I want you to think about __________ [the desired positive behavior, e.g., sleeping in my own bed alone; handling anger in an appropriate way] with those words __________ [say the new PC] with all the __________ [elicit positive visual cues], _________ [positive sounds], and _________ [positive kinesthetic sensations]." Therapist processes future template with BLS: 24 saccades. If something negative comes up, then process the negative through with whatever comes up as the target. If the adaptive resolution continues in a positive direction, continue as follows:

"Now, I want you to imagine (or pretend) in three nights from now with the same _________ [desired positive behavior]."
Do BLS.
"Now, in 1 week, . . . [same words and scenario]."
Do BLS.
"Now, in 1 month, . . . [same words and scenario]."
Do BLS.
"Now, let's pretend we are seeing yourself when you're bigger and one time when you would need _________ [desired behavior]. Imagine the _________ [positive behavior] and _________ [PC]."
Do BLS.

You can have the child draw a picture, use the sand tray, or create a clay sculpture at any point. Stay attuned to evaluate any negative associations or distortions that may emerge. The child should feel emotionally, physically, and cognitively comfortable with the anticipated event.

When the future template has been completed, the therapist then returns to reprocess another target. Once again, time management in the session dictates whether or not to begin reprocessing another target or to close the session, with a plan to reprocess another target at the next session. Closure includes debriefing the client and normalizing the experience in the session, while also preparing the client for what might occur between sessions. It is important to take the time to bring the client to a comfortable state before leaving the office, while also explaining to the child and parents what to predict between sessions.

A target is completed when the SUD is 0, the VoC is 7, and the client is reporting a clear body scan. Closure can be applied at the end of a session where there is a completed target. (For instructions on closing an incomplete session, we refer the reader to chapter 6.)

PHASE 7: CLOSURE

The Closure Phase of EMDR occurs any time the therapist needs to close a session. The goal of the Closure Phase is to choose an appropriate ending point for the session, while assisting the client in debriefing and shutting down any disturbance that arose during the session. Once the therapist has assisted the child in transitioning to a more comfortable state, the last goal of the Closure Phase is to prepare the child and parent for in between sessions.

We have also included in this chapter additional tools for unfinished sessions, teaching skills for children and parents to use between sessions, and how to use a Child/Adolescent Monitoring Form (see Appendix III) for children and parents to track progress in therapy.

Choosing an Ending Point for the Session

As we previously discussed, it is important for the therapist to manage the time available for the session, while allowing time to debrief the child and assist the child in achieving a more comfortable state in which to leave the office. If the client is reprocessing a target during the Desensitization Phase, we refer the therapist to Appendix VIII for a script for closing an incomplete session during desensitization. If the therapist has moved to the Installation or Body Scan Phase, we have included scripts in this chapter. If the client has completed reprocessing the target with a SUD of 0, and the positive cognition is installed with a VoC of 7, we encourage therapists either to allow time for a completed body scan or to end the session after completing the Installation Phase. During each step of the EMDR protocol, the therapist is anticipating what the client will need to end the session, while planning on an appropriate point to wind down from the work that has occurred during the session to allow the client to leave the session in a calm state. It is not appropriate to end a session with a client in an extremely agitated or disturbed state, and especially not in the middle of an abreaction, if at all possible. Learning how to pace the therapeutic process is an important tool for all therapies.

Tools for Assisting a Child to Debrief and Regroup at the End of a Session

There are many creative and fun tools for helping children to debrief and regroup at the end of the session. We included some techniques for closing incomplete sessions in chapter 6, but there are additional tools that can be used to close therapy at any time. We have included information on containers in chapter 4 and will further explain how to use containers as well as homework, relaxation, and visualization skills, for children at the end of a session.

Containers. Throughout the book, we have discussed the use of containers in EMDR. Even though we have discussed using containers in chapter 4 during the Preparation Phase and in chapter 6 for use in the Desensitization Phase for closing incomplete sessions, the use of containers can also be helpful for between sessions, as a mastery tool for managing intense affect, for closure, and as part of future template. Containers can be used for closure when the session is incomplete or for managing intense affect. We teach children to use containers to store their bad thoughts or scary feelings that overwhelm them until they can each be reprocessed. Any kind of small box, plastic container, lock box, or other container that can be either made in the therapy session or purchased from craft stores can be used as containers. Children are very creative, and the therapist can even have the child draw a picture of the container the child might feel he or she needs to manage intense affect or flashbacks. Children can use as many containers as they need to cope and continue functioning at home and school.

Launching Containers Into the Future. When a child is using containers to assist him or her in managing intense affect, it is helpful to ask the child to launch the container into the future and ask the child, "What do you think you will need to someday be able to deal with the things you put in the container? When do you think that will happen?" By launching containers into the future, like time capsules, the therapist indicates to the child that they will return to reprocess any issues that are put into the containers and that the therapist is predicting that the child will someday have the skills to successfully deal with anything that bothers him or her.

Tools for Between Sessions, Including Coping Strategies, if Additional Information Arises Between Sessions

Children need to be taught to use their containers to manage any intense affect that may arise between sessions and to use whatever coping skills the therapist has taught the child during sessions. Children gain confidence in their ability to manage intense affect when they have learned coping strategies.

Homework. EMDR does not require homework; however, it is helpful to encourage the child and the parent to practice any relaxation skills the child has learned in therapy and for the parent to practice any new parenting skills he or she may have learned. It is also helpful for the child to practice using his or her Safe/Calm Place and to attempt to use the Safe/Calm Place any time that the child might feel distressed between sessions.

Relaxation and Visualization Skills for Children. Children benefit from learning deep breathing exercises, visualization, and imagery skills. See chapter 9 for additional tools for teaching children relaxation and visualizations skills.

Script for Closure/Debriefing the Experience

Say to the child, "Well, we've done a lot of work today, and you're awesome. Before I see you next time, you may think about stuff, so would you draw me a picture or write something down or tell your mom and dad if you have any thoughts, dreams, or feelings that you want to remember to tell me or would be good for me to know?"

SUMMARY

In this chapter, we combined three phases of EMDR: Installation, Body Scan, and Closure. We purposely combined the three phases for several reasons. First, the flow from installing the positive cognition to body scan is very simple, while moving to closure happens naturally. In addition, the movement from installing the positive cognition to a clear body scan often happens quickly with children, and then children are just done, and the therapist needs to be prepared to close the session on a positive note to keep the child engaged in therapy. It is important for the therapist to understand the relationship between installation and body scan to be able to dance with children in a fluid and creative manner. It is our experience that children move so quickly between these phases that even seasoned therapists miss what has happened with the child in the session. Children may demonstrate a clear body scan with body language, and many do not appreciate the therapist's need to belabor the point. Kids are just done, and you can see it. Children might stand up with confidence, straighten their posture and stretch their arms out wide, and make statements like "I can do this" or "I'm not scared anymore."

Once the positive cognition is installed, the body scan is clear, and the therapist has closed the session, case conceptualization moves to reevaluating the progress on specific targets and the entire course of therapy.

CHAPTER 8

EMDR Phase 8: Reevaluation

The eighth phase of the EMDR protocol is the Reevaluation Phase. The word *reevaluation* is used in several different places during the EMDR protocol. Reevaluation is the process by which the therapist evaluates the progress in treatment on a specific target and progress in the overall course of treatment.

Reevaluation first occurs at the beginning of each session of psychotherapy, after the Assessment Phase is completed for the first time. In case conceptualization of the overall course of treatment, the therapist has the client return to reevaluate the original target memory until that target memory is completed. An ongoing process of reevaluating progress on the specific target through desensitization, installation of the positive cognition, and clear body scan continues with each session. Reevaluation continues until the target is cleared and a new target is selected and the therapist conducts the procedural steps of the Assessment Phase on the new target.

Reevaluation also occurs during overall case conceptualization, when it appears that all targets have been reprocessed, symptoms have resolved, and the treatment plan is now focused on discharge. Reevaluation of the treatment plan goals, which include processing targets through the three-pronged protocol and ending with future template for each target, occurs when the client and therapist believe that they are coming to the end of the therapeutic process. The symptoms with which the client initially entered treatment have now resolved, and the client has a plan for healthy functioning in the future. Ideally, graduation from therapy would leave the client with a plan for the future that integrates all that the client has learned from therapy. Some clients may have decided that they have made significant progress in this episode of care, and we leave the door open for the client to return for tune-up sessions. We make sure that we leave the client with an understanding that returning to therapy is not failure, but actually predictable in life. Reevaluation occurs for the client after discharge as the client is able to assess the ongoing impact of therapy in his or her daily life.

For the purposes of clarification, we will refer to the reevaluation that occurs at the end of the overall therapeutic process as *treatment evaluation*. The goal of reevaluation in EMDR in the eight-phase EMDR protocol is to assess progress in treatment, whether between sessions or at the end of treatment.

Reevaluation is extremely important in psychotherapy with children. Since it is more difficult to assess a child's progress in treatment, whether because of the occurrence of state change, in which the child simply reports feeling better, or because children are not as demonstrative of affect. No matter what the reason, it is essential to take the time in therapy to reevaluate symptoms and targets. Children may process quickly and report feeling much better, but there may be a remnant of the channel that the parent notices that the child is not identifying as a problem or symptom.

Case Study: Jeremiah

With Jeremiah whose case was discussed in chapter 5, Jeremiah reprocessed his fears of the bad news on television—and in the following session, reported no disturbance on his targets on the map. He felt significantly better, and his parents noticed great symptom reduction; however, he was still checking the locks on the house before they went to bed.

Jeremiah's case illustrates why it is important to include the parents in reevaluating the child's symptoms to make sure that they reprocessed the whole way through. Sometimes children do not identify symptoms that the parents identify.

Case Study: Brianna and the Rottweiler

As previously discussed in chapter 5, Brianna reprocessed the traumatic memories of being attacked by a Rottweiler dog, and her symptoms had cleared, and therapy was discontinued. However, Brianna returned for therapy 6 months later, when another neighbor's Rottweiler dog unexpectedly lunged at her. Brianna began to display symptoms that had been previously treated. Her clinging behavior resurfaced after the second encounter with the Rottweiler dog. The symptoms were milder and easier to reprocess than during the first episode of care.

There is new research (Zaghrat-Hodali et al., in press) on resiliency in children who have reprocessed a traumatic event with EMDR who later encounter a similar traumatic event. Initial findings suggest that the symptoms at the second traumatic event are not as severe as the initial trauma. Reevaluating the progress in treatment is important, and even when symptoms appear to have abated, similar symptoms can arise in the future, if the child experiences new stressful and/or traumatic events.

REEVALUATION PHASE

There are three components to reevaluation. One is to review changes in the environment between sessions. A second part is to assess the specific target, and a third part is to assess treatment progress. Again, we refer the therapist to chapter 3, on interviewing the child and parents regarding the child's current life situation and response to treatment. We recommend that no matter whether or not the target was completed in the previous session, or it was an incomplete session, the therapist needs to include the following steps at the beginning of every session.

Review What Is Currently Happening in the Child's Environment

At the beginning of each session, the therapist should review the current status and life situation for the child, especially in light of the treatment process. It is important to note any changes that may have occurred between sessions in the child's life. Has the family moved? Did school start between sessions? Was the child moved from a shelter to a foster home since the last session? The therapist needs to be ever aware of the impact of current environmental changes that could present as intervening variables to the therapeutic process.

Clinical Implications

If the child or parent is identifying an urgent issue in the child's life, it is important to evaluate the situation in light of the previous therapy session. The therapist always needs to reevaluate the target in light of the current circumstances in the child's life. We suggest that the therapist consider a predictable and consistent series of questions with which to begin each session. We always have the parents and child in the session, especially during the reevaluation process. We start with a general question to both parent and child: "How was your week, or how have things been since the last time we got together?" After the response, ask, "How is school? How is it going with your friends? How are things at home?" If the responses are limited or little information is offered, we might also add, "Tell me one good thing that happened since the last time I saw you," then, "Tell me one bad thing that happened that bothered you." After this series, we also explore what ramifications the previous session may have had on the child and family.

Review the Child's Response to Previous Sessions

It is also important to review the child's response to previous sessions from both the child's perspective and the parent's perspective and to briefly explore any internal or external changes in the child's behavior. Has the child started or stopped wetting the bed? Has the child been getting in trouble in school? Have the child's presenting symptoms increased or decreased? Has the child made progress since the last session? Did the symptom related to the original target change in any way? We have found that children will frequently report internal changes, while parents report external changes. It is common for children and parents to be surprised by the other's responses. Parents often focus on identifying symptoms, without offering progress in treatment, while children may underreport ongoing symptoms because their internal experience is positive. This is why we recommend interviewing parents and children together to gain a more comprehensive assessment of the child's progress in treatment. It is also helpful to discuss the Child/Adolescent Symptom Monitoring form (see Appendix III) because it makes parents think about symptoms that have disappeared.

Reevaluate the Specific Target

After reviewing what has happened to the child between sessions, the therapist next explores any new triggers or memory links that arose between sessions. The therapist should ask the child in general terms, "Do you remember what we worked on last time you were here?" However, we often find children to be so present oriented that they do not remember the last session. So we progress with a gentle reminder such as,

"You know the sleeping thing we worked on last week?" We try to use a cue word or more generic reminder to link up with the previous work; however, being more specific with children may be necessary to prompt them.

Once the child appears to have linked to the work that transpired during the previous session, we then ask, "What do you think now, and how does that bother you now?" We continue with the script for reevaluation, as follows.

Script for Reevaluation. At the start of every session after EMDR has been introduced, the therapist assesses the treatment progress and resolves previously activated traumas:

1. "Remember what we worked on last time? Did you think about it at all? Was there anything that you wanted me to know since our last session?"
2. Ask the parent if there have been any changes since the last session (i.e., changes in symptoms, new behaviors, etc.).
3. The therapist reevaluates the degree of processing of the previous target to determine whether or not the target has been resolved (SUD) = 0, (VoC) = 7. SUD of more than 0 or VoC of less than 7 is only acceptable if ecologically valid. The therapist reevaluates SUD as the child focuses on the target from the previous session. If not, what remains disturbing as the client holds the target in his or her awareness (image, cognition, emotion, sensation)? "When you go back to what we worked on last time, what do you get now?" After the child answers, the therapist responds, "When you think about that _________ [client's answer], how much does it bother you now?" (Therapist elicits SUD.) Therapist continues by asking the child, "And when you think about the thing we worked on and the thought _________ [therapist repeats client's positive cognition from the previous session], how true does that feel for you right now, from 1, 'not true at all,' to 7, 'totally true'?" (Therapist can use hand distance or other measure previously utilized with the specific client.)
4. Therapist continues with reprocessing, with all targets associated with current symptoms, until all the necessary targets have been reprocessed.

Procedural Considerations

In case conceptualization, it is important for the therapist to consider what occurred in the previous session, with an eye always on the treatment plan. Did the previous session end as an incomplete session, or was a target completed? If the target was completed with a SUD of 0, a VoC of 7, and a clear body scan, did the therapist complete a previous target memory, or did the session end with a completed future template? Depending on the outcome of the previous session, any changes in the child's life, and the child's responses to the previous target, the therapist will need to consider different steps in the EMDR protocol.

Reevaluation After an Incomplete Session. If the previous session ended with an incomplete target, the therapist needs to reassess the target to determine if the target resolved between sessions. Theoretically, a session could begin following an incomplete session with a SUD greater than 0, a VoC less than 7, or an incomplete body scan.

Subjective Units of Disturbance Greater Than 0. After the therapist assesses the target and determines that there is still a level of disturbance associated with the target, as evidenced by a SUD greater than 0, the therapist continues with desensitization. We refer the reader to chapter 6 for continuing desensitization after an incomplete session.

Validity of Cognition Less Than 7. If the child has reported a SUD of 0, the therapist then checks on the installation of the positive cognition. If the VoC is less than 7, the therapist continues with the installation phase, as described in chapter 7. Once the positive cognition is installed with a VoC of 7 or greater, the session continues by moving to the body scan phase.

Incomplete Body Scan. If the previous session ended with a SUD of 0 and a VoC of 7, but the body scan was not conducted or there was disturbance remaining in the body scan, the EMDR protocol continues with the Body Scan Phase, also discussed in chapter 7.

As discussed in several previous sections of this book, if the target was completed in the previous session with a SUD of 0, a VoC of 7, and a clear body scan, then the session ended with a completed target. This could have occurred with a past target, a present issue, or with future template.

Reevaluation After Completing a Target in a Previous Session. If the target was completed in the previous session, it is important to check the target and current symptoms and then move to future template. A script for conducting future template is included in Appendix VIII.

Instructions to the Therapist for Reevaluation. The therapist can use the following instructions for reevaluation:

1. Therapist assesses general functioning since previous session. Therapist reviews current status of any symptoms identified in previous session and explores any new symptoms: "Has anything changed since our last session?" Therapist reviews any notations from parent on the Child/Adolescent Symptoms Monitoring Form.

The therapist also queries the child about changes in symptoms or behaviors that have occurred since the last session.

2. For reevaluation, therapist obtains feedback on experiences/observations since last session. Ask child to return to target or incident from the previous session, per script. Check SUD and VoC on previous target. Check for any unprocessed material from previous session and probe for any new material that might have emerged.
3. If child appears stable, therapist proceeds with standard EMDR protocol. If child appears unstable, therapist continues with resource work. Therapist must discriminate between disturbance caused by situation/trauma and that caused by internal instability. The former should be processed, while the latter should be improved through strengthening resources.
4. Reestablish setting in office to provide for child comfort for EMDR processing. Review BLS as utilized in Safe/Calm Place and RDI exercises.
5. If SUD rating on previous week's target is greater than 0, continue to reprocess this target. If VoC rating for previous week's target is less than 7 (and does not appear to be ecologically valid), continue to reprocess this target. If previous week's target appears to be resolved (SUD = 0, VoC = 7) and there is a complete body scan, then move on to the next target on the treatment plan target list or move on to target current triggers associated with the memory addressed in the previous session.
6. Establish EMDR target and begin EMDR (Assessment, Desensitization, Installation, Body Scan, and Closure). Target old activated memories/material first. Proceed to focusing on current/recent triggers and future templates only after a specific old activated memory has been completely processed.
7. Complete as much work as time and circumstances allow, leaving adequate time for closure and debriefing.
8. Therapist schedules next session and escorts child and parent to waiting room/exit.

REEVALUATION AT THE END OF TREATMENT

The goal of reevaluation at the end of treatment or treatment reevaluation is to assess the treatment plan and determine what will need to occur prior to discharging the client from treatment.

The expectations and results for treatment outcome vary, depending on the population. I (C.S.) have observed children reprocess targets very quickly. This is especially true with children with single incident trauma, such as a dog bite or motor vehicle accident. I have discharged children from treatment after only three sessions because after reevaluation, symptoms had resolved and treatment was completed. In contrast, the population that I (R.T.) treat are more likely to be children from the child welfare system or children with a chronic severe history of trauma. These children also show significant progress in treatment but are much more likely to end treatment prematurely because of moves, funding issues, or the decision to take a break from treatment because the child has made a great deal of progress but will need to return in the future. Even though children with severe and chronic trauma history may still need to seek treatment in the future, these episodes of care can be very successful with EMDR and provide the child with a strong foundation for future treatment episodes.

Treatment Reevaluation With Single-Incident Traumas

When the plan is for discharge for a child with a single-incident trauma, we evaluate the child's current functioning in all areas of life and then proceed with assessing the child's response to the previous session, as discussed earlier in this chapter. We then reevaluate the target by asking, "Remember that thing we worked on last time? Well, when you think about it now, what happens?" We check the SUD, the validity of the positive cognition, and clear body scan, and if everything is holding, we then bring out the map. If there is any disturbance from any target on the map, we continue with desensitization. If the child is reporting no disturbance from anything on the map, we then check the original symptoms and goals for treatment. We have prescribed that the child practice the future template with future desired behaviors and report on his or her success. For example, is the child now able to sleep in his or her own bed?

If all the symptoms have resolved, we then validate the child's progress in therapy and encourage the child to continue to use all the skills and resources he or she has gained from therapy and remind the child and parent that they can return at any time in the future.

Treatment Reevaluation With Chronic Trauma

Treatment reevaluation for children with a history of chronic trauma is obviously more complicated and may include episodes of care when working with children with histories of child abuse or domestic violence, children in the child welfare system (including foster care and adoption), and children who have experienced a natural or man-made disaster, including the after effects of the disaster. For example, we have worked with the Gulf Coast relief effort resulting from Hurricane Katrina in the U.S. on training therapists using EMDR with children who, after more than 2 years, are not in stable housing and may never return to their homes or schools or neighborhoods. The aftermath of Katrina contributes to ongoing and chronic trauma for many children living in the Gulf Coast region.

The course of treatment with any type of psychotherapy is impacted by many variables, including funding, legal issues both from the court system and caregivers, and changes that occur within the child's treatment team. The child's treatment team in the child welfare system can at times change on a daily basis due to changes in case managers, foster placements, group home staff, attorneys, judges, and other professionals who have a decision-making role in the child's life. Reevaluation with these children becomes a more complicated process. When I (R.T.) work with children who are living in unstable and unpredictable environments, I must include reevaluation and containment skills in each session because each session with that child may be the last session I have with him or her. With reprocessing targets, the pace of the course of treatment also is slower and unpredictable. With some children, such as the homeless children I work with, EMDR may never reach the desensitization phase, but instead will focus on mastery and resource development and teaching the child coping and containment skills to help the child survive with the hope that the child will at some time in the future be in a more stable living environment and be again able to access care for another episode of care. After practicing for 25 years, I have had the experience of seeing children that I saw for episodes of care during the child's time in the child welfare system return as adults and begin therapy.

As a therapist in this type of mental health system, the goal of therapy may be to give the child a positive experience for whatever time he or she is in my office, with the hope that the therapy experience can buoy the child and give him or her confidence in the process in order that the child will seek treatment in the future. During each session, the reevaluation then must include a focus on reinforcing the child's hard work and participation in therapy as well as encouraging and supporting the child for whatever efforts the child has made in his or her environment. This is also why asking the parent or caregiver, whoever that might be, to give at least one example of what the child did well the previous week is very important. Taking that positive experience and installing it as a mastery experience is important to do each session. At the end of each session, I (R.T.) will install a mastery experience and also a future mastery experience to predict that the child will do well at a future task at home, at school, or in the community. For example, I typically ask the child about upcoming events or activities and discuss how the child can see himself or herself being successful in that future experience.

Case Study: Child With a History of Distress

I (R.T.) worked with a 5-year-old girl with a history of distress and school refusal behaviors. Each week, we worked on the targets that we had identified, but at the end of each session, I left time for the child to see herself being successful at something over the course of the next few days. With this 5-year-old, each week, we installed successive approximations of her being able to attend kindergarten, from going with her mom to register for school, to visiting her classroom on "meet the teacher" night, to actually going to school the first day. By the time it became the week before school was to start, when I asked about any fears about going to school, the little girl looked at me like I was making up fears that she had never had. When I reminded her of how we started working together to address her fears of school, she looked at me and said, "I don't remember that, and it doesn't matter anymore." After that, she grinned and asked to play a game, and the next week, she started kindergarten with all the other 5-year-olds.

With adolescents living in group homes, I (R.T.) will ask the teens to think about where they want their lives to be in 2 years, or 5 years, or 10 years. I discuss the issue of choices and that the adolescent can choose many different paths in the future, but that his or her current behavior and effort have an impact on the future. I have always discussed with adolescents that their past does not have to dictate their future, and any behavior including being an active participant in therapy is choosing not to repeat their past or those of some of their family members, and to choose a hero or heroine that they might want to be like in the future.

With children with chronic trauma histories, there is an ongoing dance between reevaluation, resourcing, and mastery that creates scaffolding for emotional regulation and competence on the child's part to be able to deal with the life he or she is currently living, while creating hope for a healthier future. Because children and adolescents are so present oriented, predicting a brighter future and finding resources for the child to be able to cope in the present is a process that is interwoven through the course of psychotherapy with EMDR.

SUMMARY

We want to emphasize the significance of ongoing reevaluation to assess reprocessing and to assist the client in feeling successful in therapy until discharge. Unlike the other seven phases of EMDR, reevaluation cycles through all the other phases of EMDR. During the Body Scan Phase, the therapist may first learn that the client has had surgery on his or her arm that the client did not report during Client History and Treatment Planning. The therapist must assess the significance to the client of the memory of the injury and subsequent medical care and reevaluate what skills the client may need to cope with that memory, and if the arm injury is a new target to be reprocessed, then case conceptualization indicates that the therapist start with the Assessment Phase on that memory. As the therapist considers the goals of treatment, reevaluation occurs during and between sessions, as does treatment reevaluation as part of discharge planning. It is important for the EMDR therapist to understand that even though reevaluation is the eighth phase of the EMDR protocol, reevaluation is not the last phase of treatment, but instead is an ongoing process that is part of all the other phases of treatment.

In the Client History and Treatment Planning Phase, reevaluation includes regularly checking on possible information from the child's past that may not have seemed important when the therapist was conducting a formal intake process, and discovering what is currently happening in the child's life that may be impacting treatment. Any of these variables can contribute to the need to reevaluate the treatment plan and revise and/or add goals to the treatment plan.

During the Preparation Phase, the therapist is regularly assessing what resources the child has and what resources the child needs to continue reprocessing with EMDR. Perhaps one of the most frequent contributors to children's reticence to continue reprocessing a target is that the child feels unprepared to cope with the information that is arising during reprocessing, and the child may need to learn additional tools or skills with which to continue reprocessing a target.

During the Assessment Phase, the EMDR protocol includes steps for reevaluating the efficacy of the positive cognition when the therapist checks to make sure the original positive cognition still fits or if a different positive cognition now feels more appropriate for the client.

With the Desensitization Phase, the therapist is reevaluating the progress made on the target and following the feeder memories, blocking beliefs, or other issues that are necessary for pacing the process of reprocessing a memory and successfully completing the memory.

In the Installation Phase, a type of reevaluation occurs when the therapist checks the VoC to make sure that the VoC is strengthening and holding. During this process, if the VoC is not strengthening or appears stuck, the therapist checks with the client to explore what is preventing the VoC from being a 7.

During the Body Scan Phase, the therapist is reevaluating the body sensations that the client identified during the Assessment Phase and checking to make sure that all disturbances are cleared from the client's body.

As we previously discussed, reevaluation is part of the closure phase, especially when the therapist is reevaluating the progress on a target and if the target is completed with a SUD of 0, a VoC of 7, and a clear body scan conceptualization of EMDR includes ongoing reevaluation.

CHAPTER 9

Emotional Resources, Coping Skills, and Strengthening Mastery Experiences for Children

This chapter was designed to provide the therapist with tools for teaching children skills for dealing with strong emotions and coping with the memories that arise during the course of psychotherapy and from experiences in their lives. The goal of this chapter is to add to the therapist's toolbox of skills for working with children in psychotherapy.

One office recommendation is that therapists absolutely need to be aware of children's genre, including games, books, movies, television shows, sports, and other current child activities. It is helpful to ask children about what they like and how they spend their free time when they have a choice.

GOALS OF RESOURCING, COPING, AND MASTERY

The goal for teaching children resourcing, coping skills, and enhancing mastery experiences is to assist the child in creating his or her own toolbox of skills to be used both in therapy and in daily life for more advanced coping. We suggest that with child clients, the therapist review the child's resources in each session and remind the child to use those resources at home and school. Ultimately, the measure of the effectiveness of the therapeutic process is for the child to be able to take the skills learned in the therapist's office and apply those skills in the child's life outside the office.

Resourcing, coping, and mastery skills also provide empowerment, mentalizing, positive foundation, emotional regulation, and boundaries and limits for children to learn, improve on, and practice in their lives. Each of these competencies assists children in dealing with life stressors and processing whatever maladaptively stored information needs to be reprocessed during EMDR. For the purposes of this book, we have defined *empowerment* as the ability to feel competent to make choices and to be able to advocate on your own behalf. *Mentalizing* is the ability to understand your own intentions and the impact you have on others and your ability to hypothesize the intentions of others and recognize how others' intentions impact you. A *positive foundation* is defined for the purpose of resourcing and mastery as creating a positive foundation with which children can tackle daily situations to set them up to meet the challenge of reprocessing trauma. And as we discussed in chapter 3, *emotional regulation* is the child's ability to regulate his or her own intense emotions. By teaching the child an array of skills, psychotherapy is both beneficial and fun for the child. Children even enjoy teaching their newly acquired skills to parents, siblings, and friends. We encourage therapists to teach children relaxation skills, breathing, mindfulness, guided imagery, progressive muscle relaxation, and other calming and self-soothing skills and techniques.

EMOTIONAL RESOURCES, COPING, AND MASTERY SKILLS

We have included an overview of skills that therapists can use in therapy with children and that therapists can teach to children and parents. Some of these may seem very obvious and others normal.

Relaxation Skills

We begin by teaching children about relaxation and then explore with the child current methods that the child already uses to relax. We ask the child to make a list of his or her top 10 favorite things the child can do to relax. We also explore ways the child can relax in more stressful environments such as school or day care.

Case Study: Doodling During Math Instruction

I (R.T.) worked with an 8-year-old boy who would become anxious and get an upset stomach every time his teacher began the math lesson in third grade. After ruling out any math-learning disabilities for the child, the little boy identified that doodling helped him relax and be able to pay attention. After asking the teacher's permission, the little boy had a small tablet he would get out during math and doodle while he listened to his teacher give instruction on math.

Breathing Techniques

Breathing is one of the simplest and most important techniques to teach children. I (C.S.) have children lie on the floor and put a book on their stomach so they learn to breathe from the bottom of their stomach. This works for older children, but with younger children, we might have the child exaggerate blowing up a balloon and learning to take really deep breaths and exhaling. With older children, it is also possible to teach them to learn to take longer and deeper breaths by simply counting and then increasing the count as the child inhales and exhales.

Guided Imagery

With guided imagery, we have the child choose a comfy place to sit in the office and have the child select a real or imaginary favorite place where the child feels most comfortable. We then take the child through a guided tour of his or her favorite place, as we ask the child questions that elicit all the senses about the place. I (C.S.) will ask the child to identify something that feels really relaxing to him or her and then have the child draw a picture of whatever he or she identifies. One child identified floating in the pool as very relaxing, while another child identified walking through an imaginary castle.

Containers

We discussed the use of containers in several previous chapters. We remind the therapist that containers can be used at any time the child needs the container for storing intense affect. We suggest that children also use containers at school when the child experiences intense emotion, but the opportunity for expression is not available at the time, and the intense emotion needs to be contained until later.

Containers for Storing Resources and Mastery Experiences. Containers can also be used in a positive light to include all the resources and skills the child needs to be able to cope in his or her life. We suggest that the child create a container to put in all his or her resources to have those available, as needed. Sometimes this means writing all the resources on a piece of paper to put in the container or toolbox that the child always has available. We have also encouraged children to draw pictures or create figures or symbols to represent their safe place, or resources, or people who help the child to be calm and self-soothe.

Containers are a fun and creative activity for children. I (R.T.) use Chinese food boxes for children to take with them to deposit anything they feel they need to contain, both in therapy and in their daily lives. I give some children to-go boxes to use on their own. (Different versions of those Chinese food boxes can be found at many craft stores.) Some children choose to leave their boxes in a safe place in my office and then make deposits and withdrawals to their containers each time they return for a session. A child makes a deposit in an actual container when he or she needs to contain something he or she is not ready to process, and then later, we make withdrawals from the container for processing in the therapy session. It is especially important to explain to children that whatever is deposited, that is, a dream, an emotion, a monster, a fear, or a memory, must later be withdrawn for later reprocessing; otherwise, the container will overflow and interfere with their lives.

Worry Dolls and Worry Rocks. I (C.S.) use worry dolls to help children contain their worries. Worry dolls are small figurines that are in a small container. Children can take the dolls out of the container and tell each doll a worry and place the doll back in the container. The child can use as many worry dolls as necessary. This can also be done with worry rocks. Children can pick from a basket of rocks I (R.T.) have in the office and use small stickers to write their worries on the rocks and place their worries in their containers. The worries the child identifies can also be targets for EMDR.

Get a Grip

I (C.S.) use the technique I call “get a grip” as a child-initiated time-out. Instead of having the parent give the child a time-out, I teach children to take a time-out when they feel themselves escalating and realize they may be losing control. I explain to children that getting a grip means getting control of yourself, your body, and your feelings. If children do not understand what a grip is, then the therapist can explain that a grip is like the tread on the bottom of their shoes that helps them not to slip and fall, or like holding on to a baseball so they can throw it better. The child can initiate or be reminded by the parent to go to his or her room and do any activity that is calming and come out when the child feels more composed. For younger children, I might suggest that they go to their rooms and see how many farm animals they can name or sing a song. Other children may need to discharge energy, so drawing an angry picture, snapping their fingers, or doing jumping jacks in their room in order to discharge energy. After the child feels calmer, the child can then choose to come out of his or her room.

Gifted children will often escalate and need to learn to self-soothe by using get a grip. Young children who have yet to develop the language skills to communicate their feelings may present with temper tantrums or meltdowns that arise from frustration at not being understood or not being able to communicate. For example, I (C.S.) find that gifted children may get overstimulated at birthday parties and may need to take a break and go in another room and get a grip. Once the child has identified something that he or she wants to do, then we will install the activity with bilateral stimulation (BLS) in the form of a future template.

Script for Getting a Grip. First, the therapist explains to the child the concept of getting a grip by saying, "Getting a grip is something that we use when we're feeling really frustrated or we're right in the middle of getting mad." We explain to children that this might happen when they are overly frustrated, tired, or hungry. The therapist further explains, "What you do is go to your room, or your mom can remind you that you might want to go to your room. After you go to your room, then you do something to get out your frustration or mad energy." Then we ask the child to identify an activity that the child thinks might help him or her to get a grip: "What do you think you could do in your room that would help you to calm down?" It is helpful to have the child identify several activities to choose from when he or she needs to get a grip. It is important to have the child imagine going through the get a grip process in the future: "Imagine yourself getting upset about something and then going to your room to get a grip." We then install the technique with BLS.

Get a Grip for a Positive Template. It is possible to take the child through the entire set of procedural steps of the Assessment Phase with get a grip as a future template. The therapist can ask the child to identify a situation when the child can imagine needing to get a grip and then elicit the bad thought (negative cognition), such as "I can't handle it" or "I'm going to explode," and the good thought (positive cognition), such as "I know how to get a grip," and complete the protocol. The child can then imagine all the possible complications that might interfere with his or her ability to get a grip, or the therapist can suggest possible bumps in the road and then process those through to successful conclusion.

The goal of get a grip is for the child to self-cue and learn to monitor his or her own emotions and learn to self-soothe and calm himself or herself. This process can be creative and fun for the child and gives the child a sense of competency and mastery in dealing with his or her own emotions.

Techniques for Discharging Intense Emotions

We use many different techniques in the office to teach children to more effectively discharge intense emotions and the body energy children typically experience with intense emotion. This includes things like drawing an angry picture, noticing their disturbing feelings and kicking their legs or stomping their feet in time with the BLS, letting the air out of the balloon, jumping jacks, running laps, swimming, and other appropriate physical activities for releasing energy to self-calm.

Calming and Soothing Skills and Techniques

In addition to breathing, guided imagery, and progressive muscle relaxation, we teach children other ways to help calm themselves.

Cool as a Cucumber. One calming technique is called "cool as a cucumber." The therapist uses cucumber slices and a body lotion that has been chilled to teach the child to self-soothe. The therapist or the child puts the cucumber slices on the child's eyes, and then the therapist or a parent can massage the child's hands with the cooling lotion, while instructing the child to take deep breaths and notice how his or her body feels with the cool sensations. This calm, cool feeling is then installed with BLS. After the child reports feeling calm, the therapist then uses the cool as a cucumber technique as part of a future template, when the therapist has the child imagine a situation in which the child predicts being upset and using the cool as a cucumber activity, or just the imagined memory of the activity, to self-calm.

Body Lotion. Scented body lotion can also be used to help children self-soothe. Using lotion not only provides a physical sensation, but also provides an olfactory experience. I (R.T.) have the child choose a lotion and then put a small amount of lotion in a take-home container. I will then have the child's parent massage the child's hands or feet with the lotion. This provides not only a comforting experience for the child, but also a bonding experience between the child and parent. I then install this calming experience and the bonding experience with BLS. I (R.T.) will discuss this further in chapter 11, in the section on EMDR with children with attachment trauma.

Transitional Objects. We have children create pictures of their resources or collages by cutting out calming things from magazines and creating a poster of things to hang in their rooms. This can be helpful when children are going to their rooms to get a grip. Another fun activity is to have the child use glow-in-the-dark fabric paint to decorate a pillowcase, a throw pillow, or a small blanket that the child can keep on his or her bed at night that reminds the child of his or her resources.

Any resources the child identifies during the resource development and installation (RDI) process can be painted on the pillowcase, pillow, or blanket (see instructions for RDI in the section Abbreviated RDI Protocol for Children at the end of this chapter). Whatever resources the child identifies as being comforting can be painted on a poster, pillowcase, pillow, or blanket. The child can paint pictures of people, pets, animals, symbols, heroes, or any other resource the child identifies as being helpful. In addition to decorating the different things, it is helpful to place a drop of essential oil on an object such as a pillow so that the olfactory senses are also engaged in calming the child. These resources identified in the office can be created in the school and home environments to remind the child of his or her resources.

I (R.T.) worked with a 5-year-old boy who identified Spider Man as a resource that helped him to feel strong. His adoptive parents bought him Spider Man bedding and posters for his room, and he had a nightlight and a flashlight that could help him to see Spider Man any time he wanted.

Dream Catchers. Children can also use dream catchers to help with scary thoughts, memories, and/or nightmares. For us, a dream catcher is an art project that children can do in which they create a hanging piece that is woven with yarn or thread that is hung above the child's bed. Children can use very simple art supplies to create a form that can then have thread or yarn woven or wrapped around the form. Children can also make dream catchers that incorporate the child's resources.

Rubber/Glue Rhyme. Rubber/glue is a resource I (C.S.) use for kids when they are complaining about bullies or siblings picking on them. I use an old rhyme that goes, "I'm rubber, you're glue. Everything bounces off of me and sticks on you." When I explained this to 9-year-old Glenda, who was complaining about kids on the playground, I said to her with a bit of sarcasm and body motions, "I'm rubber. You're glue. Everything bounces off me and sticks on you." Glenda giggled and said, "I can see myself with a rubber igloo around me when I'm on the playground." I then installed this as a resource with BLS and then did a future template, with Glenda imagining herself on the playground tomorrow with the kids teasing her.

Children's Songs. Using various rhymes, Metaphors, or sayings from the children's genre helps with creating and installing resources, especially if the therapist uses humor, movement, and a bit of silliness to engage the child. Using children's songs to help children remember resources is quite helpful. I (C.S.) use a song called "Mommy Comes Back" to help children in intact families who are experiencing school refusal or separation anxiety. I sing the song with the child and do BLS. I have the child imagine the next time his or her mom is going to go somewhere without him or her, and I have the child do BLS and sing the song to himself or herself. We choose characters with certain qualities from the children's genre to create imaginal resources for children. The therapist can choose characters from cartoons, television shows, movies, or whatever characters are appropriate for children.

Positive Affirmations. Another fun activity for building positive resources for children is installing positive affirmations. This is a simple process involving having children and their parents write positive affirmations on slips of paper and then pick affirmations to install with BLS. Positive affirmations include simple statements like "My needs are important" or "I am lovable." These positive affirmations are obviously potential positive cognitions, also. Once the child chooses the positive affirmation, the therapist then installs this positive affirmation with BLS. The therapist can remind the child and parent to repeat the positive affirmation outside the office. I (R.T.) suggest that families can write positive affirmations on 3 × 5 cards and hang the cards in strategic places in the home. Installing positive affirmations is also helpful in working with children in foster and adoptive families.

We have integrated various play therapy and art therapy techniques that are used to help children improve coping and self-soothing. Many of the techniques have come from years of play therapy training and experience as well as other therapists. We have adapted and/or changed pieces of the original techniques to be used in EMDR with children. We have made efforts to give credit for the technique to the creator of the technique but have not been able to identify the creator in all instances.

MASTERY SKILLS FOR CHILDREN

Children are most likely to be scheduled for psychotherapy because of emotional or behavioral concerns identified by their parents. Parents are quick to identify issues or symptoms with children but are much less likely to identify the child's strengths or accomplishments. Because we come from a strength-based model, where the treatment focuses on enhancing the child's and family's strengths, we model and teach a strength-based approach to children and families. This is integrated into each session, including asking the child and parent about something the child did well since the last session. We then strengthen and install those accomplishments as mastery experiences for children by adding BLS to strengthen the memory. There are subtle nuances between identifying a memory of a positive experience and installing that experience by adding BLS to add that experience to the child's toolbox of mastery skills, versus creating resources through resourcing by using pieces of the RDI protocol or deciding to use the extended RDI protocol and taking a full session to go through all the steps of enhancing the resource.

You can install resources like we discussed earlier or have the child identify something that makes the child feel good about himself or herself or something the child has accomplished, which is what we call a *mastery skill.* A mastery skill is something that is installed that is a memory or experience that makes the child feel competent. This can be about a time when the child learned to ride a bike, or attended his or her first day of school, or got a good grade on a test, or even had a positive experience with sports. One goal of mastery is to identify an experience that is already stored in a positive memory network and strengthen the memory with BLS. This serves several purposes, including creating a positive foundation and feeling for the child, and it helps to get the child to associate positive affect with BLS. Focusing on mastery will help the child become more confident in himself or herself and in the therapeutic process before trying to process traumas. If necessary, the therapist can remind the child that he or she can use his or her mastery experience to assist in making the child feel more confident. Installing a mastery experience is quite helpful when a child is reluctant to work on a target or explore his or her current symptoms. The therapist can also teach children mastery skills to use as resources.

You can also have a child participate in more extensive RDI protocols that include identifying mastery experiences, and we have translated the RDI protocol into children's language in the next section of this chapter.

Sometimes children may need mastery skills to cope with upcoming stressful events, such as when we prepare children to go to court to testify. In this type of situation, we might ask the child to identify a time in his or her life when the child was initially scared to do something, but in spite of the child's anxiety or fear, then did it anyhow, and was proud of what he or she accomplished. We might say to a child, "Tell me about a time when you were really scared to do something, but you did it anyway and were very glad that you did it."

Procedural Considerations for Mastery Skills

If the child becomes overwhelmed by affect, the child is most likely to attribute the discomfort to the EMDR and the therapeutic process. Like adults, children need time to integrate what is occurring in therapy without becoming overwhelmed. Teaching containers, affect management, resourcing, and mastery skills is a critical part of the process; however, we also found that therapists' hesitancy to target the most severe trauma delayed the process when the child did not need as much skill building as the therapist conducted. We have heard many therapists express angst about targeting the most horrendous traumas with child clients. This can be a huge issue for therapists. We ask therapists to consider whether it is the child who is not prepared to reprocess the target memory, or perhaps it is the therapist's countertransference issue where the therapist is not prepared to handle the child's trauma. It is not uncommon for therapists to experience vicarious trauma from the severity of the child's experiences. It is important for therapists to be always aware of their own countertransference issues with children.

RESOURCE DEVELOPMENT AND INSTALLATION (RDI) SKILLS FOR CHILDREN

Andrew Leeds (1998) first published his protocol for RDI skills for adults in 1998 to provide a template for clients to develop skills for accessing maladaptively stored memory networks, while being able to cope with the sometimes intense affect associated with the memories. Later, Korn and Leeds (2002) tested the efficacy of the RDI protocol for use during the preparation phase of EMDR to enhance stabilization of adults with complex posttraumatic stress disorder. Currently, RDI is taught in the basic EMDR training. The goal of RDI is to enhance the ability of the client for emotional regulation and improve the capacity for coping with intense affect during EMDR reprocessing.

In this chapter, we have adapted portions of the RDI protocol as originally created by Leeds for use with child clients. We also include specific directions and scripts as well as forms for the therapist for using different sections of the RDI protocol with children in the paragraphs below and in Exhibit 9.1. Also, in the last section of this chapter, an abbreviate RDI protocol for use with child clients is included as a template for therapists to use during sessions with children, which simplifies the RDI process when therapists need to be fluid and flexible working with children.

Procedural Considerations for RDI With Child Clients

In the research study we conducted with children referred for services at Childhelp Children's Center (see chapter 1), the therapists struggled with the RDI protocol with severely traumatized children and children under 7 years of age because children had difficulty focusing on the full RDI protocol because of the length of the protocol and because many children had little positive resources and/or struggled with positive affect tolerance. There are still benefits to using portions of the RDI protocol

Exhibit 9.1 RDI WORKSHEET FOR USE WITH CHILD CLIENTS – PART 1

DATE: ____________ CHILD'S NAME: ________________________

Step 1

Needed resources (qualities, capacities, strengths, needs, feelings, beliefs as identified by client): ________________________________

____

____

Resource Development

Mastery experiences and images: ________________________________

____

____

Relational resources: ____

____

____

____

Metaphors and symbols: ______________________________________

____

____

____

Client's Signature: ______________________ Date: _______________

After completing this worksheet, the therapist needs to consider the child's needs for further developing the resource. If so, continue with the next section.

RDI WORKSHEET – PART 2

Step 2

Needed resource (quality, capacity, strength, need, feeling, belief as identified by client): ____

____

____

Resource target selected (e.g., mastery experience or image, supportive person, Metaphor, or symbol): ______________________________

____

____

Image: ____

____

____

Additional details (sounds, smells, textures, etc.): ________________

____

____

Positive emotions: ____________________________________

Positive physical sensations (location and description): ____________

____

Associated positive cue words: ______________________________

____

What strengthens the client's connection to the resource (i.e., hearing words of encouragement from a supportive person, holding the resource in their hands, moving closer to the resource)? ________________

____

____

____

Client's Signature: ____________________ Date: ______________

ABBREVIATED RDI PROTOCOL

(We included this abbreviated protocol as a checklist to remind the therapist of the steps of RDI).

Step 1: Identify needed resources (qualities, capacities, strengths, needs, feelings, beliefs as identified by the client).

Step 2: Resource development: exploring various types of resources

Mastery experiences and images
Relational resources
Metaphors and symbols

Step 3: Resource development: accessing more information (working with one resource image at a time)—what do you see, hear, smell, feel (emotions and sensations)?

Step 4: Checking the resource: Check the resource by asking the client to notice how he or she feels when focusing on the resource image. Response must be positive. If not, reevaluate the resource selected.

Step 5: Reflecting the resource.

Step 6: Installing the resource: Install the resource using several short sets of BLS, four to six complete movements in each set. What are you feeling or noticing now?

Step 7: Strengthen the resource by linking with verbal (i.e., positive cue words or words of encouragement from a supportive figure) or sensory cues (i.e., feel the supportive figure's hand on your shoulder, breathe in that energy).

Step 8: Cue word or phrase.

Linking cue word or phrase with resource
Practicing cue word or phrase with disturbance

Step 9: Establish a future template.

with children. When using the RDI protocol with children, we recommend that the therapist do shorter pieces of the RDI protocol and weave different pieces through each session of therapy. It is helpful with children to use shorter sets of BLS and do segments of RDI in continued sessions. Another option is to use mastery installations for children who are not able to benefit from the RDI protocol.

Instructions to the therapist regarding RDI follow:

1. The instructions for RDI with children need to be adapted in developmentally appropriate language. RDI should only be used when the child does not appear to have adequate tolerance to utilize EMDR. If the child is unable to complete a Safe/Calm Place exercise, or if the child becomes overwhelmed during reprocessing in the Desensitization Phase, the therapist may need to focus on assisting the child to develop more advanced coping skills.
2. Initially, the child is asked to focus on a problematic current life situation or blocking belief. The child is then asked to identify the qualities (or capacities, strengths, feelings, people, pets, or other resources) the child believes he or she needs to deal with this situation or belief. If the child identifies multiple qualities, the therapist asks the child to identify the quality that the child thinks or feels would be most important to assist the child with this specific situation. If necessary, this process is repeated for each of the qualities the child identifies.
3. The therapist uses knowledge of the child's history and current social and personal resources to help identify a mastery experience associated with this quality and with positive affect.
4. If such an experience cannot be recalled, the child is asked to remember someone else dealing effectively with this type of situation or someone who embodies the desired quality. The child can be asked to identify a person who is seen as a good coach, mentor, or support figure from the child's present or past. The person can be real or imaginary and include characters from the current children's genre, including from books, TV, games, videos, and so on.
5. BLS is utilized to install the resource, and if the resource experience is enhanced, the therapist continues with two to three saccades of BLS, as long as positive feelings and associations get stronger. BLS is discontinued when the resource is optimally strengthened.
6. The BLS is stopped if the child associates to negative material. In this case, the therapist should select a different resource or resource image and determine if it can be successfully installed.

The therapist may want to encourage the child to set aside the negative material in an imaginal container before proceeding. In addition, the therapist may choose to use very short sets (two to five saccades) to decrease the possibility of activating negative material.

7. The therapist should next consider the use of a future template to verify that the resource can indeed assist the child in coping with the initially identified challenging situation.
8. In future sessions, the therapist should check resources that have been installed as well as the parent's written log for any feedback.
9. During trauma-focused EMDR desensitization, the therapist may use previously installed resources as interweaves to address blocked responses to treatment. The therapist should be aware that if he or she chooses to use RDI during desensitization, processing of traumatic material has stopped.

Scripts for RDI

Identifying Needed Resources for Child Clients. Sometimes this protocol is all that is needed by the child and does not require any installation with BLS. We suggest that the therapist first try this protocol with child clients, and if successful, no additional RDI may be necessary.

Script. "I want you to think about something that bothers you. It could be something that happened at home or school or with friends. When you think about that thing, how do you want to think or feel about it instead? What would you rather be able to do? What do you think could help you right now to do that? Let's figure out what you might need to be able to feel or act the way you want to."

Resource Development: Exploring Various Types of Resources. If a child is unable to be successful with the more general protocol described in the preceding paragraphs, the therapist can consider more detailed RDI protocols, as included subsequently. Again, the therapist is choosing one script to conduct with a child client. The therapist may need to return to teach new RDI skills during the EMDR process; however, more than one protocol at a time is overwhelming for children.

After choosing a mastery experience and image, relational resource, or Metaphors and symbolic resources, the therapist then proceeds with the steps of developing and enhancing the protocol, as described subsequently.

Mastery Experiences and Images. "Think about a time when you felt _________ [e.g., strong, safe, confident, soothed, able to tolerate your feelings]. Think about a time when you were able to act _________ [e.g., smarter, stronger, calmer, friendlier, etc.]. Tell me about a time when you remember feeling like that or when you acted like that. Can you see yourself tomorrow or next week with that _________ [e.g., stronger feeling, some type of different behavior]?"

Relational Resources (Models and Supportive Figures). "Think of people or things that would help you feel the way that you want to feel. Can you think of somebody who is like that? These could be real people like your mom or dad, grandparents . . . [identify significant adults/friends in child's life], or these could be people in books or on television that help you feel good. Are there any animals or pets that you think could help you with this?"

Metaphors and Symbolic Resources. "Is there something you can think of that would make you feel _________ [whatever resource it is] like a magic feather, or sword, magic wand, fairy, or a cool tree house? Is there anything from your drawings, daydreams, ideas, games you've played, books you like, or movies you've watched?"

Procedural Considerations for RDI Protocols With Children

Once the therapist has chosen one of the three resources listed previously, if the therapist determines that identifying the resource and installing with short sets of BLS is sufficient for the child, the RDI process for children can end here. If the therapist believes the child needs to further develop the resource, then the therapist can choose to further develop the specific resource by using the following protocols.

Resource Development: Accessing More Information. When working with one resource image or association at a time, the therapist says, "When you think about that _________ [e.g., experience, person, symbol, etc.], what do you see? What do you hear? What do you smell? What do you notice in your body when you think about it?" (Use examples and physical motions to demonstrate for the child.) "What feelings do you notice as you focus on this picture or memory?" Make verbatim notes of these descriptions to use in the following sections.

Checking the Resource. "When you think about that picture _________ [repeat description of image] and the _________ [repeat description of feelings, sensations, smells, sounds, etc.], how does that make you feel?" Then verify that the selected resource would help the child cope with the challenging situation by asking, "When you think about _________ [the target situation], how true or helpful does _________ [repeat description of the image and feelings] feel to you now, from 1 being not helpful, to 7 being completely true or helpful?" (Therapist uses whatever measurement is most applicable to the individual child and his or her development.)

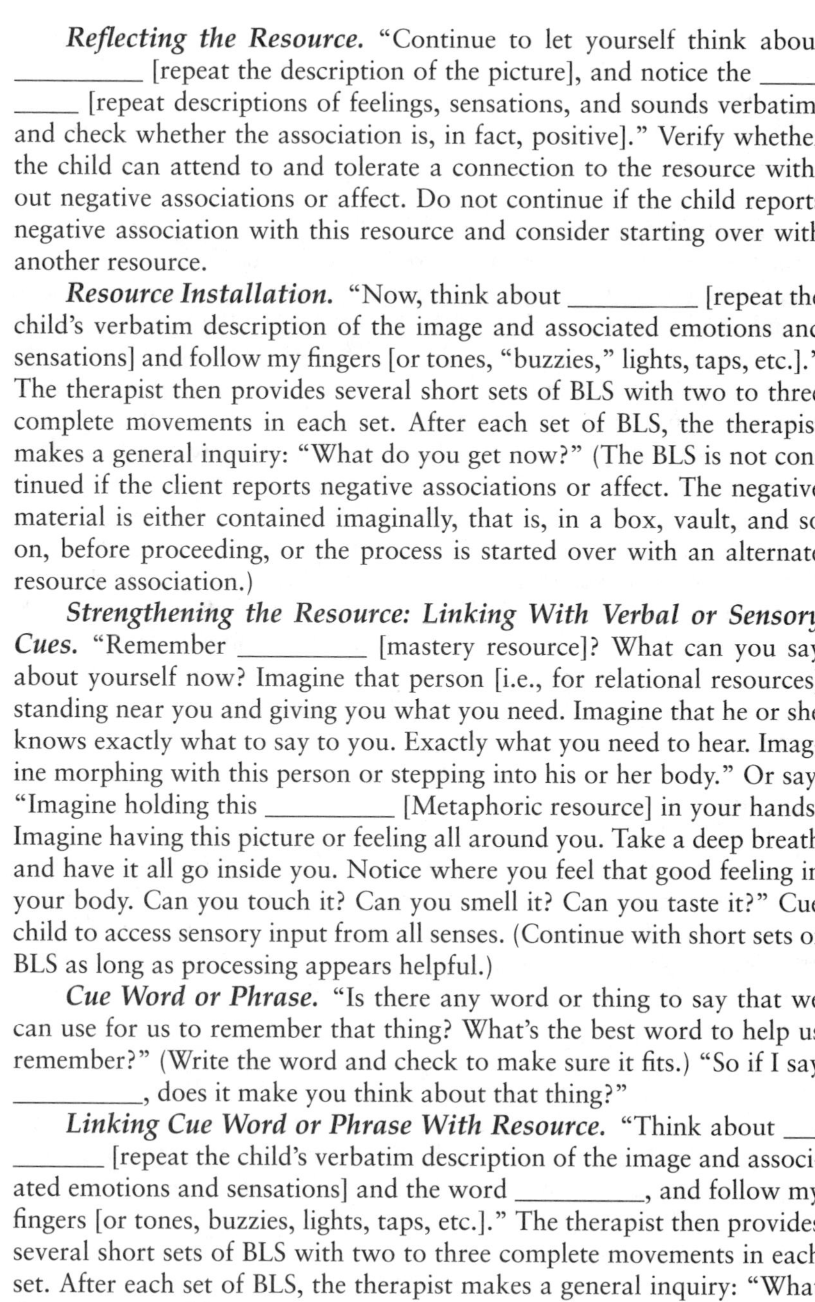

Reflecting the Resource. "Continue to let yourself think about _________ [repeat the description of the picture], and notice the _____ _____ [repeat descriptions of feelings, sensations, and sounds verbatim, and check whether the association is, in fact, positive]." Verify whether the child can attend to and tolerate a connection to the resource without negative associations or affect. Do not continue if the child reports negative association with this resource and consider starting over with another resource.

Resource Installation. "Now, think about _________ [repeat the child's verbatim description of the image and associated emotions and sensations] and follow my fingers [or tones, "buzzies," lights, taps, etc.]." The therapist then provides several short sets of BLS with two to three complete movements in each set. After each set of BLS, the therapist makes a general inquiry: "What do you get now?" (The BLS is not continued if the client reports negative associations or affect. The negative material is either contained imaginally, that is, in a box, vault, and so on, before proceeding, or the process is started over with an alternate resource association.)

Strengthening the Resource: Linking With Verbal or Sensory Cues. "Remember _________ [mastery resource]? What can you say about yourself now? Imagine that person [i.e., for relational resources] standing near you and giving you what you need. Imagine that he or she knows exactly what to say to you. Exactly what you need to hear. Imagine morphing with this person or stepping into his or her body." Or say, "Imagine holding this _________ [Metaphoric resource] in your hands. Imagine having this picture or feeling all around you. Take a deep breath and have it all go inside you. Notice where you feel that good feeling in your body. Can you touch it? Can you smell it? Can you taste it?" Cue child to access sensory input from all senses. (Continue with short sets of BLS as long as processing appears helpful.)

Cue Word or Phrase. "Is there any word or thing to say that we can use for us to remember that thing? What's the best word to help us remember?" (Write the word and check to make sure it fits.) "So if I say _________, does it make you think about that thing?"

Linking Cue Word or Phrase With Resource. "Think about ___ _______ [repeat the child's verbatim description of the image and associated emotions and sensations] and the word _________, and follow my fingers [or tones, buzzies, lights, taps, etc.]." The therapist then provides several short sets of BLS with two to three complete movements in each set. After each set of BLS, the therapist makes a general inquiry: "What do you get now?"

Practicing Cue Word With Disturbance. "Can you think about something little that happened this last week that bugged you a little bit that you'd like to have that thought or feeling with instead? Let's pretend that you can use that thought or feeling and the word _________ to make that little thing stop bugging you now." The therapist then provides several short sets of BLS with two to three complete movements in each set. After each set of BLS, the therapist makes a general inquiry: "What do you get now?"

Establishing a Future Template. "If there was something tomorrow, the next day, or next week you'd want to use this thought with, what would it be? Pretend that you're using that thing with all the smells, sounds, and feelings and the word _________. Think about that just the way you need to feel it. Now follow my fingers [taps, or buzzies]." The therapist then provides several short sets of BLS with two to three complete movements in each set. After each set of BLS, the therapist makes a general inquiry: "What do you get now?" (Continue with short sets of BLS as long as processing improves the resource.) This process may be repeated for each of the qualities the child wants to strengthen. In future sessions, the therapist should check resources that have been installed as well as the child's feedback. When the child is ready for trauma-focused work, the therapist can begin the session by first bringing in and strengthening (with BLS) the toolbox that contains the resources needed to address the traumatic material. During trauma-focused EMDR reprocessing, the therapist may use previously installed resources as interweaves (Shapiro, 1995–2007) to address blocked responses to treatment; however, any use of an interweave is considered only one channel. Processing is not considered complete until the undistorted target is accessed and associated channels are followed to resolution without distortion.

Once the child has successfully identified as many resources as necessary to participate in targeting a memory for reprocessing, the therapist can return to the assessment phase to begin with a memory. Sometimes the child may have been able to process a memory, but other memories may be overwhelming, indicating that the child may be in need of additional resources.

It is important for the therapist to remind the child during each session to use his or her resources and mastery skills both during the session and at home. If the child has drawn any pictures of resources or created any symbols of other resources, the therapist can have the child look at the picture or hold the symbol to help anchor the resource.

SUMMARY

This chapter has focused on teaching children emotional resources, coping, and mastery skills. As we have discussed, creating new resources and coping skills, while enhancing mastery experiences the child has recalled, helps create a positive foundation for children to deal with reprocessing traumatic events in therapy. These skills are especially important for children who are reluctant to address symptoms and traumatic memories in therapy. In case conceptualization, the therapist must regularly assess what skills the child possesses as well as when the child needs additional skills to cope with therapeutic and life challenges.

ABBREVIATED RDI PROTOCOL FOR CHILDREN

This abbreviated protocol is explained in detail earlier in this chapter, with scripts for each step available for the therapist to adjust according to the child's developmental and emotional functioning age. We encourage children to draw a picture of the identified resource and then keep the picture in the child's file for future use, as necessary.

Step 1: Identify needed resources (qualities, capacities, strengths, needs, feelings, beliefs as identified by client).
Step 2: Resource development: exploring various types of resources.

Mastery experiences and images
Relational resources
Metaphors and symbols

Step 3: Resource development: accessing more information (working with one resource at a time)—what do you see, hear, smell, feel (emotions and sensations)?
Step 4: Checking the resource: Check the resource by asking client to notice how he or she feels when focusing on resource image. Response must be positive. If not, reevaluate the resource selected.
Step 5: Reflecting the resource.
Step 6: Installing the resource: Install the resource using several short sets of BLS, four to six complete movements in each set. What are you feeling or noticing now?
Step 7: Strengthen the resource by linking with verbal (i.e., positive cue words or words of encouragement from a supportive figure) or sensory cues (i.e., feel the supportive figure's hand on your shoulder, breathe in that energy).
Step 8: Cue word or phrase.

Linking cue word or phrase with resource
Practicing cue word or phrase with disturbance

Step 9: Establish a future template.

CHAPTER 10

Tools for Blocked Processing and Cognitive Interweaves

We wrote this as a separate chapter because there can be many places where using EMDR in psychotherapy with children is challenging. This is where the true art of child psychotherapy and EMDR merge. It is at this point where we believe many therapists abandon EMDR and revert to psychotherapeutic models that make the therapist feel more confident. This has nothing to do with the efficacy of EMDR, but rather with the therapist's confidence in his or her own skills. Because we believe that therapists who feel confident in their own EMDR skills will be more likely to use EMDR in their practices, we have tried to weave practical tools with support and encouragement throughout this book. In this chapter we have attempted to anticipate places where therapists might struggle in using EMDR with children and offer clinical interventions that therapists can use to return the child to successfully reprocessing with EMDR.

As consultants, we regularly hear from therapists who are encountering difficulties in using EMDR with children. In an effort to provide clinical direction, we have built into this chapter an explanation for what a therapist might encounter in working with children and possible solutions for getting the process back on track. We have also included a detailed explanation of cognitive interweaves, along with examples of cognitive interweaves for children.

There are many places where therapists can find themselves struggling with the EMDR protocol, including when a child presents with blocked processing. We strongly encourage therapists to try the techniques in Shapiro's (2001) book, with the adjustments for working with children that we have provided. Finally, we have added some new ideas integrated from our practices.

BLOCKED PROCESSING

Blocked processing basically means either the subjective units of disturbance (SUD) are not going down or the child is overwhelmed by the intense emotion, which halts processing. With children, blocked processing can also present as avoidance, hesitancy, nonresponsiveness, or not engaging in treatment. There are many different reasons why a child may experience blocked processing.

Editing

During the desensitization phase, editing may be what is occurring when the child is analyzing what's coming up during bilateral stimulation and determining that nothing is changing thus restricting what they present to the therapist. Editing occurs when the child is evaluating the content of what's coming up before telling the therapist. At times this is due to not understanding the therapist's instructions while other times this may occur because the child is not comfortable reporting what is occurring. For clarification, the therapist may need to explain to the child that the child needs only to observe and report, but not edit before telling the therapist what's occurring during BLS. If the child is uncomfortable or too embarrassed to report what is occurring during BLS, the therapist may need to remind the child that it is not necessary to describe in detail what is happening in order to continue with reprocessing. *Editing* may also occur when the child reports his or her experience in general terms such as "it's the same" or "nothing" or "I'm numb." Children will say things like "I feel nothing" instead of "numb." Ask the child in a respectful way to specifically describe everything he or she is getting, or ask the child to describe specifically what "nothing" is like. The therapist can also ask the child to describe numbness or nothingness and ask where he or she feels it in his or her body.

Sometimes editing occurs when the child is trying to remember everything that happened so as to tell the therapist. This may require additional instruction, with the therapist saying to the child, "Just notice and let whatever happens happen, and just tell me what you're getting at the moment when I ask you. What do you get now?" Some children will not actually be editing but may just need to be given more instruction.

Looping

Looping is another form of blocked processing. *Looping* is when the child is saying the same thing in the same modality (i.e., cognitions, emotions, images, body sensations) at least two or three times, such as "I'm bad" (cognition), "I'm scared" (emotion), "I see my mom standing on the stairs" (image), or "My stomach hurts" (body sensation). Looping is stuck processing. Looping is not the patient reporting sequences of trauma, which are really channels of association or associative chains (Shapiro, 2001), but instead, the child is stuck, and no new channels are coming up.

If the therapist believes the child is looping, the therapist should change the speed, direction, or type of bilateral stimulation (BLS), or the therapist can ask the child to notice his or her body or notice where the body sensation is most pronounced. The therapist can also ask the child where he or she feels the negative cognition in his or her body. For example, if the negative cognition is "I'm bad," the therapist asks the child, "Where do you feel that in your body?" What are the unspoken words that the child may need to speak? Simple statements like "No!" can be very powerful. What movements does the child need to make? Is the child frozen, and does he or she need to move, stand up and feel strong, kick, and so on? The therapist can also have the child press on his or her body where the child is having the sensation to access an image or a thought or a memory. All of these actions are intended to access different aspects of the target.

Numbing

Numbing can occur when children report feeling nothing or when children begin to yawn. *Numbing* in children is an example of depersonalization, where children are still connected with the office and the therapist but not with their own experience of reprocessing the memory. If the therapist suspects that the child is numbing, then the therapist just treats that as another layer of emotion (Shapiro, 2001). Children may become sleepy or yawn or report feeling nothing when they are numbing. If the child reports that he or she feels numb or nothing, the therapist can instruct the child to just notice that or to notice where the child feels numb or nothing in his or her body.

Feeling numb or nothing can also be a form of editing when the child does not report what he or she is actually noticing because the child thinks it is unimportant or not related. If the therapist suspects the child is omitting or withholding information, the therapist can query the child, "Tell me the last thing you were thinking." Whatever response the child gives, the therapist says, "Go with that." This may happen occasionally, and the reprocessing continues, but if a child seems to be too far off topic, the child may need to be reminded of the target with instruction from the therapist. The therapist may need to suggest, "OK, I just want to check in real quick. Do you remember that thing we started with?" If the child says yes, the therapist says, "Go with that." If the child does not remember what the target was, the therapist can offer a cue. The therapist might say, "Remember that thing that happened in the car? When you bring that up, what do you get now? Go with that." Depending on the age of the child, the therapist's instructions might be simpler, with more direct instruction, such as showing the child the picture the child drew of the car accident. This is only used to return the child to focusing on reprocessing the target.

For some children, BLS creates a relaxation response. The child is neither numbing nor editing, but relaxing. One of the beauties of EMDR is that children may relax and be in a state of calmness, where new ideas or associations can emerge, while their anxiety is decreased or absent.

Avoidance/Reluctance

We assess children as being avoidant when children demonstrate behaviors that suggest that the child is doing everything but focusing on the EMDR process. As most therapists who work with children will recognize, children move around or change the subject or do something to distract the process when they do not want to do something. Children can be masters at evading the work of therapy because most children just do not want to think about or talk about what is bothering them. It is important to remember that avoidance is a hallmark of posttraumatic stress disorder. It is just more fun to play with the therapist and not think about things that cause distress. Therapists will need to be persistent, creative, and convincing in explaining why a child would want to participate in reprocessing targets.

We have had the opportunity to work with many creative therapists who have designed games and activities or used play therapy techniques to engage children in the work of psychotherapy. The talented therapist is one who can find avenues to help children participate in therapy without even knowing what is happening. We are not suggesting that therapists trick children, but instead use the power of persuasion and integrate EMDR into play activities. For example, many children will enjoy working in the sand tray, and therapists can do many phases of the EMDR protocol while having the child work in the sand tray. Targets can be identified by having children create scenes of things that bother them in the sand tray. The therapist can then take digital pictures of the sand tray creations or simply copy the child's sand tray scene onto a progress note.

It is often much more engaging to have a child identify targets in the sand tray, rather than just by talking. We have discussed various play therapy techniques that therapists can use to engage children in therapy and translate the EMDR protocol into child language throughout this book.

Children can be reticent to participate in therapy for many reasons, and the child's hesitancy can actually be a target for EMDR. The therapist can also conduct a future template on therapy, where the child can see himself or herself doing EMDR and being successful.

Our experience is that therapists who struggle with engaging children in EMDR need additional skills in working with children or would benefit from consultation. Sometimes just staffing a child's case with a colleague will help the therapist to become clearer about what the therapist needs to do in the session. We strongly recommend ongoing peer consultation to provide support for the therapist, ongoing learning opportunities, checks for countertransference issues, and to process the vicarious trauma that can occur, especially when working with children.

The ability to engage children in psychotherapy is foundational to working with children. It is important to differentiate between clinical skills versus the EMDR methodology. As we discuss in chapter 1, where we summarize our research findings, therapists who had experience in working with children and knowledge of child development were much more successful in using the EMDR protocol with children. Training in EMDR alone is not sufficient for therapists to be able to use EMDR with children. This is also true of therapists who work with dissociation. Additional training in dissociation is imperative to successfully treating dissociation in children.

Dissociation

Dissociation occurs when children are not only numb to the process, but also lose the connection with the therapist and the office and essentially separate from their body. When this happens, the child is no longer engaged in therapy. We will discuss working with children who dissociate in chapter 11.

It is important to note that dissociation not only blocks processing, but most likely stops processing altogether, and may leave the child feeling retraumatized from the therapy experience. Once the therapist has assessed that the child has dissociated, it is important to stop BLS and ground the child in the office. There are many techniques for grounding children and dealing with children who are dissociative; these will be discussed in chapter 11 as well.

We would encourage therapists not to avoid working with children who dissociate, but instead to realize that most therapists who work with trauma are also working with some degree of dissociation. It is important for therapists to have some skills and comfort in working with children who dissociate.

Abreactions

An *abreaction* occurs when a child begins to relive the traumatic event with all the thoughts, emotions, and body sensations of the original experience. The goal of therapy is not to cause an abreaction, but abreactions can occur as part of reprocessing a target with EMDR. It is the therapist's responsibility to keep the therapeutic process moving and not allow the child to stay stuck in the memory.

It seems as if some therapists may avoid or be vicariously traumatized by the intensity of an abreaction. This is most likely due to therapist issues, both from personal discomfort and lack of training, and not due to the therapy process. It is important for therapists to understand that abreactions are not a bad thing, but instead can happen when conducting therapy.

Abreactions are indicators that the therapist has identified the correct target and that the target resonates for the child. Some children may have abreactions but not dissociate. Therapists need to be cognizant of the difference between abreactions where the child dissociates because he or she is overwhelmed and abreactions where the child is able to work through the intense experience and resolve the memory. The former is blocked processing, while the latter is effective processing.

Therapists can be supportive and encouraging to a child who is experiencing an abreaction by offering the child a pillow or a blanket and encouraging words such as "Just notice. You're here in the office, and it's not happening now. Can you hang with me? Let's keep going through and come out the other side of the tunnel. Keep going. Good job!" It is not necessary to say all of that, but choose portions as necessary to support the child. The therapist must continue to actively monitor the child's progress and at times may ask the child, "What do you need to continue to work on this memory?" Sometimes it is helpful to remind the child that it is like going through a dark tunnel: If we stop in the middle, we will stay stuck in the dark, but if we keep coming, we will come out the other side.

Abreactions are more manageable and can be normalized when the therapist has prepared the child for abreactions and explained that this can be part of the process. It is important for the therapist to explain to the child in language the child can understand that sometimes the child may experience strong emotions or body sensations, or stuff that reminds the child of what happened. If this occurs, the process is working, and the therapist and child can handle it together. We explain to children that they have already survived the experience and that they were very courageous and brave when it happened. Now we just have to reprocess the leftover feelings from the experience. I (C.S.) explain to the child that sometimes when we do EMDR, this is part of the process, and we are going to go through the feeling, and he or she is going to finish the memory and feel better. This is not a demand characteristic, but instead, we explain the possibility that abreactions can happen, and if they do, the therapist knows what to do and can help the child move through the abreaction and feel better.

Abreactions can be traumatizing to a child if the child relives the traumatic experience during therapy and dissociates at the same time. Part of the therapist's attunement to the child is to make sure that the child is staying connected with the therapist while reprocessing the event. If the child experiences an abreaction and dissociates, the therapist can use techniques to reconnect with the child and help the child calm himself or herself and self-soothe. The therapist can then explain how the brain works to protect the child from things that are overwhelming and demystify the experience so that the child does not experience retraumatization from an abreaction.

Therapists who understand abreactions and feel confident in their own clinical skills in dealing with abreactions tend to be successful at helping children work through and cope with abreactions when they occur.

Intense Emotional Reactions

Children can also experience intense emotional reactions when they are concerned about future events. Some children may have a strong emotional experience that is not evident to the therapist. Children who experience an intense emotional reaction may then refuse to continue in therapy. Therapists will need to also consider that a child's reluctance to participate in therapy may be due to an unpredictable or unanticipated intense emotional reaction. Sometimes children experience scary feelings or strong emotions that the therapist is unaware of, but the evidence is the child's unwillingness to participate or continue in therapy or EMDR.

Clinical Implications for Therapists Working With Blocked Processing

It is important for therapists to have sufficiently prepared the child for processing, while creating a safe environment that is focused on the child's needs. Attunement to the child and awareness of when the child may need to take a break and use a container to continue at a later time are important clinical decisions for the therapist. These decisions must be made based on the child's needs and pacing in therapy, rather than on the therapist's discomfort. We certainly attend to the child's needs but also continue to check in where the child is with the processing.

Therapists' Responses to Intense Emotional Reactions. Therapists who come from a more cognitive or behavioral foundation may find it more difficult to respond to abreactions or intense emotional reactions in therapy. It can be surprising to witness the intensity at which children express their emotions and memories; however, the cathartic effect of EMDR reprocessing is invaluable. It is the therapist's responsibility to explore his or her own comfort with intense emotional, behavioral, and physical reactions. We have encountered children with extreme anger, sadness, and even physiological reactions such as vomiting or urinating. In consultation with therapists, I (R.T.) ask therapists to consider, "What can happen in a therapy session that you can't handle or are not prepared to handle?"

Blocking Beliefs. A *blocking belief* is an underlying belief that may interfere with processing. Blocking beliefs are often not obvious, and the therapist may need to come back and explore why the memory is not reprocessing. For example, some children believe that "big boys don't cry." If a child is trying to process the emotions associated with a memory when his dog died, the memory may start looping because to fully reprocess the memory, the child has to address his belief that "big boys don't cry."

Another clinical tool for assisting children with blocked processing is the therapist's use of cognitive interweaves.

COGNITIVE INTERWEAVES

Cognitive interweaves are used to jump-start (Shapiro, 2001) blocked processing when the previous approaches have not worked. With cognitive interweaves, the therapist introduces new material without relying on the child to provide it. It is a light touch to elicit certain information from the child's neuronetworks. The therapist initiates cognitive interweaves through questions or instructions that elicit thoughts, actions, or imagery. Cognitive interweaves should be used selectively so the child's own processing system can do the work, which allows full integration of information and is empowering to the child (Shapiro, 2001).

In addition to cognitive interweaves, we also suggest that the therapist consider slightly different types of interweaves.

Motor Interweaves

A motor interweave can be used when the therapist assesses a need for the child to move in order to facilitate reprocessing. This is different than cognitive interweave in that the therapist suggests that the child might want to actually make the movement or take the action. Since children's memories are often stored in sensory-motor memories, finishing a thwarted or frozen action can help to reprocess the memory through to adaptive resolution. For example, a little boy who remembered being molested by an older adolescent needed to stand up and physically feel himself push the older child away and say, "No, you aren't allowed to touch me that way."

Sensory Interweaves

Sensory interweaves can be used when the therapist assesses a need to weave together a body sensation and a memory. I (R.T.) started working with a child who was remembering an event when her arm was broken and she connected with the image of the child's dad twisting her arm. The little girl then became stuck on the body sensations in her arm, but because of her age and developmental level, she was not able to make the connections. In this case, I offered a sensory interweave to assist the child in making the links. For example, if the child is reporting body sensations that appear to be stuck, the therapist can wonder with the child about the possibility that the feeling the child is having in his or her arm could be a similar feeling to the one the child experienced when the child's father broke the child's arm. In that situation, I (R.T.) said to the child, "I wonder if your arm is hurting because you are remembering what it felt like when your dad twisted your arm and you needed to get a cast on it?" It is important for the therapist not to offer interpretations or suggest information that has not been discussed, but instead to offer interweaves that might help the child link together two pieces of information to move the child off of the stuck spot.

Educational Interweaves

Educational interweaves are used to help give children information they do not have because of maturation, level of development, or life experience. I (R.T.) use this type of interweave to help children link information that is not making sense hypothetically because the information the child needs to understand the information is missing. Sometimes this is because what the child experienced is so far outside the range of normal experience that there would be no way for the child and/or parent to make the links. This happens quite often with foster and adoptive children. For example, I (R.T.) was working with a child who was with her birth mother until age 4, in foster care until age 7, and then adopted. This child struggled with unusual eating habits and had phobias related to certain kinds of food, especially ham. As we explored the child's fear of ham, she described the anxiety she experienced when she would see "shiny ham." Because the shiny ham issue seemed strange to the child and her adoptive parents, I offered the possibility that because ham comes in food boxes given to families in need and this child's birth mother was very low functioning and, per the records, often gave the children spoiled food, it was possible that the child had been given spoiled ham. The child discussed how she examines ham each time before she eats it, including the color, smell, and feel of the ham. We hypothesized that this could be one possibility for explaining the anxiety about shiny ham. Neither the child nor her adoptive mother knew that ham was often put in food boxes but did think that shiny ham is often an indicator that the ham is spoiled and thought that this was a reasonable explanation for the child's concerns. Once we targeted the child's image of shiny ham and reprocessed the associated sensations she experienced, she seemed to create a coherent narrative to explain her concerns and was validated that her concerns had a basis in reality and that she was now able to make good choices about eating fresh food. The anxiety abated about the shiny ham.

We have no way of knowing if this is what actually caused the child's anxiety about shiny ham; however, once we created a reasonable explanation for her anxiety and used the shiny ham interweave, the child's anxiety decreased. By offering this new information, which most people would not know, the child no longer struggled with eating ham, and in fact, some of her other food issues improved.

With educational interweaves, we have theorized that it is not possible to verify the touchstone event that contributed to the symptom presentation, especially with children who have been in foster care and/or adopted, because these children most likely have no one to provide a coherent narrative of their life experiences; therefore we may need to create a reasonable explanation for the child's symptoms, given what information we have, to give the child a template with which to understand and process the experience. We caution therapists not to offer conclusions about what might have happened such as "you are having this experience because you were sexually abused as a child." Instead, we are suggesting that the therapist use the information that is available about the child and common information to wonder about a possible explanation to create a coherent narrative for the child. In the end, the therapist is helping the child connect the dots but is not creating the dots.

Narrative Interweaves

If a child experiences blocked processing because the information he or she is getting is not making sense, I (R.T.) might wonder with the child about the possibility that a third variable could explain the reason why the child is having the experience. I use this type of interweave very often with foster and adoptive children when the child's history is unknown or has gaps in it. For example, I worked with a child adopted from China who knew nothing about the first 9 months of her life, with the exception of what the workers at the orphanage told her adoptive mother. With this child, we wondered about what it would be like for a baby from China to leave everything she knew—language, foods, smells, and people—and go with a stranger on a plane for 14 hours to a place where she did not understand the language, where she did not know the smells or tastes of the food, and where she was given a bottle for the first time, when she had only been given cups in the orphanage. We wondered about how this might feel for that baby, and the child responded, "That poor baby. She had to be so confused." My response as the therapist was "Go with that."

The goal of this narrative interweave was to combine all the facts we had to wonder about what that experience was like for the child. This can be useful for clients of all ages but is frequently helpful to children for whom we have minimal to no information about their pasts.

Cognitive Interweaves With Children

Instructions to the Therapist. A cognitive interweave is the elicitation of an adaptive perspective by the therapist that is offered when reprocessing is stuck, when the child is looping, or when time is running out and it is necessary to expedite the session so that the child does not remain in a highly activated state. Cognitive interweaves can also be used to help children generalize positive associations beyond the original target, which can be difficult for children.

Cognitive interweaves for children fall mainly under the categories of safety, responsibility, and choice/empowerment. Usually, cognitive interweaves are a question such as "Are you safe now?" (safety), "Well, whose job was it?" (responsibility), or "Are you making better choices now?" (choice/empowerment).

When utilizing a cognitive interweave, it is important to make sure that the cognitive interweave that is chosen resonates for the child and stimulates the child's own internal resources. When using a cognitive interweave, the therapist uses the least amount of information and the fewest questions to help guide the child to find an answer drawn from the child's own internal wisdom.

The therapist may use Socratic questioning to access the child's own logic to resume the child's own natural processing, for example, "If your friend was feeling the same way, what would you tell one of your friends?" If the child responds, the therapist continues, "Go with that." The goal of a cognitive interweave is to provide the least amount of therapist intervention to nudge the continuation of processing.

Examples of Scripts for Cognitive Interweaves for Children. When a child is stuck at a SUD of 3 or less, the therapist can say to the child, "What would it take to get it to be a zero?" (Or use an alternate phrase for the type of measurement the child has identified for measuring SUD.) So if the child says, "I need to feel safe," the therapist says, "What would it take for you to feel safe?" If the child responds with a realistic statement, the therapist then proceeds with further sets of BLS by directing the child to "Go with that." If the child responds with an irrational or unrealistic statement, the therapist then goes through a series of questions to guide the child to an adaptive response. For example, a child might respond, "I could fly away." The therapist may need to assist by saying, "That sounds fun, but what would need to happen for real?"

Once an adaptive response is elicited from the child, the therapist proceeds with further sets of BLS by saying, "Go with that." The goal of the therapist's intervention, again, is to help to resume reprocessing and then stay out of the way.

Examples of Cognitive Interweaves to Restart Processing With Children

The following sections detail types of cognitive interweaves and examples of how to utilize them, when appropriate.

New Information. When the child has insufficient information, such as poor education, little experience in an area, or developmental capabilities that do not give the child enough information to process, then the therapist offers the following to assist the child with processing:

CHILD: I did something bad.

THERAPIST: Kids have to be taught how to get mad in the right way. It's a grown-up's job to teach kids this and show them how to do it. Nobody is born knowing how to do that. Did anyone teach you?

CHILD: No.

THERAPIST: Think about that.

[BLS]

"I'm Confused." The child has the information, but the therapist uses another way of getting to that information.

CHILD: I could have stopped him.

THERAPIST: I'm confused. Are you saying a little boy can stop a very big grown-up from hitting another grown-up?

[BLS]

"What if It Were Your Best Friend?" The therapist can use anyone the child feels lovingly protective of who would be an appropriate replacement in the incident.

THERAPIST: If this happened to your best friend, what would you tell her?

CHILD: I tell her, "It's not your fault. Your mommy should've taken care of you."

[BLS]

Ask the Child. The SUDS is not coming down or the validity of cognition is not going up; the therapist has attempted other ways to get processing moving, and the therapist is not sure what interweave might be helpful. The therapist can ask the child directly for the interweave.

THERAPIST: What would it take to make that thing be only this upsetting [using hands or other appropriate measures]? What would it take for the SUD to go from a 3 to a 0? What would it take to make that ________ __ [positive cognition] stronger?

[BLS]

Change Pictures, Perspectives, and Personal Referent. The purpose of this type of cognitive interweave is to give the child distance, a different perspective, or a sense of empowerment in a way the child may not have thought about. For example,

THERAPIST: When you think about kids who are mean to you, think about the kids on a black-and-white movie screen. Or when that teacher is yelling at you, think about her at the end of a long, long hall. How loud does she sound now?

CHILD: Quieter and far away.

THERAPIST: Think about that.

[BLS]

THERAPIST: What's the difference between then and now?

CHILD: I'm bigger.

THERAPIST: Think about that.

[BLS]

Metaphor/Analogy. Impact therapeutic lessons through stories, songs, poems, movies, TV shows, or stories of other children's struggles.

THERAPIST: Harry Potter didn't have his parents. How did he handle his loneliness at Hogwarts?

CHILD: He talked to his friends and looked at a picture of his parents.

THERAPIST: Think about that.

[BLS]

Alternatively, when a child does not know how to handle another child's insults, use a story about the old rhyme "I'm rubber and you're super-glue. Whatever you say bounces off of me and sticks to you."

THERAPIST: Think about that.

[BLS]

Socratic Method. Using the Socratic method of cognitive interweaves is about asking the child a series of questions that shapes the child's perspective and/or leads the child to come to a new conclusion. The following example depicts a child irrationally worried about his house burning down:

THERAPIST: How old are you?

CHILD: Ten.

THERAPIST: That's pretty old.

CHILD: Yeah.

THERAPIST: Has your house ever caught fire before? [*make sure you know the answer is no*]

CHILD: No.

THERAPIST: How old is your mother?

CHILD: I don't know. Pretty old. Maybe thirty-something.

THERAPIST: Has her house or houses ever burnt down? [*again, make sure you know the answer is no*]

CHILD: No.

THERAPIST: Think about that.

[BLS]

Alternatively, gifted kids often worry about nuclear war or getting diseases.

THERAPIST: Less than 1% of children get deadly cancer. Did you know that?

CHILD: No.

THERAPIST: So if the weatherman told you there was less than 1% of rain today, how likely do you think it would be that it rained today? Would you bring your umbrella?

CHILD: No. I guess not.

THERAPIST: Think about that.

[BLS]

Designate Appropriate Responsibility. This type of cognitive interweave is the root of the issue of misattribution of responsibility. The goal of this interweave is to get the child to move on from looping on "it's my fault" and taking responsibility for things that are not the child's responsibility to have the child begin to appropriately assign responsibility.

THERAPIST: Who is supposed to take care of kids, grown-ups or kids?

CHILD: Grown-ups.

THERAPIST: Think about that.

[BLS]

Let's Pretend. Using this type of cognitive interweave helps the child think about other positive ways of change and can reduce fear.

THERAPIST: Let's pretend you could say anything you wanted and not worry about what would happen. What would you say?

CHILD: I hate you.

THERAPIST: Imagine saying that.

[BLS]

Alternatively, consider the following script:

THERAPIST: Let's pretend you were 10 feet taller; what would you do?

CHILD: I'd stomp on him and run away.

THERAPIST: Imagine doing that.

[BLS]

Consider the following:

THERAPIST: Do you know somebody, either real or imaginary, who could handle dealing with things without his or her parents being there?

CHILD: Like maybe Harry Potter?

THERAPIST: Think about that.

[BLS]

After the cognitive interweave is initiated, do only 24 saccades of BLS to check in quickly to determine if the cognitive interweave worked to restart reprocessing. If the child rejects the cognitive interweave, be open to trying others.

Cognitive Interweaves for Current or Future Issues

Cognitive interweaves can also be used for stuck processing associated with current or future issues.

Assimilation. Assimilation helps to decrease strong emotions and give new information to develop positive future behaviors. For example, the child is still fearful, even though the perpetrator is in jail:

THERAPIST: Can he hurt you now?

CHILD: No.

THERAPIST: Think about that.

[BLS]

Verbalizations and Actions. The therapist can prompt the child with either verbalizations or actions to express or practice future behaviors.

THERAPIST: What would you have liked to say to him?

CHILD: I'm gonna tell on you.

THERAPIST: Imagine that.

[BLS]

THERAPIST: Now say it out loud.

[BLS]

SUMMARY

This chapter was written to provide support and guidance for therapists who are trying to use the EMDR protocol with children and have run into blocked processing. Because we have encountered therapists who give up on EMDR with children because the therapist does not know how to work with blocked processing, we decided to provide detailed explanations to provide therapists with the encouragement to keep going.

First, it is important for therapists to understand what blocked processing is and what is contributing to the blocked processing. Often, there is more than one issue contributing to the blocked processing, including editing and numbing, and there are therapeutic tools to work with blocked processing. Therapists need to remember to change direction and modalities of BLS, skills for accessing and underaccessing, to address blocking beliefs, to target feeder memories, and to use cognitive interweaves for blocked processing. These same skills can be used with children with modifications and languaging changes as described in this chapter. Therapists need to have tools and techniques to work with blocked processing to help children move beyond that stuck place and continue reprocessing.

Finally, therapists need to be aware of their own issues related to working with EMDR and, more important, the vicarious trauma that can occur from working with children with trauma. Therapists need to seek consultation and support and continually recognize the need for self-care. Seeking training, support, and consultation helps therapists hang in there and find the benefits of using EMDR with children.

CHAPTER 11

Specialty Topics on Using EMDR With Children

This chapter is written for therapists who have learned the basic Eye Movement Desensitization and Reprocessing (EMDR) protocol and are interested in expanding their skills in using EMDR in individual treatment with children. In this chapter we will explore the advanced application of EMDR with other clinical, emotional, developmental, and behavioral issues, in addition to using EMDR with children who experienced trauma. As therapists who have worked with children collectively for more than 55 years, we have found EMDR to be quite effective with many childhood issues with which children present in therapy.

This chapter is organized into headings of specific childhood diagnoses, issues, or presenting problems, with recommendations for procedural considerations and adjustments to the EMDR protocol. Unless indicated otherwise, the EMDR protocol follows the eight phases, as discussed in chapters 3–8, with additions or modifications, as indicated subsequently.

We have discussed the Client History and Treatment Planning Phase in chapter 3. With that template in mind, the therapist begins the process of creating a hypothesis about what the child is experiencing and what is driving the current symptom presentation. Young children are often brought to therapy by parents who are concerned about clinical, emotional, behavioral, regulatory, and situational issues. Some parents may have been referred by their pediatrician after the pediatrician had ruled out medical issues as accounting for the child's symptoms. If the child has not been assessed by a pediatrician, it is important to consider if the child needs to be referred to a pediatrician or child psychiatrist for further evaluation to rule out any concurrent or contributing medical conditions. With childhood issues, it is important to also assess the etiology for the presenting symptoms within a developmental framework.

With each type of issue, it is essential to assess the range of development that would be expected given the child's chronological age. If the child is developmentally in the range given for the child's age and the parent has unrealistic expectations given the child's age, therapy would focus on parent education and training.

Once parenting issues and developmental issues have been ruled out and the therapist has assessed that mental health issues are at the root of the child's symptoms, then therapists can continue with the EMDR protocol. During the Preparation Phase, as we discussed in chapter 4, children may need skill building and resourcing to cope with specific symptoms and diagnoses. For example, most clients will benefit from learning relaxation and breathing skills; however, children with poor frustration tolerance will benefit from learning the "get a grip" exercise. Psychotherapy with children is most improved when children are taught resources and mastery skills such as emotional literacy, affect regulation, skills for dealing with intense affect, and those skills we explored in detail in chapter 9.

In addition to preparing the child for working on issues in psychotherapy, each childhood issue may require subtle changes or additions to the EMDR protocol, while some areas require more significant modifications. For additional resources, the EMDR community has created specialty training in many of these areas for adult clients. Lists of specialty providers and training opportunities can be located on the EMDR International Association Web site (http://www.emdria.org).

PARENTS, PARENTING SKILLS, AND ACTIVE PARENTING

In psychotherapy with children, case conceptualization must include the parent. We see the parent as playing an integral role in the child's success in therapy. The parent's own issues, the parent's parenting skills, and the parent's ability to enact his or her parenting skills have a great deal to do with the child's issues. I (R.T.) explain to parents that we are cotherapists. I only see the child for sessions in my office, while the parent is involved with the child 24 hours a day, 7 days a week. Because of this, it is the parent who must be involved with the child's work outside the office.

This can be a very difficult issue for parents. Some parents may have a good idea of what to do but need validation from the therapist. Other parents may have no idea how to handle the situation and will need training and coaching. The therapist may need to teach the parent about using behavioral skills in working with the child. We commonly refer to parenting classes and offer reading materials to parents. We recommend that parents read *Growing Up Again* (Clarke & Dawson, 1998) and books by Dr. T. Berry Brazelton such as *Touchpoints, Birth to Three* (1992) 2nd ed., rev. (Brazelton & Sparrow, 2006) and *The Earliest Relationship* (Brazelton & Cramer, 1990), and *Parenting From the Inside Out* (Siegel & Hartzell, 2003). We also recommend that parents reference Dr. Bruce Perry's Web site (http://www.childtrauma.org) and the Zero to Three Web site (http://www.zerotothree.com) for additional information on parenting.

In addition to parent training, we assess the parents' relationship with the child and consider any attachment issues that need to be addressed. Additional information on working with children with attachment issues is included later in this chapter. Frequently, parents do not know how to play, so we may coach the parent on how to play with the child. Many parents only interact with children when the parent is giving instructions or teaching, not when just relaxing and playing. We may suggest that parents give the child 5 minutes of special time, for which the child chooses the activity and the parent has to do whatever the child wants to do. We also teach positive reinforcement skills and natural and logical consequences in parenting.

GENERAL CATEGORIES OF CHILDHOOD CONCERNS

We delineated these general categories based on the etiology of why children present for therapy, even though many children can present with symptoms that fit under more than one of these arbitrary categories. The symptoms with which child clients present for mental health treatment can include both internalizing and externalizing issues. At times, children will have symptoms that do not rise to the level of a specific diagnosis. For specific criteria regarding differential diagnoses, please consult the *Diagnostic and Statistical Manual of the American Psychiatric Association*, 4th Edition, Text Revision (*DSM–IV–TR*; American Psychiatric Association, 2000) and the *Diagnostic Classification of Mental Health and Developmental Disorders of Infancy and Early Childhood Revised* (DC 0–3 R) (Zero to Three, 2005).

Clinical Diagnoses of Childhood

Attention-Deficit/Hyperactivity Disorder (ADHD). One frequently encountered diagnosis of childhood is Attention-Deficit/Hyperactivity Disorder (ADHD), where children can present with inattentiveness, with hyperactivity, or with a combined type of attention deficit and hyperactivity. Unfortunately, many children are diagnosed, especially by school personnel, as presenting with ADHD, when the children may actually be suffering from other medical and psychological issues that look like ADHD but are not. After clear diagnosis has been determined, EMDR will not necessarily resolve ADHD, but a portion of the child's hyperactivity may decrease if the hyperactivity is related to anxiety and/or PTSD. Some children diagnosed with ADHD may have concurrent PTSD or have experienced a significant traumatic event. It is important to be aware of the possibility that children with difficulty focusing and/or hyperactivity may be presenting those symptoms as a response to trauma. Some children may have an underlying ADHD diagnosis that has been exacerbated by a traumatic event, while other children with ADHD may have experienced distressing events that are a result of the child struggling with ADHD. For example, children with ADHD often have a history of unsuccessful moments in academic or social situations. Children with ADHD have often experienced negative feedback from frustrated parents, family members, or teachers. These distressing experiences and events are all potential targets for EMDR. Because children can have many stressing events that contribute to anxiety, difficulty functioning, and hyperactivity, it is important to use some type of tool to collect targets for EMDR. We find it is helpful to have the child complete a map of targets, as we discussed in chapter 5.

Case Study: Gordan and ADHD

I (C.S.) once worked with a young boy named Gordan who was diagnosed with ADHD, and after coaching him and helping the parents to learn more effective parenting skills, the child was doing well and discontinued therapy. After several months, Gordan's parents brought him back to therapy because his hyperactivity had increased significantly, and Gordan's parents were trying to determine if Gordan needed his medications increased. Even though Gordan refused to do a map of his targets, Gordan did want to write a story about his worries. In a few words, Gordan wrote about a child in his classroom who had sexually assaulted Gordan in the boy's bathroom at school. After targeting Gordan's trauma, Gordan's hyperactivity returned to the previous level, and he did not require an increase in his ADHD medication.

Children With ADHD and Coexisting Issues. In addition, children with ADHD may also present with coexisting sensory integration issues and tics. We discuss working with sensory integration issues and tics in another section of this chapter as well.

During therapy with children with ADHD symptoms, therapists must be willing to move around a lot and change modalities in therapy. Children with ADHD can potentially be very challenging in therapy, and it is important for the therapist to be aware of his or her own responses to the child. If this is occurring in therapy, this is most likely reminiscent of what occurs with friends, teachers, and others in the child's life. Those social experiences can also be sources of trauma that cause anxiety, which in turn tends to exacerbate the hyperactivity. This cycle of asynchrony with people and the world around the child is a very appropriate target for psychotherapy as well as suggestive of the child's need for skill building and resourcing. We will use the relationship in psychotherapy and the parent–child relationship to exemplify what might be happening outside the office and have the child practice noticing and trying new behaviors. For example, we say to the child, "When you did __________ [behavior], I felt __________. Was that what you wanted me to feel, or did you mean something different?" This gives the therapist additional information as to how others react to the child and provides an opportunity to practice new responses and to install those more appropriate behaviors with bilateral stimulation (BLS).

Children with ADHD can have difficultly transitioning and may ask many questions without waiting for answers and then correct anything the therapist says. In the therapist's office, children with ADHD can be very aggressive and try to control the environment in what oftentimes seems to be the child's effort to minimize his or her anxiety. We find it is helpful to teach children with ADHD relaxation skills, emotional regulation tools, and boundaries. I (C.S.) do a great deal of coaching with children with ADHD. This is when teaching resource development and mastery skills is very important for children struggling with ADHD issues.

Sometimes after targeting the traumatic experiences and teaching new behaviors and skills, we have found that it has been possible to reduce medications for children with ADHD.

Tic Disorders. Tics are a neurological disorder that can be caused by many things, including infection, disease, trauma, or as the side effect to a medication. First, it is necessary to have the child see a pediatrician to assess the possible causes of the tics and rule out any serious medical issues. Once that is done, EMDR can be used to target the anxiety around the tic, which can assist with reducing the frequency and intensity of the tic.

Case Study: Sam and a Facial Tic

I (C.S.) worked with a happy 9-year-old boy named Sam, who had a facial tic. His tic behaviors would escalate in frequency and intensity in stressful and social situations. We targeted the first time another child noticed his tic and how he felt. After reprocessing this incident, we targeted more recent times in which someone else had noticed his tick. We then contemplated future times in which others might notice the tic and the child's response to someone else noticing. The child's negative cognition was "I can't control myself." The child's positive cognition was "I can deal with what people say." This helped reduce the tic tremendously. Sam was then better able to handle his tics in stressful and social situations.

Disorders Associated With Stressful or Traumatic Life Events. Children may experience stressful life situations or events from which clinical issues arise, including adjustment disorders, acute stress disorder, and at the extreme end, PTSD and dissociation. Children may initially present with symptoms suggestive of an adjustment disorder, where the child is struggling to adjust to a specific life situation or event. Children with acute stress disorder are responding to an extreme stressor, with symptoms that are of an acute nature and have occurred within 4 weeks of the traumatic event. If a child has experienced a recent event defined as a traumatic event that happened within the last 3 months, it is important for the therapist to consider whether or not to use the *recent event protocol* (Shapiro, 2001) or to follow the eight-phase protocol. The decision to use the recent event protocol is made depending on how the child has stored the memory of the event. Using the recent event protocol is not always necessary with children because children are so present oriented. The impact of the passage of time and memory consolidation for children are not the same as for adults. Often, just targeting the event or the symptom that arose from the event is sufficient for child clients. If, however, that does not work, using Shapiro's recent event protocol can be helpful. We have provided the recent event protocol in child language in Appendix VII.

Case Study: Elena and Her Recent Event

I (C.S.) worked with a 5-year-old girl, Elena, 1 month after the World Trade Center was bombed on September 11, 2001. She had developed school anxiety that was exhibited when she was supposed to get on the school bus. Elena would begin screaming and crying and hanging on to her mother. When I interviewed Elena, she said that she was upset after watching the news and seeing the airplanes hit the two towers over and over again. This made her worry about going to school and being separated from her mother. I had Elena describe what she saw on television, and she reported that the worst part was the first plane hitting a tower, and she drew a picture of the incident. Her negative cognition was "I'm in danger." Her positive cognition was "I'm safe." We reprocessed that incident, and she felt much better. I then had her tell me a story of everything that she saw on television from start to finish, and I had her draw pictures of everything. We reprocessed each picture from beginning to end, until there was a subjective units of disturbance (SUD) of 0. This only took about 25 minutes. We then addressed the present stimulus, which was Elena's worry about not being with her mother. On further exploration, it became clear that Elena's mother was recovering from her own depression, and I discussed depression with Elena and did some attachment repair work for Elena to feel connected and safe.

Elena's symptoms quickly abated; however, if the child's symptoms continue for more than an additional 4 weeks, the child could eventually meet the criteria for a diagnosis of PTSD. Even though the diagnostic criteria for acute stress disorder and PTSD require a traumatic event, children may have extreme responses to a traumatic event that is less severe than described in the *DSM–IV–TR*, but the child may respond with severe symptoms. This is a common occurrence when children experience medical procedures. Children may respond with symptoms that would meet the criteria for PTSD after having surgery to have tubes put in their ears. It is important to not place so much emphasis on the situation or event, but rather on the fact that there is an event, and the child is responding with symptoms from the event. In some cases, it appears that the child has experienced a traumatic event, but neither the parent nor the child are able to identify the event.

Case Study: Ean and the School Bus Accident

I (R.T.) met with a 7-year-old boy who displayed classic symptoms of PTSD, but we were unable to identify the traumatic event, until the parents learned from the school that Ean's bus had passed a severe traffic accident, where Ean witnessed the bloody victims of the traffic accident out the window of the school bus. Ean was not able to relay what he had seen, and the school bus driver was focused on maneuvering through the traffic and did not see what the children on one side of the bus had witnessed. Ean did not connect witnessing the car accident with his nightmares, hypervigilance, fears of riding in the car, or anxiety from hearing sirens. After reviewing Ean's experiences and checking with other children on the bus, the parents were able to glean enough information that when we explored this with the little boy, Ean then talked about the bloody people he had seen out the window of the bus. It is important to consider that the severity of the event may not be interpreted as traumatic to an older child or adult and that it may take some detective work to determine what the child has actually experienced.

I (R.T.) have found that often there are events that children witness that are unknown to parents. For example, I have met with many children who have been in a classroom with other children and witnessed another child having a seizure and emergency personnel coming to the classroom or the playground. With other young clients, the child may have witnessed the school staff conducting a restraint on a classmate who was physically violent in school and on the playground.

No matter what the diagnosis, the therapist should use the standard EMDR protocol, with a focus on reprocessing the situations or events that are underlying the clinical symptoms. (We discuss, in chapter 1, the research on using EMDR with children presenting with symptoms consistent with PTSD, both in an individual and a group protocol.) If the child is diagnosed with acute stress disorder because it has been less than 4 weeks since the child experienced the traumatic event, the therapist may need to determine if the standard protocol is appropriate or if the therapist needs to use the recent event protocol.

Anxiety Disorders/Obsessive Compulsive Disorders/Generalized Anxiety Disorders and Phobias. We would encourage therapists who work with clients with any anxiety or related disorder to pursue specialty training with providers who present specialty training on using EMDR with anxiety disorders in adult clients. Shapiro (2001) also described a phobia protocol. Children with anxiety-related disorders will most likely have a touchstone event driving the anxiety. Sometimes it is difficult to determine what the missing piece is for the child, but it is important to ask the child the first time he or she remembers thinking or feeling that way. Sometimes the event will appear related, while other times, the event may seem to have nothing to do with the current manifestation of the anxiety.

Case Study: Stella and Needles

I (C.S.) worked with a little girl who came to therapy due to a needle phobia. Stella would get light-headed and faint when she had to get a shot, even if she was lying down. Despite the fact that we targeted the first time that this happened and the worst time, the SUD did not go down. With Stella, we had to trace her thought process of the origins of her feelings, which eventually led to the first time that Stella fainted. As it turns out, the first time Stella fainted was in a science class, where her teacher was explaining how germs get in the body. After Stella fainted in front of her class and was embarrassed by what had happened, Stella then began to generalize to the fear of anything entering her body, including needles. Once we targeted Stella's memory of fainting in science class, Stella's needle phobia improved. We continued to target other triggers for Stella, until her anxiety decreased.

What is different about using EMDR with phobias or anxiety attacks is that it is important to target the actual instances when the child had an anxiety attack and the associated body symptoms. The remainder of the eight-phase protocol needs to be applied in the treatment of children with any anxiety-related disorder, including the manifestations of the anxiety disorder as targets. We recommend that therapists consider the *phobia protocol* given by Shapiro (2001).

It is important to teach children ways to handle their anticipatory anxiety about having another panic attack. This is part of the skill building that is part of the preparation phase of EMDR. Children also need to be educated about anxiety and what the body does in response to a real or imaginary threat.

As with any EMDR target, it is important to have the child float back to the first time he or she remembers thinking or feeling that way, and any time he or she almost felt that way (see the discussion of the floatback technique in chapter 3). Then, it is important to have the child recount the time this was the worst and the last time that it happened. It is also important to have the child reprocess any secondary traumas that occurred as a result of an anxiety attack, including fainting or being ridiculed.

We also suggest that therapists target the child's memories of what happens to the child's body when he or she is anxious. Does the child's heart race, does the child's hands sweat, or does he or she feel light-headed? We would encourage therapists to educate the child about the fear of the fear and then targeting the fear of becoming anxious.

Once all the previous events and current symptoms have been targeted, it is important to do a future template, where the child sees himself or herself starting to feel anxious and using resources to successfully calm himself or herself and avert the anxiety attack.

Performance Anxiety and Test Taking. After ruling out learning disabilities, ADHD, or medical conditions, the therapist should gather information regarding anxiety-provoking situations at school and at home and then regarding test taking. Next, the therapist should list the current stimuli that trigger the anxiety.

Making a map is particularly helpful to ensure that the therapist targets all the possible aspects of the test-taking anxiety. Pay particular attention to what a teacher, tutor, parent, or child may have said to the child regarding his or her learning disabilities. The therapist can use mastery skills and resource development and installation (chapter 9) to reinforce times when the child felt successful in school. If the child cannot remember any positives associated with school, the child can choose another situation he or she feels good about. And again, reprocess the earliest and worst, and run a movie of the future taking a test.

I (C.S.) have had parents bring in spelling tests the child had completed but done poorly on. I have the child retake the test in the session and have the child report when he or she was feeling nervous, and I applied BLS in the moment to reprocess the anxiety in the in vivo experience of test taking.

Symptoms on the Dissociative Continuum. Therapists who treat children with dissociative symptoms need to be aware of the current research and guidelines on working with these children, and we refer you to the *Guidelines for the Evaluation and Treatment of Dissociative Symptoms in Children and Adolescents* (International Society for the Study of Dissociation [ISSD] Task Force on Children and Adolescents, 2003) for additional information. That being said, we suggest that children often present with dissociative qualities, especially when the child has experienced any kind of distressing or traumatic event in his or her life. On the continuum of dissociative disorders, children are naturally imaginative and use fantasy a great deal, and it is important for the therapist not to pathologize the child's presentation but consider the continuum of normal development in children. However, some children dissociate as a response to traumatic events, including extreme and chronic abuse. Therapists need to learn about dissociation and gain an understanding about what dissociation looks like in children. Some degree of dissociation is evident in most children with trauma histories, but with EMDR, we do not target dissociation directly. Dissociation is a symptom of a trauma in a child's life, and in case conceptualization for treatment, dissociation is a brilliant survival response to anything that threatens the child's survival. We make note of any dissociative symptoms with which the child presents such as a glazed look, as if the child is looking off into space. According to the ISSD Task Force for Children and Adolescents (2004), "An important goal of therapy is for the child to learn increasingly adaptive and flexible ways to manage affect and to integrate past, current, and new experiences so that development is not compromised" (p. 134). Children may also look like they are daydreaming or are startled when the therapist talks to them or moves, suggestive of a trance or derealization. Some children will act out the dissociation by taking on an animal persona.

Case Study: Mylie and the Deer

I (R.T.) worked with a 9-year-old girl who had experienced extreme abuse and would become a deer when she was overwhelmed. I soon realized that this child's presentation was more than just playing. The child would look around the room in an alarmed and hypervigilant state, as she walked on all fours and jumped around the room when she was startled. The child became a deer and could not process the trauma history. With this child, I would have her talk about what a deer would need to relax or sleep. We would then create a narrative of a relaxed deer and install the positive experiences of being a deer. The child then was able to understand what would scare the deer and cause the deer to be worried, and she built a safe area where the deer could remember, but not get hurt. The child began to move in and out of being a deer much more quickly, and it appeared that she felt more powerful, both as a child and as a deer, until she did not need to be the deer very often at all. The deer was also silent, as we know deer to be, so she became the child voice of the deer to interpret what only she could hear from the deer. Once the child's foster parents could accept why the child needed to be a deer and say to her, "It looks like something scary might be happening because the deer is here. Can you explain to us what is happening?" the child began to talk more openly with her parents and explain her experiences and feelings. Initially, this child was completely dissociated and would be surprised as to why she would get in trouble for acting like a deer and then for lying about it. When the parents began to understand that the child was not lying, but instead dissociating, the parents learned from the child how they should act when the deer was present. As the parents began to create a safety zone for the deer, the barriers between the child and the deer persona began to soften and come down. The child became aware of the deer, and the deer learned about the child. Eventually, the deer became part of the child, and she protected the deer from harm with the help of her new family. As she felt more safe, both internally and externally, this child's intelligence and creativity became more evident, and she was successful in school and in attaching to her new parents.

There is interplay between trauma and attachment trauma as it relates to the development of dissociation in children. Theoretically, dissociation is part of normal development but becomes problematic when it changes the course of normal development and causes difficulty in the child's life. Children who experience distress or abuse in their relationships with their primary caregivers often find survival and attachment at odds, thus causing distress for the child. To cope and survive, children often dissociate. Children may experience depersonalization, derealization, and psychic numbing, without presenting with separate personalities. At the extreme end of the dissociative continuum, research suggests that early attachment trauma with an intelligent and creative child can lead to severe types of dissociation and possibly dissociative identity disorder.

It is important that therapists assess for dissociation and consider to what degree the child is using dissociation as a coping mechanism, especially in current circumstances. Children may also present with bland affect, numbing, and even sleepiness. Sleeping can be a form of dissociation, especially with children. When experiencing overwhelming distress and emotion, children will begin to get sleepy and yawn. This is part of the flight–fight–freeze response. Dr. Bruce Perry (2006) writes that in children, the dissociative continuum includes rest, avoidance, protection, and compliance, in which the child experiences a sense of detachment and depersonalization, and then dissociation, which includes this blankness and noncommunicative response from the client, in which the client appears either frozen or displays behaviors such as fetal rocking and sleep. When children stop processing and fall asleep, many therapists will stop EMDR; however, we encourage the therapist to help the child ground himself or herself by reconnecting with the therapist and the office. Grounding techniques may include the therapist stomping his or her feet or making other body movements, or the therapist can gently toss a pillow to the child in an effort to have the child reconnect to his or her body and the safety of the therapist's office.

When using EMDR with children who dissociate, the therapist needs to spend a great deal of time front loading with skills and techniques during the preparation phase before proceeding with any desensitization of targets. It is important to teach the child and parents about dissociation and tools for affect regulation and managing intense affect in order that the child can stay connected during therapy. The goal is to increase the affect regulatory capacity of the child, and part of this is dealing with attachment trauma and creating new healthy attachments in the environment.

EMDR With Children With Attachment Disorders. In case conceptualization in working with children with attachment trauma, it is important to follow the eight-phase protocol because it is concise and thorough. During client history and treatment planning, the therapist needs to consider that even babies are capable of "pathological mourning" (Bowlby, 1999); therefore the therapist needs to follow the steps we discussed in chapter 3, with several additional modifications. As with any client, it is important to assess for concurrent disorders, including PTSD, anxiety, and depression. It is also important to consider what has happened to the child, including prenatal drug exposure, exposure to domestic violence, multiple caregivers, multiple moves, medical interventions, and previous relationship disruptions in the child's life. It is helpful to use an assessment tool to comprehensively collect information because reporters may not think to tell you. We encourage you not only to ask the child and the parent, but also to collect data from medical charts and hospital birth records, if available.

Attachment and Dissociation. It is also important to consider that for children with attachment trauma, there is almost always an element of dissociation. Furthermore, there is often sexual exposure or boundary violations of some kind, with sexually acting out behaviors, including excessive masturbation (assess and educate parent about what is typical and healthy for children and what behaviors are of concern). The therapist needs to explore the extent of the child's sexual acting out and consider risk factors and safety needs. There is more information on working with children with sexually reactive or trauma-reactive behaviors later in this chapter.

Parent/Caregiver Attachment History. It is important also to assess the parents' attachment history or the attachment history of any caregiver. Use a genogram that explores relationships in the child's family. If there is no parent available, ask the foster/adoptive parents, or have the child explore what stories he or she has heard about the child's family history. During this process of exploring relationships in the child's life, it is important to note attachment traumas and other traumas such as surgical procedures, number of caregivers, and so on. I (R.T.) use mapping that is focused on caregiving and nurturing relationships as a way to conceptualize attachment issues as relationship trauma from a grief and loss perspective. EMDR with children with symptoms of attachment disorders focuses on treating attachment disorders as relationship trauma.

By addressing the child's relationship trauma and incorporating the parent or adoptive parent as cotherapist, EMDR can teach attunement, nurturing, awareness of child's needs, and skills an adoptive parent needs to parent children with attachment symptoms. These skills can be taught to the parent and the child during the preparation phase of EMDR.

During the Preparation Phase, as with any other client, it is important to consider what resources the child has and what he or she needs. Who are possible attachment figures—both real or imaginary? What trauma does the child potentially have from that earliest relationship, and are there currently any receptive attachment environments in the child's life? With children with attachment trauma, it is important to consider including the healthiest attachment figures in the child's life in treatment, if at all possible. This caregiver can become part of the child's resources, even if the caregiver is a group home staff member.

It is also important to install mastery skills and several Safe/Calm Places for the child. Even if the therapist's office is the only safe place in the child's life, the therapist can ask the child to notice how he or she feels in the office. I (R.T.) may provide the child with a transitional object, if appropriate, such as a notebook to write in or a blanket for nurturing. I have children put a blanket around their shoulders to give themselves an imaginary hug when they feel upset or uncomfortable. The purpose of any type of transitional object is to create a sense of object permanency with the therapist. This can be difficult with children in the child welfare system, who move often and may change therapists frequently; however, it is important to conceptualize what the child needs to feel like there is someone safe and caring in his or her life, even if the therapist is only in the child's life for a short period of time. This will be discussed further when we explore episodes of care for children in the child welfare system later in this chapter.

It is also important to teach mindfulness, emotional regulation, emotional literacy, and body awareness to keep the child's body engaged in the therapy. These are some examples of skills and resources children can learn to use during the preparation phase. Children can also be taught to use their current selves to nurture younger selves. This can be included as part of creating a coherent narrative or as a cognitive interweave during the later phases of EMDR. It is possible to ask the child, "If you could take care of that part of yourself that was sad or hurt, what do you think that part of you would need to feel better?"

Case Study: Stormy and Her Younger Self

I (R.T.) worked with a 12-year-old girl, named Stormy, who was placed in her adoptive home at age 10, after being with her abusive family until age 6 and then moved back and forth from foster homes to her biological family for 4 years. Because the child never felt stable, she was always moving and was not able to allow herself to attach to her adoptive family. During the therapeutic process, this child decided that she would take her adoptive mom and her 12-year-old self back to get her 6-year-old self. During a session in which the child worked on a negative cognition of "I'm not safe," she decided to pack up her 6-year-old self and bring her 6-year-old self to the present to share her room and her new family. Once the child felt herself join with her traumatized 6-year-old self, she felt empowered to make new choices to be safe and to attach to her new family.

In working with children with attachment issues, the therapist needs to process the child's memories of attachment traumas with important focus on the body scan phase of EMDR. Since attachment trauma often happens in that earliest relationship, the memory is often stored in the body, and the therapist needs to assist the child in achieving a clear body scan. Clearing the affect and body sensations helps the child resolve the memories that are stored from infancy and early childhood. This is also true with future template. It is important to work with the child and parents on the child's feelings of being parented: "What does it feel like in your body when your mom takes care of you? Just notice that." Installing positive body sensations with nurturing from the parent as replacement for the brain stem–based fear of being parented is particularly helpful with EMDR. The therapist can provide simple food, such as Cheerios, to the parent to feed the child, and as the child is being fed by the parent, the therapist has the child notice the positive experience of being fed, while using BLS. This is a mastery experience that can be strengthened as a resource with EMDR. It is also possible to have the parent put body lotion on the child's hands or feet. We keep bottles of lotion in the office and have the parent put the lotion on as a nurturing experience and install this experience as a resource with EMDR.

One additional resource to install is helping the child create a coherent narrative with a foster and/or adoptive parent. I (R.T.) assist adoptive families in creating a coherent narrative for what might have happened to the child and then target the worst part of the narrative for the child to grieve and reprocess the memory. I do not tell the child what to think, but instead ask questions such as, "What do you think it would have been like for a baby in an orphanage in Romania with so many babies and so little money to care for the babies?" Whatever the child reports we use to create a coherent narrative. We also ask the parent to provide whatever factual information the parent knows about the orphanage and tell us what the parent felt when bringing the child to a new home and what the parent hypothesized about what the experience might have been like for the child. We weave what the parent knows, what the child reports, and possible information that I (R.T.) have from working with adoptive families for 20 years to create a story that the child believes is a close approximation to what might have happened in his or her earlier life. I then will ask the child the questions of the procedural steps to target the history that the child has created. Once the child has processed through this history, I ask the child and parents to create a new story as a resource and install how the child found a family that loved and wanted him or her. This new story becomes a resource to allow the child to attach and create a new history.

Children with attachment issues who are being adopted need to reprocess the trauma that originated from early relationships and grieve what they lost to be able to attach to a new family. At times, I may actually ask the child, "What can you give up and what do you need to hold on to?" Children may say, "I can know my mom loved me but couldn't take care of me." "Just notice that." When using EMDR with attachment and adoption, it is important for the therapist to reprocess the child's traumatic losses and clear the grief, and then install the claiming of the new family. The therapist has the child focus on being a member of the family, which is about claiming the adoptive family as the child's own. When working with adoptive children, *claiming* is the psychological process associated with the legal process of adoption. Even though not all children who are dealing with attachment trauma are being adopted, treating attachment trauma is oftentimes necessary before working with even young children who are being adopted.

It is important for therapists to consider that attachment traumas may underlie many emotional and behavioral issues with which children present for therapy and to always consider the impact of healthy attachments on the child's life.

EMDR Phases of Treatment With Sexually Reactive and Trauma-Reactive Sexual Issues. Children who are referred because the child is sexually acting out require unique case conceptualization considerations for therapists. I (R.T.) work with children referred for sexualized behaviors, both by their parents and by the child welfare system. After years of feeling very frustrated at processing these issues in therapy, I found that EMDR gave me the tool I needed to successfully treat children who were sexually acting out by using EMDR as the template for treatment and weaving into phases of the EMDR protocol psychoeducational information, relaxation and emotional regulation work, and urge reduction as well as all the tools I had previously been using to work with children with these issues. This is by no means simple or brief clinical work, but by using EMDR as the template for treatment, psychotherapy can work, with results appearing very early on in treatment. Because this is a complicated treatment issue, I have organized the additional pieces I add to the EMDR eight-phase protocol during case conceptualization with sexually reactive and trauma issues.

Client History and Treatment Planning. During this phase of treatment, I am conducting the same process as discussed in chapter 3, with several additions. I spend more time in exploring any early grief and loss issues, separation from primary caregivers, and who has cared for the child since birth, including baby-sitters, relatives, and other possibilities. I ask the parent when the parent first noticed the behaviors. I also explore how the behaviors have been addressed when the parent has noticed the behaviors. For example, did Dad find the 5-year-old girl and her 6-year-old cousin playing doctor in the child's bedroom and then spank both girls? If so, I consider that this is possibly a trauma for the child, and the child is confused. Remember, children who are trying to figure out something will perseverate and obsess about the issue and reenact the situation over and over in an effort to understand what happened. Is this reenactment behavior? The reenactment behavior gets reinforced because it feels good and then can become an issue of urges that the child feels unable to stop. Remember, sexual behaviors are normal, and both the therapist and parent need to understand what normal development is and what is beyond normal development. There are always cultural and religious beliefs involved as well. It is important to explore any possible accidental exposure to sexually explicit information, media, sleeping arrangements, older siblings, religious issues, movies, parents, and so on.

Case Study: Eleanor and the Bambi Movie

I (R.T.) worked with a 4-year-old girl who had started demonstrating sexually inappropriate behaviors with her dolls, peeking in when adults were changing, and looking under bathroom stalls in public restrooms. Her parents were divorced, and her mother accused her father of sexually abusing Eleanor. After interviewing Eleanor and her parents, I discovered that Dad had previously put in a movie for Eleanor to watch while he took a shower. The movie was labeled "Bambi," and Dad walked away to take a shower but found out on his return that the movie was not a movie about a deer. Unfortunately, Dad had other roommates who had left the movie on the television stand, and Dad did not bother to prescreen the movie before playing it for the 4-year-old. This child was inadvertently exposed to sexually explicit media, even though the parent had not intended to hurt the child.

It is important to explore what boundaries are in the home. Are bathroom doors closed, and do people knock before entering? Is the home developmentally informed and aware, without being too rigid? Parents may not realize that the child is aware of and curious about sexuality.

Children can be exposed to sexuality by covert means that can create sexually reactive behaviors, even if the child has not been overtly sexually abused. No matter what the origin of the inappropriate behaviors, the therapist can use EMDR to treat the child's urges and install replacement behaviors.

Preparation. During this phase of treatment, I am working with the child to see if we can use thought-stopping, relaxation, and replacement behaviors for the child to learn to distract himself or herself. What rules are in the house about this behavior? What is the safety plan in the house? I have included an example of a safety plan that I ask families to complete when there is concern about a child sexually acting out and possibly hurting other children.

Some children may confuse love and sex. This can occur overtly or covertly, as discussed previously. If the therapist assesses that the child cannot differentiate between love and sex, the therapist may have to provide psychoeducational information about the differences between the two and about boundaries and appropriate behaviors for children. Children who have older siblings may be exposed to behaviors that younger children mimic.

Assessment, Desensitization, Installation, and Body Scan. When identifying targets for reprocessing with sexually reactive children, I ask the child to discuss what happens right before the child feels like sexually acting out. Once the child describes what happens, I have the child float back to the first time the child remembers feeling that way. This becomes the touchstone event that we use to reprocess. It is very important to have the child pay attention to body sensations. Some children are embarrassed and need encouragement to process the memory. Some children began sexually acting out after they were caught touching themselves or playing doctor with another child, and the event is now stored maladaptively. Because many memories may be embarrassing for children, it is possible to have the child identify the event without describing everything that happened. I simply ask the child to bring up the image that represents the worst part of the event and then continue with the procedural steps of EMDR. Many children will identify a negative cognition as "I'm bad" or "I'm bad for having those feelings." In processing targets with sexually reactive children, the therapist may need cognitive interweaves that educate the child about physical responses and normal body sensations, and this may require that the therapist assist the child in differentiating having a feeling or body sensation versus acting on the feeling. It is important for the child to come to the resolution that the feeling or body sensation is not wrong, but it is the behavior that, at times, is inappropriate. I find that I may have to ask the child to consider alternative or replacement behaviors that can be installed instead of sexually acting out.

Future Template. After reprocessing past events and current triggers, I ask the child to image a time in the future when the child experiences the urge to act out and then sees himself or herself making healthy and appropriate choices. Again, use the protocol for the future template, and install new, healthy behaviors that are developmentally and age-appropriate for the child. This will help the child to make new choices when experiencing the urge to act out sexually.

Case Study: Maddie and Her Success With Reducing Sexually Reactive Behaviors

A 10-year-old girl was brought to my (R.T.) office for therapy by her birth mother. Maddie presented with severe temper tantrums, defiance, severe mood instability, poor school performance, sexualized behaviors, and a suspected history of sexual abuse from a grandfather that is believed to have occurred until the child was 2 years old. The child had been treated for the last 7 years by various mental health professionals, and the child had been prescribed a series of medications that did not improve the child's presenting symptoms. The last therapist concluded that the child had symptoms consistent with an attachment disorder and recommended the child be seen by a mental health professional with expertise in working with children with attachment issues. I learned that the child was the eldest child of four siblings in a family that consisted of her mother, stepfather, half-sibling, and two stepsiblings. After conducting a comprehensive client history and treatment plan, we began working on skills for the child to use when she felt overwhelmed. After learning relaxation skills and thought stopping and the get a grip technique, the child began to identify situations that were triggering her tantrums. The child was being humiliated by a boy on the bus, and we later found that a neighbor girl had been initiating sexual behaviors with the child. We used future template for the child to imagine herself being successful ignoring the boy on the bus and desensitized the feelings she had about herself when the boy teased her. The bad thought was "I can't handle it," and her good thought was "He's just a stupid boy. He is the one with problems. I can handle it." The child imagined herself using an imaginary magic wand to put a bubble around herself so she could not hear the boy when he was teasing her. The child was especially sensitive to teasing from other children, and we began to target past events of teasing and install mastery experiences when she was successfully ignoring other children. The child tended to focus on the times she got in trouble and not the times when she was able to ignore another child and walk away. Therefore, at the beginning of each session, I would ask her for examples when she had been successful calming herself and not being triggered. After the child experienced success with current symptoms with EMDR, she was much more willing to target more potent issues. We then began to target the child's sexualized behaviors. We explored what triggered the feelings. After working with learning boundaries and reading books about private parts, the child began to explain the funny feeling she would have in her body that would make her want to sexually act out, even though she knew it was wrong. The child identified a toolbox of things she could do to stop her thoughts and distract herself until the body sensations went away. We focused on installing future templates and mastery experiences, when the child would see herself being successful. We continued by targeting her uncomfortable and "funny" body sensations as well. During a session when the child was targeting the body sensations she would get in her privates, she began to respond, "I can go play the piano." My response was "Go with that." During the next set of BLS, she said, "I don't feel that feeling when I'm playing the piano." Again, I responded, "Go with that." She then began to report many instances where she had drawn a picture or read a book or left the situation with another child and felt like she was not responsible for her body sensations, but that she now had choices when she felt the body sensations. We also targeted the child's grief that she was the only child who did not biologically belong to her stepfather, who was very loving and cared for the child. We processed her grief and then worked on her relationship with her biological father in order that she could grieve and then allow herself to feel a secure attachment with her stepfather. As we continued to reprocess the child's targets, while installing mastery experiences for the child to use when she was triggered, the child began to verbalize her feelings, instead of having meltdowns, and began to perform in school and achieved her first report card with all As. I also worked with the family to educate them about attachment and trauma and teach them more positive parenting, in which they would praise the child when they saw her struggling but not having a meltdown. We focused on her strengths and accomplishments, while allowing her to choose consequences when she made unhealthy choices.

Using EMDR to treat children with sexually reactive and trauma-reactive behaviors can be very successful when the therapist treats the origins of the child's behaviors and the associated urges the child experiences, while then installing resources and replacement behaviors for when the child feels the urge to act out sexually.

Children With Traumatic Medical Conditions. We have used EMDR with children who must endure medical procedures and with chronic medical conditions or injuries. We not only use EMDR to target the traumatic and intrusive memories of medical procedures, but also for children who must endure ongoing medical issues such as treatment for cancer, diabetes, and burns. Case conceptualization with children with medical trauma or conditions follows the eight phases that we have discussed in the chapters of this book, with mapping to identify targets for reprocessing. We also use resourcing and future template to assist children in preparing for medical examinations and treatments. I (C.S.) have used EMDR with a child with a traumatic brain injury. We believe this case is important in that we demonstrate an example of when the parent narrative is helpful in using EMDR with children.

Case Study: Darren's Near-Drowning

I (C.S.) had been called by a priest to go to Phoenix Children's Hospital to do some EMDR with the parents of a 2-year-old boy who was in a vegetative coma from a near-drowning 2 days earlier. The boy, Darren, was not expected to live. The doctors were preparing to remove life support. I did EMDR on the parents, which helped them to become calmer and clearer about their decisions and helped them remember more positive things about Darren than only focusing on the last 2 days.

After the life support was removed, the doctors gave the parents permission to take Darren home to die. However, Darren did not die, and the parents began to take care of his medical needs at home. A senior EMDR child therapist suggested I do

EMDR on the toddler. I was reluctant because the child was having seizures, but I discussed this with the parents, and they agreed that it might help.

When I saw Darren, he was lying on the couch with his arms rigidly pulled up to his chest, his legs outstretched and stiff, with his gaze affixed off to the left, occasionally blinking and rolling his eyes. We decided to do a parent narrative similar to that written about by Lovett (1999). The mother sat behind Darren and tapped his shoulders, telling the story of his near-drowning. Although she had not been there, she recounted the story in the way she imagined it had happened. We chose a negative cognition in words that Darren might have actually used: "My not safe." The positive cognition was "My safe."

As his mother told the story and it approached the actual fall into the water, Darren's body visibly stiffened and arched. He writhed around when she talked of the helicopter transport and the events in the hospital. She continued with the story, interweaving "My not safe" until she reached the part of the story when Darren was brought home and taken care of. At that point, she began to say, "My safe." Darren noticeably relaxed, his arms loosened for the first time on his chest, and he fell asleep. The mother and I were amazed.

Darren continued to improve, and the parents actively pursued medical care as well as alternative healing. I came back 2 weeks later, and the mother reported that one of the difficulties they were having was getting Darren to all of his medical appointments. Because his muscles were stiff, it was hard to get him in a car seat without causing him pain. The mother agreed to do the parent-narrative form of EMDR again. This time, she told the narrative of a recent doctor's visit, starting with trying to get Darren into a child car seat. She continued to describe Darren's distress all the way through the doctor's visit and all the way to the ride home. Again, Darren's mother wove the negative cognition, "My not safe," throughout the narrative, until he was coming home, at which time she changed to the positive cognition, "My safe." We then did a future template of a doctor's visit using the positive cognition "My safe" throughout. At the end, Darren was relaxed and looked directly at his mother for the first time.

Over the years, Darren continued to progress. He vocalized, laughed, and would look at his parents, and he would cry when his mother was sad. He could eat some. He loved the sound of birds and clearly responded to the environment. His muscles in his legs were still stiff, but he was obviously no longer in a coma.

Darren recently passed away at 7 years old. It was unclear why, although he began losing weight for no apparent reason. Darren died in his mother's arms, and despite the struggles, he gave his parents much love and joy.

Because Darren was nonverbal and in a vegetative state, I (C.S.) used the parent narrative to reprocess Darren's memories of the event, yet we encourage therapists to ask the child, if at all possible. It is also important to discuss the treatment with the physician prior to beginning EMDR because reprocessing can be soothing and relaxing, but I have also seen EMDR to be overstimulating for the client. Since affect regulation and self-soothing are difficult to teach and monitor with clients with head injuries, I suggest that the therapist begin with a safe place protocol that is done very slowly and with brief sets of BLS. As the therapist proceeds, it is important to be attuned to the client, who may react with vocalizations and unusual body movements. It is best to proceed prudently and cautiously, until the therapist and parent are comfortable that the process is benefiting the client.

Early-Onset or Juvenile Bipolar Disorder. Children who present with severe mood instability along with irritability and extreme behavior issues need to participate in a thorough assessment process as part of the diagnostic process. Children who meet the criteria for a diagnosis of early-onset bipolar disorder or juvenile bipolar disorder also need to participate in an extensive diagnostic process to rule out other diagnoses or identify concurrent diagnoses because many children are misdiagnosed with ADHD and oppositional defiant disorder (ODD). Even some children who test gifted may present with a severe mood instability, low frustration tolerance, and difficulty self-soothing that resembles early-onset bipolar disorder. Medical issues, along with the child's trauma history, current levels of stress, and a family genealogy that explores the possibility of relatives diagnosed with bipolar disorder, must be thoroughly explored during the intake process as well. Making a diagnosis of early-onset bipolar disorder should not be taken lightly, and it is important to rule out concurrent issues.

Children with early-onset bipolar disorder also need to be referred to a pediatric psychiatrist for evaluation; however, during the assessment process, children can still benefit from self-soothing and calming skills. Once the child has been evaluated, and the treatment team is confident that a diagnosis of early-onset bipolar disorder is accurate, the child will most likely be prescribed psychotropic medications to improve mood stability.

As the team works to improve and stabilize the child's mood, the therapist can begin the mapping process with the child to identify experiences that may have been traumatic for the child, including what has happened to the child as a result of the extreme moods and irritability. Many children who have early-onset bipolar disorder have a history of getting in trouble with adults, along with a difficulty in social situations that has caused the child to feel like a bad child or that no one likes him or her. As is appropriate for the child's developmental level, we encourage therapists to explain bipolar disorder to children and to help children understand why they have encountered certain responses from others, for example, "You know how you told me that people seem to get mad at you a lot? Well, can you tell me what people seem to get mad at you about?" Most children will say, "I'm always in trouble, and I don't know why" or "I get in trouble because I get mad a lot." Some children will openly discuss what happens, and others will want to pretend that it does not happen. It is my (R.T.) experience that children with early-onset bipolar disorder tend to be very creative and bright children. Exploring the secondary issues that arise for a child with early-onset bipolar disorder is important, and those experiences can be targeted for reprocessing with EMDR. It appears to be a vicious cycle of the child presenting with the symptoms of early-onset bipolar disorder and then getting in trouble at school and home, and even sometimes getting kicked out of school, so that the child feels angry or hurt, and this distress exacerbates the mood instability and irritability. We recommend that therapists use emotional mastery and resource skills to help children stabilize and that any traumas be reprocessed with EMDR when the child has been successfully prepared for the desensitization phase.

Parents need to become educated about early-onset bipolar disorder and be offered resources and additional parenting skills, for example, handouts from the National Alliance for the Mentally Ill (http://www.nami.org). We also recommend that assistance be provided to the child's school to help the teacher and school personnel prepare improvement-focused educational resources for the child. Therapists can also offer guidance and information for school personnel who are writing individualized education plans for children diagnosed with early-onset bipolar disorder. Additional information on juvenile bipolar disorders can be found on the Juvenile Bipolar Research Foundation Web site (http://www.jbrf.org), the organization that also published the Child Bipolar Questionnaire.

Therefore case conceptualization when EMDR is used to treat children diagnosed with early-onset bipolar disorder requires thorough assessment, both psychologically and psychiatrically, while working through the phases of EMDR to treat the various dynamics of dealing with bipolar disorder at such a young age.

Clinical and Behavioral Issues

Trichotillomania. *Trichotillomania* is both a clinical and behavioral disorder and is defined as an impulse control disorder that typically has an event associated with the onset of symptoms. Trichotillomania is diagnosed with clients who pull out body hair, including scalp hair, eyebrows, eyelashes, and hair on any part of the body. In addition to obvious hygiene and physical presentation issues, trichotillomania can cause conflict in relationships and social situations. In case conceptualization with using EMDR to treat children with trichotillomania, we rule out other disorders by referring to a pediatrician, who can assess for medical issues and consider the use of any medications, if necessary. Medication is not necessarily the treatment of choice; however, given the time that it takes to get an appointment with a child psychiatrist, we refer the parent while we try therapeutic interventions, knowing that the appointment with the psychiatrist can be canceled if the interventions are successful. Once any other medical conditions are ruled out, the next step in therapy is to determine when the symptoms started and what situations or events might have occurred at that time. The symptoms have often escalated because the parent is so disturbed by the child's symptoms that the parent's response increases the pressure to stop and causes an added level of shame for the child. It is important to work with the parent to help the parent cope with the child's trichotillomania and to teach the parent not to react, but to simply observe and encourage the child.

Children with trichotillomania may have a critical internal or external voice. The external voice can be from a parent, teacher, coach, or older sibling. The critical external voice is so loud that the child feels constantly put down and incompetent. This critical external voice may become internalized and then the child can become self-critical and perfectionistic. With the EMDR protocol, it is important to find the touchstone event and then target what the current stimulus is that leads to hair pulling. As with the standard EMDR protocol, it is important to do the future template, but we add a replacement behavior for the child to imagine doing in the future that is comforting and soothing.

Case Study: Chloe's Experience With Trichotillomania

Nine-year-old Chloe was brought in to see me (C.S.) because she was pulling her eyelashes out. Chloe's mother said this had begun after school had started, when her new art teacher yelled at the class. By Chloe's report, her art teacher was very critical and yelled constantly. The mother had spoken to the art teacher and the principal and the yelling had stopped, but the eyelash pulling continued. Mother said in passing that Chloe's dance teacher last year also had yelled at the students but that it was not an issue anymore since the parents had taken Chloe out of dance class 6 months ago.

Chloe was a bright, pretty girl but had difficulty expressing emotions. Chloe's mother described her as a perfectionist who kept her room ultraclean and loved arranging her pen and pencil collection. Chloe's mother was very anxious and critical of Chloe's eyelash pulling.

The first step was to reassure Chloe's mother that her daughter would be fine and that it was important for her to be calm and supportive of Chloe's efforts. The next step was to teach Chloe about emotions and how to express them. I recommended the American Girls book Feelings. *We targeted the first, worst, and most recent times the art teacher had yelled. Her negative cognition was "I'm in danger." Then, we targeted the blocking belief "I have to be perfect." We also targeted the mother's critical voice. And finally, we targeted the times she tended to pull her eyelashes out when she was relaxing, watching TV, or right before she fell asleep. This reduced the eyelash pulling significantly, but she still had a pulling episode once a week. Finally, I returned to her original cognition and asked her, "When was the first time you felt 'I'm in danger'?" And Chloe promptly said, "When my dance teacher told us she was going to kill us with a hammer." We successfully targeted that incident, and the eyelash pulling stopped.*

It is our experience that children with trichotillomania and other impulse control disorders do not realize that they are exhibiting the behavior in the moment, and it is not until later that the child notices, or the child notices when confronted by someone else. This can also be true with children with self-abusive behaviors.

Self-Abusive Behaviors, Including Picking. Children with self-abusive behaviors can include children who pick at open wounds or who create wounds by picking. As with trichotillomania, it is important to assess the degree of anxiety and depression that the child is experiencing and to rule out other medical issues. Self-abusive behaviors and picking can cause secondary medical issues, including infections and scarring, that are extremely stressful for parents. It is important to explore the first time that the child and parents remember the child picking and to address the touchstone event and then process current stimuli.

Children With Chemical Dependency Issues. Children under the age of 10 do not typically present with chemical dependency issues; however, we included this topic to suggest that readers who work with children and adolescents with substance abuse issues learn about Popky's (2005) DeTUR model protocol to get additional information on using EMDR to treat substance abuse.

Behavioral/Developmental Issues of Childhood

Sensory Integration Disorders. Sensory integration disorders, including sensory integration dysfunction (SID), are not a clinical diagnosis but need to be assessed when treating children. Sensory integration issues can be seen as one symptom of obsessive-compulsive disorder or in children who have autism or Asperger's disorder, and sometimes in children who are also intellectually gifted. Sensory integration disorders are often identified by occupational therapists. This section is not about SID; rather, our goal is to bring to your attention the impact of sensory integration difficulties when using EMDR. If you are interested in learning more about sensory integration, we encourage you to read *The Out-of-Sync Child* by Kranowitz (2005).

Sensory integration is the process of taking in, processing, and responding to sensory input. The primary function of our brain is to process sensory information, and some individuals have strength in specific senses. Since BLS is sensory input, it is important to determine the client's most effective sensory input function and to assess for SID. It is important to assess sensory functioning and the client's sensory preferences to facilitate processing, especially related to the selection of BLS.

Case Study: Michelle and Her Sister Alyssa

In a previous case study, we discussed a little girl named Michelle, who had lost her hand in an accident. I (C.S.) also worked with Michelle's sister Alyssa, who had witnessed the accident. Because Michelle did so well using the tactile stimulation, I made the assumption that Alyssa would respond as well to the tactile stimulation. But after noticing that Alyssa processed very slowly and with great difficulty, I spoke with Alyssa's mom, who reported that Alyssa had sensory integration issues as an infant and needed to be spun in circles to calm down, and Alyssa could only learn to read if she heard the words spoken out loud. Because of this, I tried the auditory stimulation with Alyssa, and she processed quite quickly. This does not imply a sensory integration dysfunction, but rather that Alyssa had a strong sensory preference. Once I became aware of it, changing the type of BLS improved Alyssa's response to EMDR.

This is not just an issue for children, but for adults as well; however, many adults have accommodated for sensory integration and will be more able to articulate why a certain type of BLS is uncomfortable. This does not mean that when an adult client states, "I'm a visual learner," eye movements will work best for the client or that each client has only one type of sensory preference when it comes to BLS, but instead, this is just one more thing for the therapist to consider with clients.

If the child has experienced sensory integration issues, the events associated with having sensory integration issues can actually be traumas. I (R.T.) worked with a little girl who refused to wear shoes to school because she only wanted to wear flip-flops because she reported that shoes bothered her feet. This child would get in trouble at school because she was supposed to wear some type of tennis shoe for her physical education classes. Her parents would also get very angry with her. Once we targeted the first time the child felt uncomfortable wearing shoes and educated her parents about sensory integration issues, the child was able to choose shoes, and mornings were no longer traumatic for the child and her parents. Sometimes children do not remember when the discomfort started, but we can target the discomfort itself with the child selecting an image of the worst time the shoes bothered the child and then with a negative cognition of "I can't stand the feeling of the shoes" and a positive cognition of "I can feel it, but it's OK." For some children, there is a missing piece that is associated with the sensation of the shoes that contributed to the initial distress. For days when she had physical education classes at school, the parents bought her a pair of shoes that she could tolerate wearing, if only for her physical education class, and then she could put on her flip-flops after class.

There are self-report checklists included online or in *The Out-of-Sync Child* (Kranowitz, 2005) to assess symptoms suggestive of sensory integration challenges.

Case Study: Amanda's Feelings

I (R.T.) worked with a 5-year-old named Amanda, who was brought to therapy by her adoptive mother, who had adopted Amanda at birth. Amanda's mother knew that both of Amanda's parents were diagnosed with schizophrenia. Amanda was referred for therapy by her developmental pediatrician because the pediatrician had diagnosed Amanda with SID, psychoses NOS, and possible Asperger's. Amanda's mother was concerned because Amanda had many fears, including the fear of using the toilet in public, which was preventing Amanda from doing many things, including going to kindergarten. Amanda was a beautiful child who always had to wear socks and wore layers of clothes, even in the Arizona heat. Amanda could not tolerate water on her face or certain clothing against her skin, or certain textures of food. Amanda had many fears and was easily agitated and would become very anxious. After mapping targets on a whiteboard in the office, Amanda began to create elaborate drawings with her bare feet on the whiteboard. Amanda would also sing and had a most beautiful voice and was taking voice lessons. We began with Amanda's first target of using the toilet in public. Since I had a bathroom in my office suite, I asked Amanda to tell me why she did not like to use the toilet, even if her mother was with her. Amanda reported, "The toilet goes boom." I asked Amanda to help me understand, and she had her mother flush the toilet, while we stood in the hall outside the office, and as the toilet bowl emptied, Amanda said, "Listen." As the tank emptied, there was a clear boom *sound at the end, before the tank began to fill again with water. Amanda reported that the worst part was the sound of the* boom, *and her bad thought was "I'll go down the toilet." The good thought was "I'll be OK." We continued through the procedural steps and then targeted the* boom *sounds, while Amanda's mother stood in the bathroom and repeatedly flushed the toilet, as requested. Amanda walked up and down the hall of the office with the NeuroTek "buzzies" in her socks, and she would stop walking when she would be ready to tell me what happened now. After about 15 minutes, Amanda took out the buzzies and told me the* boom *was not scary anymore. We went into the bathroom, and she stood on the toilet next to me as we both made funny faces in the mirror. She then decided she could use the toilet, so I waited outside. Amanda quickly began to identify all the sounds that were associated with fears and how desensitizing the sounds alleviated her fears. Amanda was extremely sound sensitive and began to put the buzzies to her ears. I learned that Amanda could hear her feelings and that by targeting sounds, Amanda's fears dissipated. At our last session, Amanda told me about how she had used refrigerator magnets I had given her to play with against her ears, and she had devised a way to cover her ears with the large round magnets and move the magnets back and forth, creating BLS, with sounds alternating in her ears. She described the sounds as like putting a shell to your ear and hearing the ocean. Amanda then decided to throw the magnets to the bottom of the pool during her swimming lesson and to dive to the bottom of the pool to see if the magnets sounded like the ocean when they were underwater. Amanda managed to not only put her face in the water, but be able to participate in her swimming lessons. Amanda was very proud of her accomplishments and was using BLS in many ways when she was fearful. Amanda's sensory integration issues resolved as she learned to relax and use BLS on her scary thoughts.*

With children, it is not always possible for therapists, as adults, to understand how the child is experiencing the distress and what may be at the root of the child's presenting symptoms; however, this does not prevent us from helping the child to resolve the issues at the root of the problem. As therapists, we do not need to understand, but it is important for the target to resonate for the child. With attunement to the child and observation skills, we can see that the child has accessed the experience in a manner that the child has constructed, and then we follow the child as he or she reprocesses the event. The evaluation of the success of the desensitization is in the change in the child's symptoms, as reported by the child, the parent, and the teachers.

Pervasive Developmental Disorder. Pervasive developmental disorders (PDD) include diagnoses of autistic spectrum disorders, Asperger's, pervasive developmental disorders, childhood disintegrative disorders, and Rhett's. When working with children with different types of pervasive developmental disorders, the therapist can use the full protocol to target associated behavioral issues and stressors the child experiences. EMDR does not resolve the disorder but certainly can assist with reducing symptoms and teaching self-soothing and calming behaviors and mastery skills, as we have discussed in previous chapters.

One school psychologist we worked with used EMDR in a school setting with a child diagnosed with autism. After the 8-year-old girl had exploded in the classroom due to a conflict with the teacher, the psychologist worked with the child on the worst part of the incident, and the child identified the negative cognition of "I can't let go of how that teacher treated me." The child's positive cognition was "I can learn to let go." After three sessions focused on desensitizing the image, the mother noticed that the girl was being much calmer at home.

It is important to assess the impact of BLS on children with any type of PDD because the BLS can be stimulating for the child and end up agitating the child. It is important to experiment with the different types of BLS to find one that is calming to the child.

If the child with PDD also has concurrent speech issues and/or mental retardation, the full protocol will need to be adapted to meet the child's developmental levels, as has been cited in previous chapters.

Children With Cognitive Challenges. Children with cognitive challenges, including mental retardation, can benefit immensely from EMDR. In fact, it is my (R.T.) assessment that EMDR is the treatment of choice for children with cognitive challenges because EMDR does not require the client to have advanced verbal skills or insight. Children will process in their own unique ways, which make the most sense to them. The proof is not in the insights that the child gains, but in the improvement in functioning and behaviors that is evident once targets have been processed with EMDR.

Case Study: Andrew and Needles

I (R.T.) worked with a 4-year-old boy, Andrew, who was diagnosed with moderate mental retardation and was nonverbal, with the exception of guttural utterances. He was brought to therapy by an adoptive parent, who reported that the boy would pass out every time he was taken for medical care. Since the child suffered from a chronic medical condition, the child would frequently get injured when he would faint and fall. In therapy, I had the child draw pictures of the things that made him really scared before he would faint. I had his adoptive mother offer suggestions for the negative cognition, and when she said, "I'm scared," he looked at both of us in a manner that suggested we captured his thought. She then suggested several positive cognitions, and he again made eye contact when his foster mother said, "How about, I'll be OK?" After assessing how much this bothered him (SUD) and where he felt the scared feeling in his body, he pointed to his head. I then asked him to think about the picture and the words I'm scared *that he felt in his head and to hold the buzzies. He would put the buzzies on the picture as well and then stop and look at me. At first, I thought he did not understand, but then I took a chance and said, "Take a deep breath, and how about drawing me another picture." He would draw energetically with many colors and then take the buzzies in his hands and place them on the picture. I would have the child take a deep breath and then turn the page and draw what came next. With each picture, the boy would draw with intention a picture that I could not understand, but the little boy seemed to be invested in the drawing. What I observed was a child who was drawing with a purpose. Even though I could make no sense of the drawing, he seemed to know. Eventually, he was done; he took a deep breath and smiled at me. The foster mother reported that at home, the child was no longer afraid when his foster sister gave herself an insulin shot and that he had managed to go to the medical doctor without fainting. We continued by targeting the sound of the trash truck and the sound of the vacuum cleaner, until he was calm with both.*

Regulatory Issues. Young children are often brought to therapy by parents who are concerned about regulatory issues such as sleeping, eating, and toilet training. Some children will have symptoms that do not rise to the level of a specific diagnosis but present with symptoms associated with self-regulation like sleeping, eating, self-care, social skills, communication skills, and motor skills.

There are several possible scenarios for explaining the child's lack of regulatory success when the child is not making developmental gains, as would be predicted given the child's age. First, the child may have developmental issues and need to be referred for an assessment by a pediatrician and participate in developmental evaluation. A second issue can occur when the child has never mastered a skill that the child should have been able to master, given the child's age, and the therapist needs to assess if this is an issue related to the child's anxiety or sensory integration issues. A third occurs when the child has been making anticipated developmental gains but has reached a plateau and is no longer making developmental gains. A fourth scenario can occur when the child had previously mastered the skill and has regressed. Any of the three latter scenarios may indicate a stressor in the child's life, or even a possible trauma.

For example, if the parent brings a 3-year-old in because of toileting issues, the therapist must first determine if the child is within the range of normal development and if the parent is feeling pressured to toilet train the child for some reason, or if the child is making appropriate developmental gains and the parent needs to be educated, or if the child had previously mastered toilet training and has now regressed. The first two are developmental issues that require parent training, while the latter may indicate a situational stressor or trauma in the child's life.

EMDR Behavioral Approach to Treating Regulatory Issues in Children. After taking a history and understanding what is going on in the child's life, we would first target whatever stressors or traumas were identified in the child's history. If sleeping is the manifestation of the trauma, then we would complete a map and work through the EMDR protocol. A child may manifest sleep disturbances when there are changes in the child's environment, including people entering or leaving, or changes in the child's routine. For example, if the child has a new day care, or parents have divorced and the child has new sleeping arrangements, or there is a new family member, or the child is experiencing changes at school, any of these situations can contribute to sleep disturbance. These situational issues can be targeted with the EMDR protocol.

If there is no identifiable stressor or trauma, we would look at what is going on internally for the child and what the family has tried so far to address the symptom. What has worked, or partially worked, and what has not worked? For example, if the child has anxiety about sleeping in his or her own bed, the therapist will need to target the anxiety with the child. We will use a systematic desensitization type of process, with gradual steps, in the treatment process.

Case Study: Cynthia's Bedroom

I (C.S.) provided treatment for a 7-year-old girl named Cynthia, who had always struggled with sleeping. Her sleep disturbance became more severe when the family moved to a new home and the child could hear street sounds outside her bedroom. We tried to target the first time, but she could not remember the first time; she could, however, identify specific things and times that scared her. Cynthia was afraid of her bedroom window, so we targeted her bedroom window, and this helped her a bit, but she still was afraid of sleeping in her own bed. As we reviewed what happened with Cynthia, she noted that she began getting anxious at dinnertime, when she began thinking about going to bed at night. We targeted her thoughts about going to bed, including her negative cognition of "I'm going to have to go to bed in 2 hours, and I'm not safe." Her positive cognition was "I'm having dinner, and I'm safe now." After installing that positive cognition, she was not freaked out at dinner anymore, and the time between dinner and bedtime was not as stressful for the child and her family. When it came to bedtime, her mother sat on the end of the bed instead of lying down with her, and we targeted the negative cognition of "My mom's not lying down with me, so I'm not safe." The child eventually was able to process to a positive cognition of "My mom's still here. I'm safe." I used gradual steps of the child's mother moving to the doorway, the hallway, then generalizing the child's positive cognitions to "My mom's in the house, and I'm safe." We then moved to generalizing to the child's parents, and then grandparents, and then the baby-sitter, and the child could believe, "There's somebody here to take care of me. I'm safe." The child eventually was able to sleep in her own bed without the distress and meltdowns associated with bedtime. This child needed to be taught relaxation skills and was able to use the relaxation skills to calm herself when she became distressed. With sleeping, I was able to use steps of successive approximations to desensitize the child's negative beliefs, until we desensitized all the child's concerns, and she was successful in sleeping in her own bed.

A systematic behavioral approach to EMDR with children can be very successful, especially when treating regulatory issues. We recommend a combination of systematic desensitization with EMDR, along with parent training and positive reinforcement in the home, as a comprehensive approach to working with children. No matter what type of self-regulatory issue the child presents, the therapist can assess the child's issues and target any maladaptively stored information in order for the child to be able to return to the normal developmental trajectory.

Selective Mutism. When using EMDR with children who present with selective mutism or children who have decided to stop talking for some reason, the therapist must find ways to communicate with the child at the onset of therapy. The therapist can use play therapy, art therapy, or drawing to find a bridge to interact with the child. It is important not to focus on the child's lack of speech because by the time the child has come to a therapist's office, the child probably has been queried and ridiculed on more than one occasion about the child's lack of vocalizations.

As part of case conceptualization, it is important to determine if the child was previously verbal and what might have occurred around the time that the child stopped talking. Sometimes the traumatic events are obvious, while other times, the therapist may have to piece together a series of events that contributed to the child's current mutism. Therefore, during the client history and treatment planning phase, the therapist is interviewing the child and parent about the child's developmental history, including mastery of communication skills. Was the child verbal until her dad was deployed to Iraq? In addition, it is important to determine if the child speaks in some settings but not others. Does the child speak to other children, but not adults? Does the child speak at home, but not at school? Does the child talk to her dolls when no one is looking? Or has the child stopped speaking altogether?

In my (R.T.) work with children with selective mutism, I have found that many children stopped talking when other children made fun of them, and especially when they were teased about their speech. For example, one child stopped talking in preschool because another child told her that she was too little to talk in school. Another child was told by a boy on the playground that she talked funny. Another child stopped talking after he tried to read a book in reading class and other children laughed at the way he tried to sound out words. Each of these incidents, which seem minor to an adult, had a tremendous impact on that individual child. It is important not to assume that the incident is too minor to have caused the child to stop talking.

It is also important for therapists to assess for any possible speech issues that may have been an issue before the child stopped speaking. Did the child have difficulty forming the *R* sound? Did the child have a speech utterance issue? Is the child very shy or anxious?

Finally, my (R.T.) greatest successes have been when I have established a working therapeutic relationship with the child and, during the course of a lighthearted interaction, simply asked the child, "So, what made you decide to stop talking anyhow?" No matter what the child's response, I will say, "Oh, I see." Following that, I will ask the child if he or she would like to target that incident so that it does not bother the child so much anymore. I try to downplay the emphasis on talking and focus on resolving memories that are disturbing or stressful.

In my (R.T.) experience, once the traumatic events have been reprocessed, then children will start talking in more areas of their lives, and eventually, the selective mutism is resolved. With one caveat, I will add that it may be difficult for children to begin talking, even if they choose to, because teachers, family members, and especially other children will overreact to the child's new speech. For this reason, I ask the parents to make arrangements for play dates with classmates in a comfortable environment so that the child with selective mutism can begin slowly to talk with other children. I also may suggest that the child be taken to the classroom with the child's teacher when no other children are in the classroom and that the child begin talking with the teacher on a one-to-one basis. Any steps that can be taken in order that the child's new speech is not such a surprise to others, which results in discomfort for the child, are important because the attention alone can make the child stop talking again.

Case Study: Bethany and Selective Mutism

Several years ago, I (R.T.) was asked to try EMDR with a 7-year-old with selective mutism. Bethany taught me a great deal about children and EMDR. Let me begin with the end. When Bethany finally started talking after 8 months of working together, I asked her why she stopped talking, and she replied, "Because a boy on the playground said I talked funny." If only I had asked her first and targeted that memory with EMDR! Thank goodness Bethany was a very patient and tolerant little girl.

Initially, Bethany was referred to me by a child welfare agency for the treatment of trauma and the selective mutism. I was told that the last time anyone knew that Bethany had spoken was when she called 911 after she found her mother overdosed on the sofa in her home. I thought the target was fairly obvious. Bethany was in foster care by the time I met her, and she was transported each week by taxi, which often left her in my office for hours, and then a new driver came every time. This part was traumatic for both of us, but that is not the point of my case study. It was just Bethany and I trying to work together regarding what she needed from therapy. Bethany and I had very little assistance from any other adults, with the exception of several telephone calls I had with Bethany's foster mother.

After building rapport and eating lunch each week, we began to write to each other on a clipboard. In the beginning, Bethany spelled everything phonetically, and then we also played charades to see if we could understand each other. At the time, Bethany was in first grade but presented as very bright and expressive. At this time, I was focused on the client history and treatment planning and preparation phases. We explored resources and installed mastery experiences about when she felt good about herself.

I then learned that this little one started answering the phone, even though she still did not talk anywhere else, so I put her on my phone in my office and then went to my waiting room phone and got on the same line. I ran back and forth from my office to the waiting room and did the entire EMDR protocol with the child talking on the phone, writing, or drawing. Finally, we targeted the 911 call and the police and emergency personnel coming to her home. I later learned that no one realized she was hiding in a closet in the home for many hours after she called 911, and they only took the other children out of the home, but not Bethany. I thought I was so smart and had a second target. So Bethany decided to reprocess this target by hiding in the closet in my office, while I sat outside the door with the tactile "buzzies" wires under the door for bilateral stimulation (BLS). She opened the door when I stopped the buzzies and then closed the door each time we continued with BLS. She would even slide notes under the door to respond when I asked her, "What happened now?"

Eventually, she came out smiling and did not close the closet door again. At the foster home, she started communicating more by ordering at restaurants and running to answer the phone, so we targeted ordering at a restaurant and then went to a restaurant for her to order lunch. I tried to use ordering in restaurants as a master experience and congratulated Bethany on her success. I made an agreement with Bethany that we could go to a nearby restaurant, and if she ordered, I would pay. The first time we went to the restaurant, she would not order, so we returned to the office. The second time, she ordered, and I bought her lunch. On our way back to the office, I asked her why she stopped talking in the first place—and she looked at me like I was so very dense. Once we targeted what the boy said on the playground, she did not stop talking.

I am not sure if targeting all the other events helped, but once we targeted the memory of the boy on the playground, Bethany did very well. She was held back in first grade, which made her angry, and rightfully so because it turned out that she was very bright but just had stopped talking, which later became another target.

I learned from this 7-year-old that I need to always ask the child for the target, at least initially. Since learning from this little one, I always ask the child for targets, no matter how old the child is—even tiny ones can draw, or set up the playroom, or use puppets or sand tray to communicate the image that bothers them or worries them or scares them, and the image can be real or imaginary. It does not matter what I think, but what the child knows to be true for him or her. I would encourage you to ask the child, look for the missing piece about why he or she stopped talking, and keep going with EMDR.

SITUATIONAL ISSUES UNIQUE TO CHILDREN

Testifying in Court

I (R.T.) work with children who may have to testify in juvenile or criminal court. Before providing any type of treatment, I check with the prosecuting attorneys or juvenile court attorneys regarding treatment and have the attorney agree to the treatment. Next, if there is sufficient time, I follow the eight-phase protocol to process any past or present issues. If there is not time to follow the eight-phase protocol, I teach the child resourcing and containment skills to contain past and current issues to return to after the child's testimony. After teaching the child skills, I then have the child focus on any anticipatory anxiety about testifying. If possible, we take the child to see the courtroom and talk with the prosecuting attorney to desensitize the environment. If necessary, I may do the EMDR with a future template in the courtroom; however, I can do the future template in vivo in my office. I will use the future template protocol to have the child imagine what it will be like to testify and then run the future template until it is processed. Next, we add potential fears that the child might be imaging about the future testimony. I will ask the child, "What is the thing you are worried about the most regarding the event?" It is helpful to continue to ask the child about what concerns he or she has about the future and reprocess the child's anticipatory anxiety until the child no longer has any fears about the future event and the child can see a positive outcome to the event. If necessary, I might offer some possible things that could happen that the child has not considered. By saying to the child, "What if this happens?" I am focused on desensitizing the child to potential stressful events that could happen in the courtroom.

I (R.T.) have had children referred from Mother's Against Drunk Drivers (MADD) who have had to testify in criminal court, oftentimes against their parents. I have found that preparing children for testifying in court by using a future template is very helpful not only to prepare the child, but also to give the child resources to not be traumatized by the process. Each time I have the opportunity to work with the child before the child testifies, I ask the child to run the video of himself or herself testifying and imagine any additional sources of distress that may have arisen between sessions. Sometimes children decide they need additional reinforcement or a safe place. For example, one young man could not identify a real safe or calm place in his life, so he chose instead to use the figures in a video game and create a fortress where he could be safe if he felt uncomfortable, especially when testifying. Each session, he added reinforcements to the fortress, including security dogs, an alarm system, armed guards, and an invisible laser system to prevent intruders. The child practiced going to his safe fortress every day, so by the time he testified, he saw himself going to the fortress and answering the questions in court from the fortress. The child eventually testified against a family member and was very successful. He left the stand feeling supported and courageous.

Children who must testify against family members or deal with stressful situations within their own families often struggle with identifying resources and support systems to help them cope with the circumstances in their lives.

Dealing With Divorce

There are many issues children face when their parents divorce. The issues of loss are huge. Children experience the loss of life as they have known it. Their living environment will change, the amount of time they spend with each parent will change, their relationships to family and friends may change. There is a variety of ways children deal with these changes. But it is when children develop disrupted daily routines, such as a significant change in sleep concentration or eating habits for longer than 2 weeks, that parents need to seek outside help.

EMDR works well with children in dealing with their sense of loss and safety, and of power and control, in a divorce situation. It can also help with their mistaken sense of responsibility and self-blame, which can result in anger at themselves and/or their parents.

Again, the child should pick the target. Many times, the child's target is a symptom, something worrying or bothering the child. The symptoms may be representative of the larger issues in a divorce scenario. Some children worry about throwing up in their bed at their father's new apartment, while others have panic attacks prior to boarding an airplane to visit their mother. Other children may be angry and scream at their friends in school. Whatever the child identifies is how the trauma is stored.

Case Study: Tessa and Her Parents' Divorce

I (C.S.) worked with 8-year-old Tessa when her parents were divorcing. Her big worry was moving out of the house she had always lived in. Tessa's negative cognition was "I don't want to leave. I don't have a choice." Her positive cognition was "I'll deal with it." Tessa was very upset, and her SUD was an 8. It took only 15 minutes for Tessa to reprocess, and then her positive cognition evolved into "I might like my new room better. This could be exciting to decorate my room. I can choose how my room looks."

So children will process in the ways that naturally fit for them. Sometimes it is very concrete, and sometimes it is a Metaphor. But always, it is in the way that is healing and empowering for them.

Motor Vehicle Accidents

Generally, when processing motor vehicle accidents, the standard protocol is sufficient in reprocessing for children. What is different for children compared to adults is what they may remember. Often, they remember sensory things or things they were doing just prior to the accident. So being a good detective is again essential.

Case Study: Devon and the Motor Vehicle Accident

I (R.T.) worked with 2-year-old Devon and his family following a motor vehicle accident in which one of Devon's siblings was killed. Since Devon's verbal skills were limited, I asked Devon's mother, who was in the car, to recount what she remembered happening right before the accident occurred and to draw the picture on the whiteboard. As Devon's mother drew the picture and talked about the song that they were singing right before the accident occurred, Devon grabbed his mother's hand and my hand and rocked back and forth, with the buzzies in his socks. Devon then erased the whiteboard and began to sing a new song. Following that session, Devon no longer had any bowel or bladder issues and began to sleep in his own bed again. Later, when the psychiatrist who was conducting the independent medical examination of the child called my office, she asked for the child's intake because the psychiatrist was not able to identify any evidence of trauma or distress in the child. The psychiatrist was stunned to learn of the 2-year-old's participation in EMDR.

If a child has been involved in a motor vehicle accident, the child may present with symptoms consistent with trauma and need to reprocess the memories of the accident and any medical interventions that followed. Some children will also need assistance to ride in a motor vehicle again without feeling anxious, and the use of future template to help the child feel that riding in a motor vehicle again is OK can be very helpful.

Child Abuse

Physical and Sexual Abuse. Targeting children's experiences of physical and sexual abuse is not explored in detail in this chapter because we believe that we have discussed these issues throughout the book. Child sexual and/or physical abuse and neglect can be successfully treated with the EMDR protocol if the therapist is also cognizant of current stressors in the child's life and addresses any dissociative symptoms and other symptoms that have arisen from the traumatic history.

Foster Care. Children in the child welfare system typically have experienced abuse and neglect prior to being placed in foster care and then must cope with changes in caregivers, schools, friends, sleeping arrangements, and life changes as a whole. The original events that brought the child into care need to be targeted with EMDR, in addition to the stressful events that occur from being in foster care. There are many events that arise from being placed in foster care, and it is important to assist the child in coping with the stress of foster care. There are many unique issues that arise from being in foster care; however, we have only included several examples in this chapter. One is the *episodes of care* that may occur with treating children in the foster care system. Episodes of care occur when the child participates in a period of treatment, but before treatment is completed the treatment is discontinued for a period of time. Children in foster care often experience moves and instability, along with poor-quality mental health services. The therapist may begin to engage the child in treatment, and then the child is moved or changed to a new therapist because of distance, funding, or the child welfare system. This makes treatment extremely difficult, and therapists must work from the perspective that each session may be the only session or last session that the therapist has with the child. Because of this, it is important to conceptualize each session as a complete session by undertaking smaller treatment goals that can be completed within one therapy session. In addition, it is important for the child to have some connection to the therapist by possibly having a transitional object such as a blanket, notebook, or stuffed animal. I (R.T.) will often tell the child the story from the movie *E.T.* to let the child know I will be with the child, even when he or she is not in my office. Because of the transitory nature of foster care and the child welfare system, therapists must consider EMDR as part of episodes of care that include a great deal of resourcing and skill building, while providing the child with resources to cope with current life circumstances. It is very helpful to teach children to use containers for past traumas in order that the child can continue to function in the here and now and someday return to reprocess the maladaptively stored information. This does not exclude using EMDR to reprocess traumatic memories but changes case conceptualization to meet the child's needs. If the therapist targets a past event, it is important to prepare in advance for the desensitization session, including preparing the child and the home environment to be supportive of the child. When targeting the event, it is important to target manageable pieces of the event and then add a positive template for the child for when the child leaves the therapy session. It is helpful to remind the child, "You worked really hard today, and it is important that you feel proud of yourself for your hard work." It is helpful to leave the child with a reminder that therapy is difficult and that the child was courageous in the process. If each session ends with a positive template for the child, the child will be able to manage these episodes of care, while being able to participate in future therapy opportunities.

Children in foster care will often experience additional traumatic events while in foster care that can include visitation with parents or other family members, which may be stressful if the parent is the alleged perpetrator of the abuse. Using containers and future templates to help the child cope with these visits is very important.

Being in foster care also creates difficult social and educational challenges that can be addressed through EMDR. EMDR can be used with many of the issues that arise from foster care, and teaching children containment tools, mastery, and emotional literacy, along with processing events as the child can tolerate, seems to help insulate the child and create some resiliency for the child, who has to continue through the unstable and oftentimes stressful experience of being raised in foster care.

Case Study: Sebastian and His School Lifeline

I (R.T.) worked with a 10-year-old boy, Sebastian, who had been acting out in his foster home. When exploring with Sebastian what was bothering him, Sebastian reported that he had been given a school assignment to write his lifeline, with one event for each year of his life. Sebastian was very upset because he could not remember his life before his foster home. In therapy, we created a lifeline for Sebastian based on what was reasonable to predict had happened to Sebastian for each year of his life. For example, we discussed what Sebastian had probably done during his first year of life. We knew his birthday and that he learned to crawl during the first year of his life, and during the second year of his life, he learned to walk. With each year of his life, we used the BLS to help Sebastian work through his sadness about not being able to remember his life, and then Sebastian created his own history. Sebastian did his lifeline assignment in therapy, and then we installed the feelings of accomplishment that Sebastian felt once he completed his lifeline. Sebastian said, "I felt like I wasn't good enough to do the lifeline, but now I feel like I'm as good as all the other kids." We then used a future template to install Sebastian seeing himself presenting his lifeline to the class and feeling courageous and strong for all that he had accomplished in his life.

EMDR can be used very effectively with children in the child welfare system if therapists conceptualize EMDR in sections that would constitute episodes of care. Episodes of care can be used to treat all children who present for therapy but is especially important to provide good therapeutic care for children living in very transient environments.

Educational Issues

EMDR With Gifted Children. This section explores the unique issues that gifted children face and how EMDR can be integrated in therapy to assist gifted children.

Gifted children can struggle with emotional and sensory integration issues. For the purposes of this chapter, giftedness is defined as the population of children who have tested in the 97th percentile or above in the quantitative, qualitative, or nonverbal areas on standardized assessment scales. This in no way suggests that children who score in the gifted range are a homogeneous group. There is as much range of variability within that 3% as in the general population. So many gifted children can be gifted in many areas intellectually and emotionally but often come to therapy due to difficulty with anxiety, depression, emotional regulation, and other emotional and behavioral symptoms. Gifted children can present with an asynchrony between their intellectual level and emotional level. This can present as an 8-year-old who understands things intellectually as a 19-year-old but emotionally as an 8-year-old. It is this asynchrony with which many gifted children struggle; however, not all gifted children encounter difficulty because there are many gifted children who never enter a therapist's office because those children are gifted in all areas, including emotionally, athletically, and artistically.

How do they deal with the discrepancy between intellectual and emotional functioning? How does a child who understands the realities of nuclear development in Iran but is emotionally an 8-year-old put that into perspective? How can he or she filter and regulate that emotionally?

Targeting their fears and drawing pictures of the fears can be useful. If the SUD does not go down, then using a cognitive interweave that focuses on actual probability can help. For example, if a child is worried about getting cancer and dying, the therapist can use known information to put probabilities in perspective. If the child is worried about getting cancer, the therapist might say, "Less than 1% of children get cancer. If the weatherman said there is less than a 1% chance of rain today, would you bring an umbrella?" "No." "Then the likelihood it would rain is small, right?" "Right." "So, how likely is it that you will get cancer and die?" "Not likely." "Go with that."

Children with giftedness can also struggle with regulating their intense emotions, be very sensitive, exhibit sensory integration issues, and grapple with interpersonal relationships and functioning in social environments. Gifted children often appear to feel things more deeply; they hear things that people are saying and understand it intellectually but have a strong emotional response because of the discrepancy between their intellect and their emotional intelligence. Sometimes this creates a high degree of anxiety because younger children think concretely, even though they are able to think about things far beyond their age. Gifted children are also able to consider intellectual issues like war and peace and have a strong emotional reaction to these issues, but yet, given the children's age, they are not yet able to think abstractly and consider gray areas. With EMDR, the therapist may need to target the child's intense emotions.

Case Study: Wally and His Intense Emotions

Wally is a highly gifted little boy who struggled with transitions and meltdowns. When Wally was working on the computer and he was asked to do something else, Wally would have a terrible temper tantrum. So I (C.S.) had Wally target one time when his mother asked him to come to dinner and identify the negative cognition. Wally's bad thought was "I'm not finished. I can't let this go." His good thought was "I can finish this part and come back to it after dinner. I can let it go for now." After reprocessing this target with Wally, in one 15-minute session, Wally was able to return to the next session with no reported instances of tantrumming, and this had generalized to all areas of transitioning in his life. Even though his mother had told him repeatedly that he could go back to his computer after dinner, Wally was never able to make use of that, until he experienced the body shift of feeling comfortable with the thought that he could wait and come back to the computer and that he could handle it.

Gifted children also have difficulty in social interactions because they are often moved up in grade and have to interact socially with older kids. Sometimes these most brilliant children have no social intelligence and no common sense. Sometimes these children are unable to make good decisions about what is appropriate and what is not. So we have a child with a higher intelligence than most adults but the maturity of a child.

Case Study: Andy and His Computer Graphics

I (C.S.) worked with a young boy in early adolescence who was extremely gifted, so he had been moved up two grades in school. Andy was the age of a typical seventh grader but was a sophomore in high school. When Andy first got a cellular phone, he took an inappropriate picture of himself and then sent it to the phones of all the kids he knew in high school. Needless to say, Andy was suspended from high school for something that is comical but very immature. So I (C.S.) used resourcing to install common sense in the form of "I can stop and think about consequences for my behaviors." We worked on consequences and using his intelligence to predict if–then situations. In this situation, I had Andy think about things like "I think this is funny, but other people might not appreciate my humor." We targeted the worst part of the incident, which was getting a disapproving letter from the principal, and the bad thought, "I wished I hadn't done it." Andy's good thought was "I can stop and think before I act." Andy was able to reprocess his shame and embarrassment about the situation and learn to use more impulse control skills to help him maneuver in social situations.

Besides dealing with impulsivity and judgment issues, gifted kids pick up things more sensorially such as lights, sounds, and touch. Gifted children sometimes have sensitivity to tags in shirts, seams in socks, lights that are too bright, or sound that is too loud. No matter what sensory area a child struggles with, the therapist can identify targets for reprocessing with EMDR. This is all part of educating kids about what it is like to be gifted. I (C.S.) often discuss with children and families emotional intelligence, based on the book by Goleman (1995). Even though it is important to support children in enriching their intelligence, it is really children who understand themselves and others emotionally who are able to make common sense decisions and be successful in their lives. I think that it is very important to teach parents about loving the child for who he or she is versus how smart the child is and that all children haves gifts and talents.

One final but important topic to process with children who are gifted is to help them to understand that they can explore choices because they have so many talents. This is the time to "pick from the banquet table," so you can make choices, but eventually, people have to make choices because there is only so much time. I have them image the things they really like and have those all on the banquet table, and they notice what things they spend longer savoring and then decide if that is something they want to invest more time in. This is often a source of distress and anxiety for gifted children because they are so bright and so talented in so many areas that the child struggles to pick one topic.

School Refusal Behavior. Children can display school refusal behavior without meeting the criteria for any specific diagnosis. School refusal behaviors can have many origins, so a thorough client history is important. Areas to consider while assessing the child are developmental and temperamental issues, the classroom environment (i.e., the physical building, the teacher, social interactions and bullying), changes in the child's life (such as moving or a parent being away), cultural pressures (i.e., Japan's intense focus on school, grades, and longer school hours), family dynamics, the anxiety of the parent or attachment issues, and how the behavior has been handled up to now.

Target what the child identifies as a worry or a reason not to go to school (e.g., "My mom might forget to pick me up"; "The teacher yells"; "Kids don't like me"). Depending on the child's ability to handle emotion during processing, you may have to do mastery skills to help the child tolerate anxiety or any strong emotion (see chapter 9). Developing a future template after reprocessing the earliest and worst incidents is important to develop the ability to actually go to school and handle it.

The therapist then can use the run-a-movie technique and have the child imagine immediate concrete successes in going to school in small, specific time increments: "Imagine walking up to the classroom tomorrow with your mom" and "Now imagine walking into your classroom."

If the child cannot handle the emotions during reprocessing, tell a story about an imaginary character, such as Winnie the Pooh, who is struggling with a similar issue. Create the story showing the fictional character problem solving the issues to teach new skills. I (C.S.) use a book titled *Annie's Stories* by Brett (1986), which helps therapists tell narrative stories to help children address personal issues. The use of a third party experiencing the anxiety helps the child manage the child's emotions while he or she is learning new skills.

Next, develop a plan with the parent alone on how to practice the new skills. For instance, taking the child to school when no one is there is helpful to begin the in vivo experience. You can install visiting the school with BLS. The therapist then coaches the parent on what behaviors the parent should reward and ignore. Sometimes the parent may need some resource development himself or herself to be able to firmly and lovingly walk away.

Case Study: Brian's Difficulties With Preschool

I (C.S.) saw Brian because he had difficulty going to preschool, and he cried hysterically all the way to school in the car. Brian had difficulty processing his anxiety, so I (C.S.) had his mom tell Brian a story about Winnie the Pooh going to preschool and how he would cry all the way there. Brian's mother would try to comfort him, but nothing seemed to work. Brian's mother remembered that Winnie the Pooh liked to play with Piglet.

So she told Brian stories about the steps of Winnie the Pooh going to school. She explained that first she would take Winnie the Pooh to the door. She then suggested that Winnie was supposed to hug his mother, turn around, and find one fun toy to look at in the classroom. Winnie the Pooh was then to look at Piglet and his other playmate Tigger, smile, and go toward them and not look back. Brian's mother told this story while tapping his knees. Brian's mother then retold the story while she and Brian were riding in the car. Brian was able to follow the directions and successfully join his preschool class. Brian's mother followed through on her instructions to hug him and turn and walk resolutely out the door.

It is also helpful to involve teachers and other school personnel in the plan to guide the child once the parent has left. Having the teacher present as caring and matter-of-fact in bringing the child into the classroom gives the child support, while not encouraging the anxiety or rebellion.

SUMMARY

In this chapter, we have provided an overview of using EMDR to work with children who have symptoms of specific mental health disorders, trauma, stressful life experiences, and educational issues. This chapter was written to assist therapists in using EMDR in case conceptualization with each child who presents for treatment. It is our experience that by using the eight phases of EMDR as the treatment model, while interweaving techniques from other treatment methodologies for working with children, therapists can treat many common issues with which children present for psychotherapy.

We conclude this chapter with a comprehensive case study provided by one of our colleagues that demonstrates how EMDR can be used with children with multiple issues who may be involved in episodes of care because of an unstable life that started with abuse and neglect and then proceeded through the child welfare system, until the child finally found a forever family. The efficacy of pieces of the EMDR protocol over the course of several years is illustrated beautifully with this child.

Case Study: Daniel's Episodes of Care in Child Welfare

Daniel is an 11-year-old boy who was removed from his home by Child Protective Services (CPS) at the age of 3 years due to sexual abuse. The youngest of six biological siblings, Daniel's father is reported (by a biological sibling case manager) to have duct taped the older siblings to force them to watch him sexually abuse Daniel. His mother would observe the abuse and comfort him when it was over. Following his removal, Daniel lived in four different foster homes before he was adopted at the age of 5. This adoption lasted 3 years but was disrupted due to the adoptive parents' concern that Daniel was bullying and sexually inappropriate with a younger sibling. After two more foster placements, he was placed in a therapeutic foster home with the current family. He is reported to have been in therapy since the age of 3, although CPS could not provide documentation of this as Daniel's foster homes were scattered throughout the state.

Daniel's diagnoses included ADHD, PTSD, reactive attachment disorder (RAD), and bipolar disorder. He was prescribed four psychotropic medications, but Daniel had made little progress with his RAD specialist in the past 2 years. The RAD specialist had concerns that Daniel's early trauma contributed to what he described as "dissociative rage." When Daniel's rage was triggered (and the specialist was unable to determine triggers), Daniel would escalate from a hyperactive/agitated state and throw stones at people. He had broken the windshield of the family car as well as damaged another vehicle by throwing stones out the school bus window. He had been suspended from the school bus. The therapeutic family reported that they were worn out from his behavioral acting out and aggression and concerned for their younger child's safety. In addition to the aggression, Daniel presented with symptoms of lying and stealing and instigating ("constantly annoying") other children in the home. Members of the Child and Family Team (CFT) expressed concerns that "he is going to kill someone." The CFT was requesting "one or two sessions on EMDR before we move him to another temporary home in another county."

This writer assessed Daniel and was heartened by his foster father's strong commitment to the boy. His Child Dissociative Checklist (CDC) score, while indicating some dissociation, was not as pathological as this writer would have expected. Although he appeared to have fragile ego strength, he was able to participate in drawing a safe place and reported that he liked the BLS and was able to strengthen his Safe/Calm Place visually and kinesthetically. When this writer explained EMDR, Daniel reported that he wanted to stop hurting people.

After explaining EMDR to the CFT, the family agreed to keep Daniel in their home for 6 months to give him ample time for stabilization before working through some of his early trauma. This writer began seeing him weekly. He participated in safe place, anchored with olfactory and kinesthetic cues. He learned controlled breathing and progressive relaxation. He participated in guided visualization (enhanced by BLS) replicating the first and second years of the life cycle's bonding and attachment. This writer has found that often, children will spontaneously begin to report targets during/after this process. However, this was not the case with Daniel. He remained extremely resistant to any activities designed to identify targets and any activities designed to identify elements of EMDR assessment. He was educated on emotional literacy and became adept at reporting his feelings.

He made a body map and learned to identify body sensations. He sat in his foster father's lap while listening to Metaphorical stories to help him with some of the PTSD symptoms, particularly avoidance. He participated in bonding and attachment work with his foster father, including mutual gaze, multisensory massage, and narrative therapy. At home, he practiced mindfulness and emotional communication. Over time, Daniel's symptoms dissipated, and he was reported to be no longer stealing, no longer lying, and to be using his mindfulness and future template visualization ("I can control myself") on the bus. The school stopped making reports. His CDC score was significantly lower. His foster father reported wanting to adopt Daniel, but the foster mother was too concerned about his sexual abuse history and approaching adolescence (there had been no reports of any sexual reactivity since the disrupted adoption).

This writer attempted to begin desensitization with current, less emotionally charged material in order for Daniel to get the feeling of EMDR processing. However, he continued to be extremely avoidant and would state, "I don't know what you are talking about" and "This is stupid" or "You are stupid." He practiced visualizing a safe room where he could bring his "little angry part." While doing this, he would curl up in a fetal position, hugging a stuffed animal, and pull a blanket over his head. Often, he appeared not to be able to speak, so he would answer in sign language. One of the more interesting things he reported in communicating with his little angry part was a memory of his biological father "throwing stones at us kids whenever he got mad."

After 8 months of preparation, a breakthrough came for Daniel when this writer learned about his desire to help other children. The therapist suggested that they design an EMDR game to teach other children how EMDR works. Daniel was very excited about this idea. Then they made up a Metaphorical story about a bunny whose story line paralleled Daniel's target of "losing my adoptive family" and the pain that had caused him. Daniel was able to identify all of the assessment data. He had difficulty with a positive cognition, becoming visibly agitated and insisting "it was my fault, I'm bad," but was able to process (within two sessions) to completion on a positive cognition of "I did the best I could." He remained avoidant around any early targets but was able to process recent targets of some of his manipulative behaviors and attempts to control adults. He also appeared proud of the game he had "invented."

At the recommendation of this writer, Daniel made a life book with the help of his foster family. He was educated age appropriately on the importance of a coherent narrative, with a past, present, and future. In sharing the book with this writer, it was pointed out to him that he had no pictures in his book of his biological family. Then I asked him if he could draw a picture of what he remembered of his family. After a few weak attempts at distraction (pointing out lint in the carpet), he drew a picture of stick figures—a terrified child running from an angry figure who was standing next to a wheelbarrow filled with rocks. The father figure is holding a hotdog, and Daniel took great care to amplify and label the hotdog. The target was "Father hurt/scared me." He identified the negative cognition as "I am the worst kid in the house" and the positive cognition as "I'm a good kid, and I am loveable." The validity of cognition was 3. The emotion was frightened and unloved. The SUD was 8, and in reaction to the body scan, Daniel reported, "I can only feel it in my head. I am so scared I am making myself run." What was interesting about this session was Daniel's somatic responsiveness. In drawing the picture and identifying thoughts/feelings/sensations, he appeared as he frequently does when distressed: talking fast and unable to sit still. Following this session, in which he verbally expressed rage at his biological father, jumping up and down on the paper drawing, he became increasingly able to identify body sensations and finally appeared visibly relaxed, heavy in his foster parent's arms.

In the next session, the foster parent reported, "He is more steady, he is more reflective, he's less hyper, doesn't talk so compulsively, he looks like he is sitting and thinking." The foster parent reported that during the week, Daniel's school had called to report that "something is wrong with him; maybe he is getting sick" due to his lack of usual hyperactivity. On reevaluation, Daniel reported that he had been having a recurrent memory that scared him and asked if this writer wanted him to draw a picture of it. He drew an image of his biological father pointing a gun at his biological mother, who was lying on a couch. In processing through this target, Daniel processed rage with his biological father and responsibility and safety issues. He could only bring it down to a SUD of 2 and reported that to bring it down to a 0, "I'd have to stop thinking about it all the time, how he hurt me and made me lose my mom." Daniel went on to process grief/loss issues over his biological mother and siblings and appeared to be making continued progress.

Although his progress in therapy was hindered by issues brought about when a potentially adoptive home that he was transitioning to ended in disruption (due to systems issues and not caused by Daniel's behaviors), Daniel has remained behaviorally and emotionally stable during the disruption and a recent move to a "forever family" out of the area that he reports is "just what I wanted; I think they love me." The new family reports that they are committed to continuing his EMDR treatment.

CHAPTER 12

The Future of EMDR With Children

This book was written to summarize all that we have learned from the professionals who created Eye Movement Desensitization and Reprocessing (EMDR) and began using EMDR with children as well as from our colleagues, our research, our students, and the children in our lives. As therapists who have spent a great deal of time learning and improving our practice of EMDR with children, we were encouraged to write about our research and our practices to encourage other therapists to use EMDR with children. The main goal of this book was to help therapists improve their practices of EMDR by teaching them how to use EMDR with young children to ultimately to help children.

We have attempted to make the book readable and practical for audiences of all levels. We wrote for the therapists who are returning to their offices and trying to use EMDR with young children for the first time after they completed their initial training in EMDR. We also wrote for the more advanced practitioners who have been practicing for years but needed to be encouraged and supported in using EMDR with children. We have also written this book for therapists who see children from 0 to 100 years because those maladaptively stored memories often originate from childhood, no matter what the age of the client sitting in the office.

Throughout this book we have attempted to answer specific questions about EMDR and the art of psychotherapy with children. How do you work with children in an Adaptive Information Processing model? How do you case conceptualize working with children? How do you change the languaging when using EMDR with young children, without omitting steps of the protocol? What does it take to use the EMDR protocol with children? We have no doubt EMDR can be used with young children and used successfully, but how do you teach therapists to do so? Can EMDR be used with children with various clinical, developmental, behavioral, and educational issues, in addition to being used with children with single and chronic posttraumatic stress disorder (PTSD)? Can you document your clinical outcomes in a treatment study? Can you demonstrate fidelity to the EMDR model with young children? How do you integrate Adaptive Information Processing (AIP) theory into your practice of providing psychotherapy with children and begin to use EMDR when you have been using other types of child psychotherapy? In this final chapter, we have provided a theoretical foundation for case conceptualization with EMDR in child psychotherapy with goals for future study and research.

ADAPTIVE INFORMATION PROCESSING AND EMDR IN CHILD PSYCHOTHERAPY

As explained in the first 11 chapters of this book, with EMDR, Shapiro (1989a, 1989b) devised a therapeutic process by which the therapist guides the client through a series of procedural steps to access the maladaptively stored information. By accessing those memory networks, the EMDR protocol focuses on reprocessing the accessed information so that the client can proceed with the healing process. With child clients, the healing process is impacted by the child's level of development and mastery of developmental tasks.

Theories of developmental psychology have attempted to explain how humans develop physically, socially, emotionally, and educationally. But, these theories stop short of suggesting the development of psychopathology in children and few offer treatment suggestions for when the trajectory of the normal course of human development veers off course.

The combination of all the fields of human development including cognitive development, learning and memory, development of human behavior and emotion, attachment theory, and behavioral theory are all combined to create a comprehensive theory of Adaptive Information Processing to explain human development and the development of psychopathology that guide the use of EMDR in psychotherapy. With this assessment of the child's development and range of competencies in different areas of development, the therapist's next task is to assess how the child constructs reality. What is the child's experience of being in the world? Therapists who work with children in psychotherapy must consider not only the child's development but also how the child constructs their own reality, how the child learns, what the child needs from the therapeutic relationship, and the therapist's role in the treatment process. With this information driving case conceptualization in using EMDR with children, therapists can help children reprocess memories that have been maladaptively stored and move that information to adaptive resolution thus restoring the healthy course of development in children.

HOW THERAPISTS CONCEPTUALIZE TREATMENT WITH CHILDREN

In conceptualizing psychotherapy with children, the therapist must understand the impact of human development, how children construct reality, how children learn, and the impact that other relationships including the relationship with the therapist may impact how the child constructs reality. This is a process that unfolds during treatment.

How Children Construct Reality

It is important as a therapist to consider how the child constructs reality and how the child tends to respond to stressful life events. Deciphering the child's unique construction of reality requires the therapist to become attuned to the child and learn how the child expresses their internal experiences and responds to external experiences. Child therapists may be inclined to construct reality for the child rather than learning how the child constructs reality. There is a very fine line between teaching children and constructing reality for them. In play therapy, the therapist is theoretically observing and interacting with the child in a manner to understand the child's experiences and help the child come to a healthier place with the issues first presented in therapy. With other types of child treatment, it is often the therapist and at times the therapist with the parent who are constructing reality for the child.

How Children Learn

We suggest that therapists consider the active involvement of the child learner at different stages of development important for understanding psychotherapy at different ages and stages of development. There are many variables that influence how children learn. The uniqueness of the child and the child's belief in their responsibility and motivation for learning, interwoven with the unique characteristics of the therapy and the dynamic, social, and interactional process of learning impacts the process of psychotherapy. Where does the therapist enter the child's world to intervene in the process? Does the therapist believe that treatment should be facilitated by the therapist or that the therapist should allow the child's natural development to unfold in a nonjudgmental environment free of adult intervention?

Another aspect of the learning process involves the "zone of proximal distance" (Vygotsky, 1978). In order to successfully engage the child in psychotherapy, the therapist needs to consider what might impact the child's interest in the treatment in order to successfully engage the child in therapy. Many children want to avoid any reminders or discussions of the traumatic event, which is one of the hallmark symptoms of PTSD; however, children are more likely to be interested in symptoms reduction. By targeting a symptom rather than a traumatic event, children may be more interested in actively participating in therapy because the child can realize the benefit of treatment. Nightmares are a very common symptom identified by children. By targeting the child's nightmares and reducing the intensity and frequency of nightmares, children often feel empowered and are willing to engage in targeting more difficult symptoms and events.

A second way to consider the zone of proximal distance in engaging a child in treatment is creating a mastery experience with EMDR. When an individual is challenged with a task slightly above what the individual has already mastered and the individual successfully completes the task, the individual gains confidence and is then motivated to attempt more challenging tasks. In using EMDR in psychotherapy with children, allowing children to have repeated small successes with reprocessing with EMDR appears to assist children in gaining confidence in the therapeutic process and empower to tackle more difficult targets as the child experiences a sense of mastery over difficult and stressful life experiences.

The child's confidence in the therapeutic process is also facilitated by the relationship with the therapist.

The Relationship Between the Child and Therapist

It is important to understand that in psychotherapy with children, the interplay between the child and therapist impacts the therapy process and ultimately the outcome of treatment. The therapist needs to allow for the establishment of a therapeutic bond with the child. We discussed the therapist–child relationship in chapters 2 and 3, and in our research we found that therapists who had not developed a therapeutic bond struggled to engage the child in therapy.

The Therapist's Role in Psychotherapy With Children

When using EMDR with children, therapists may find that they experience EMDR as more directive while play therapy is more nondirective. We suggest that case conceptualization in EMDR with children can include both directive and nondirective roles from the therapist depending on the phase of the EMDR protocol and the individual needs of the child. Developing rapport may be more nondirective for the therapist, while assessment, psychoeducational training and skill building, and reprocessing traumatic events may require a more directive role from the therapist. Therapists providing therapy to children must be able to remain fluid in their interactions with children in order to weave together the child's needs, the treatment goals and the pieces of the EMDR protocol. For example, allowing a child to create the image in the sand tray and distill a negative cognition or bad thought may require education, support, and encouragement from the therapist while some children will freely create the image in the sand tray if the therapist is simply observant and aware of the child's presentation.

It has been our experience in working with child therapists who have previously been trained and practice play therapy, that integrating EMDR into psychotherapy with children may feel uncomfortable because the therapist is no longer an observer but directs the course of therapy. In a study conducted by the authors (Adler-Tapia & Settle, in progress), evidence of the therapists' impact on the treatment process was documented.

With an understanding of Adaptive Information Processing theory and the array of theories that capture the various types of human development as the underpinnings for psychotherapy, we have summarized the current treatment modalities that guide psychotherapeutic methods in treating children.

THEORETICAL ORIENTATIONS OF PSYCHOTHERAPY

Theoretical orientations that have attempted to explain the development and treatment of psychopathology are typically adult models based on the assumption that the client has developed a certain set of skills with which to participate in therapy.

Research suggests more than 120 orientations to psychotherapy including, Behaviorism, Cognitivism, Cognitive Behavioral, Existential, Family Systems, Feminist, Gestalt, Humanistic, Psychoanalytic, Analytical, Psychodynamic, and Transpersonal to name a few of the more popular research theories. Many of these theories combine to create an array of mental health treatments primarily focused on working with adult clients; however, there are but a few therapies that have explored the psychological treatment of children.

THEORETICAL ORIENTATIONS AND PSYCHOTHERAPY APPROACHES WITH CHILDREN

In this book we have included references to specific psychotherapies for children that we believe are significant to the treatment of children with the belief that the skills from each treatment modality can be used in an overall treatment conceptualization through the use of the eight phases of EMDR.

With child psychotherapy, there is some agreement in the mental health community that children communicate and process through play and recently some agreement that children can be impacted by trauma that can be treated with psychotherapy. But how do you treat a young child who is growing and developing and changing very rapidly?

Play Therapy

There are many types of play therapy that include play therapy as developed by Anna Freud, Clark Moustaskas, and Virgina Axline (1964) and later expanded in various forms including Theraplay and Sand Tray work.

Virginia Axline and Nondirective Play Therapy. Virginia Axline wrote about nondirective play therapy in 1979 when she suggested ways to work with children with emotional and behavioral issues. Axline developed basic principles for play therapy that guide the therapist's role in working with young children. Nondirective play therapy occurs when the therapist allows the child to lead the process with only limitations to ensure safety and appropriateness in the therapy environment where the therapist provides acceptance of the child. Axline's first book, *Dibs: In Search of Self* (1964), focused on Axline's treatment of a child through Rogerian-type treatment that allowed the child to guide the treatment process.

The techniques that are included in play therapy can be incorporated in EMDR treatment with young children even though EMDR includes more directive and psychoeducational interventions with children. Play therapy techniques within an EMDR template create a very effective and efficient treatment of young children. This is also true of the techniques of Theraplay.

Ann M. Jernberg and Theraplay. In 1967, Ann Jernberg developed Theraplay as a treatment approach that combined play therapy with building healthy relationships between children and parents (Jernberg, 1979; Jernberg & Booth, 1999). Theraplay is based on the belief that parent–child interactions are developmentally necessary and an integral part of treatment. Unlike most play therapy, Theraplay actively engages the parent in the therapeutic process.

As we discussed previously in this book, there are many ways to integrate parents into the therapy process within an EMDR template and relationship-based treatment interventions are effective especially during the Preparation Phase of EMDR. Working in a parent cotherapist model provides ongoing support and guidance for the child when the child is not in the therapist's office.

Including the parent in the treatment process is also part of Daniel Hughes's treatment methodology.

Daniel Hughes's Dyadic Developmental Psychotherapy. John Bowlby and Mary Ainsworth's work with attachment led Daniel Hughes to develop the Dyadic Developmental Psychotherapy (Hughes, 1997, 1998, 2007) for treating children.

Dyadic Developmental Psychotherapy focuses on integrating attachment therapy that includes parents and children in clinical interventions focused on improving attachment in parent–child relationships and healing child trauma. Hughes writes that treatment includes safety, self-regulation, self-reflective information processing, traumatic experiences integration, relational engagement, and positive affect enhancement. Hughes also writes that he incorporates cognitive-behavioral interventions in the treatment process.

Trauma-Focused Cognitive Behavioral Therapy (TF-CBT)

Trauma-Focused Cognitive Behavioral Therapy combines cognitive therapy, behavioral therapy, and family therapy in a specific treatment protocol focused on psychotherapy with children who have experienced trauma primarily from abuse. TF-CBT was developed jointly by Esther Deblinger, PhD, codirector of the New Jersey CARES Institute at the University of Medicine and Dentistry of New Jersey's School of Osteopathic Medicine, and Judith Cohen, MD, and Anthony Mannarino, PhD, who are the medical director and director of the Center for Traumatic Stress in Children and Adolescents at Allegheny General Hospital, in Pittsburgh. According to the authors, TF-CBT includes four components of treatment including exposure, cognitive processing and reframing, stress management, and parental treatment. In a brief entitled *Trauma-Focused Cognitive Behavioral Therapy: Addressing the Mental Health of Sexually Abused Children* (Cohen, Deblinger, Mannarino, Wilson, Taylor, et al., 2007), TF-CBT includes "components" that can be summarized in the word "PRACTICE." TF-CBT includes psychoeducational training and parenting skills, relaxation techniques, affective expression and regulation, cognitive coping and processing, trauma narrative, in vivo exposure, conjoint parent and child sessions, and enhancing personal safety and future growth (2007, pp. 4–5).

With TF-CBT, the process of cognitive coping and processing includes "exploration and correction of inaccurate attributions about the cause of, responsibility for, and results of the abusive experience(s)" (Cohen et al., 2007, p. 5). This therapeutic process continues with the *trauma narrative,* which is described as "gradual exposure exercises, including verbal, written, or symbolic recounting of abusive events. . . . In vivo exposure," which entails "gradual exposure to nonthreatening trauma reminders in the child's environment . . . so the child learns to control his or her own emotional reactions" (Cohen et al., 2007, p. 5). For additional information and training on TF-CBT, therapists can learn more by accessing a Web-based training program titled TF-CBT Web at http://tfcbt.musc.edu/.

THE EMDR TREATMENT MODEL AS A TEMPLATE FOR A COMPREHENSIVE APPROACH TO CHILD PSYCHOTHERAPY

In using EMDR with children we suggest the integration of play therapy techniques as explained by Virginia Axline and Clark Moustakas along with Theraplay techniques, tools from Dyadic Developmental Psychotherapy (Hughes, 2007), along with the foundations and techniques from attachment therapy, and TF-CBT that are integrated into case conceptualization of psychotherapy with children throughout the 8 phases of the EMDR protocol. We encourage therapists to use all of the clinical skills and tools to create a therapist's toolbox that can be integrated into the EMDR 8-phase treatment protocol. We are not suggesting that all other clinical skills or training be abandoned but instead suggest that therapists consider organizing treatment and case conceptualization as a comprehensive process with the 8 phases of EMDR.

The chapters of this book have focused on explaining the detailed and integrated skills therapists need to provide psychotherapy to children through case conceptualization with the EMDR protocol. The use of play therapy techniques and skills are beneficial throughout the EMDR protocol. While the use of exposure, cognitive processing and reframing, stress management, and parental treatment included in TF-CBT are all important to the EMDR protocol, with the EMDR methodology cognitive reprocessing following how the child has maladaptively stored the traumatic and stressful events. EMDR allows the process to unfold in a coherent narrative that originates from the child rather than one that is created in therapy as it is in TF-CBT. The focus in EMDR is what is originating from the child through the phases of the EMDR protocol. TF-CBT also includes psychoeducational techniques and parent trainings along with stress management and relaxation skills that are also taught during the 8 phases of EMDR. The final phases of EMDR focus on reprocessing the event to a healthy and adaptive conclusion with the future template focused on in vivo exposure for future success to assist the client with learning new skills, reliving anticipatory anxiety, and envisioning a positive future.

While incorporating the most effective techniques, strategies, and clinical tools of all the psychotherapeutic interventions for children, EMDR creates a comprehensive treatment approach to working with children's issues. By creating specific treatment protocols and teaching therapists to use EMDR with young children and adhere to the protocol, the research needs to explore the efficacy of EMDR in treatment outcomes studies and in comparative studies with other types of child psychotherapy.

EMDR With Children as Evidence-Based Practice

Why is it necessary to document research on EMDR with young children? Research studies that explore the efficacy of EMDR with young children are necessary to support the use of EMDR as evidence-based practice so as to pursue additional research funding and, more important, to find financial support for training and treatment. Public funding for research, training, and treatment in the United States is often based on guidelines from federal organizations such as the Substance Abuse and Mental Health Services Administration. Once EMDR is afforded the rating of evidence-based practice, the use of EMDR with young children is more likely to be subsidized by public funding and private funding such as third-party insurance payors. In the end, the research on and status of EMDR as evidence-based practice with young children will increase the likelihood that more children will be able to receive EMDR therapy. Again, our goal has always been to help the children.

We do not need to defend the use of EMDR with children or explain why the literature published to date is not comprehensive. We need to explore from an objective perspective where we are with EMDR with children and the path we need to take to collect evidence to support the use of EMDR with children. To do this, we need to explain EMDR so others can see why EMDR is so important for children so that people will ask themselves why they have not been using EMDR with children all along. As with any new treatment modality, we need to create a standard protocol that can be taught to others and replicated through fidelity assessments. We then need to conduct controlled studies that evaluate the outcomes of using the treatment in therapy and then conduct comparative studies that compare EMDR treatment with other methodologies considered to be evidence-based practice.

So can we do EMDR with young children? Can we teach others to do EMDR with children? Can we conduct research on EMDR with children to evaluate the efficacy of the EMDR treatment protocol? Can we explain the mechanisms of EMDR that enhance treatment outcomes? And finally, can we compare EMDR with other efficacious treatments to assess the benefit of EMDR therapy for children?

WHAT REALLY MATTERS: THE CHILDREN'S STORIES

We have included comments from two children who wanted to share their opinions about EMDR. What the children wrote is included exactly as they wrote it.

At age 10, Nina was reportedly not adoptable after experiencing tremendous and extensive abuse. After being assigned to work with me (R.T.) in therapy, Nina agreed to try EMDR. Today, at age 15, Nina is successfully adopted and on track to be the first person in her biological family to ever graduate from high school. Nina and her new family agreed that they wanted Nina's story included in this book to encourage other children and therapists.

> *My name is Nina, and when i first started EMDR it was amazing! i started to notice that i wasn't as self mutalted as i normally was. I was more open to other and I wanted to be around other people, and thats all thanks to Dr. Tapia who introduced EMDR to me. For me EMDR is like my drug . . . it helps to keep me saine and rational. When im in my state of mood when i start to go downhill my life is really messed up. Then i just kind of work it out with EMDR and i watch my problem pass me by. After all that work, yeah sure i feel really exhausted, but it was all worth it. thanks Dr. Tapia*

Mari has been in foster care since 2 years of age, and after many homes, she found an adoptive family at age 4. Unfortunately, this adoptive family was not safe for Mari either, so she was removed and reentered the foster care system at 8 years. She was moved to several placements before she found a forever mom. Mari has her own opinions about EMDR and recommended EMDR for her new sister.

> *EMDR is something to help with problems. I like EMDR because it calms me down. There is a bridge and you have a person on*

the bridge. You move the person to the number on the bridge to show how big the problem is. From 1 to 10. Mari age 12

THE END IS JUST THE BEGINNING

This book is just a beginning. We strongly believe that as more and more therapists begin to feel confident in their ability to use EMDR with young children, and as the public becomes aware of the benefit of using EMDR with children, both in individual and group therapy, the need for training and consultation will grow. With this growth, we need to convince therapists to use the entire protocol with even young children and strive to adhere to the EMDR protocol. The ultimate goal of using EMDR with children is to change the trajectory of children's lives in order that children's futures are healthier and happier. The end of this book is anything but. This is just the start of advanced training for therapists working with children to pursue the recognition of EMDR as evidence-based practice for adults and children. As part of a worldwide effort to change the trajectory of children's lives, we change all of our futures.

Appendices

APPENDIX I

Consent/Assent for Treatment Form

CONSENT FOR TREATMENT OF MINOR

This is an authorization for ____________________ (therapist name) to provide treatment and/or diagnostic services to my child/adolescent, __________________________ (name). By signing this Consent for Treatment, I certify that I legally have custody or joint custody of my son or daughter and, thus, can legally consent for treatment of my child.

____ _______

Parent/Guardian signature Date

CHILD ASSENT FORM

I understand that my parent or guardian may consent for my treatment; however, I have also been asked to give my assent for my own treatment. By signing below, I realize that the therapist listed above has elicited my own assent for treatment.

____________________________ ________________________

Child's name Birth date

____________________________ ________________________

Sign your name here Witness

APPENDIX II

EMDR Client History/ Treatment Planning Form

(This form is completed in addition to the clinician's standard intake form.)

1. What are the parent's current concerns and goals for treatment? ("*I know my child will have been successful in treatment when* __________.")

   ____
   ____
   ____

2. Themes: (What themes are presented by child/parent related to responsibility, safety, control/choice?)

   ____
   ____
   ____

3. Symptom assessment: Does child/parent have any indication as to precursor of symptoms? How long have symptoms been present? Are there any times when symptom(s) are not present?

   ____
   ____
   ____

Clinician's Name ________________________ **Date** ____________

Clinician's Signature ________________________________

4. Identify traumatic experiences as reported by parent only. Therapist asks child to wait in playroom while interviewing parent regarding targets: What is the worst trauma experienced by the child per parent report? Assess for currently activated traumas, including traumas/triggers most closely related to current distress or symptoms. Note any additional traumatic experiences spontaneously reported by the child. List triggers, that is, people, places, things, and so on which activate traumatic memories, cause distress or symptoms, or lead to avoidance.

___

___

___

5. Identify traumatic experiences as reported by child. (Therapist asks child to rejoin session and interviews child per target identification script. Child may not identify any of the responses that the parent has identified.) Therapist also completes assessment tools (for child 8 years or older) during this process. (Parent is asked to wait in the waiting room and complete assessment tools if child is comfortable with parent leaving.)

___

___

___

6. Identify mastery experiences presented by the child. ("*Tell me something that you are proud of that you have done. Tell me a time when you felt really good about yourself.*")

___

___

___

NOTES:

___

___

___

___

___

Clinician's Name ______________________ **Date** ____________

Clinician's Signature ______________________________

APPENDIX III

Child/Adolescent Symptom Monitoring Form

CHILD/ADOLESCENT SYMPTOM MONITORING FORM

Date_____________ *Child's Name* __________________________
Parent Completing Form _____________________________
Therapist ____

Symptoms	Day by Day (Following Therapy)						
	Day1	Day2	Day3	Day4	Day5	Day6	Day7
Stomach aches							
Diarrhea/Constipation							
Sleep Disturbance							
Behavioral Problems							
Tantrums/Acting Out							
Crying							
Avoidance Behaviors							
Agitation							
Urination/Bowel Problems							
Refusal Behavior							
Anxiety							
Change in Eating Habits							
Headaches							

Note: 1 = minimal, 2 = moderate, 3 = severe

Other symptoms possibly related to treatment:

Symptoms	Day by Day						
	Day1	Day2	Day3	Day4	Day5	Day6	Day7

Note: 1 = minimal, 2 = moderate, 3 = severe

Additional Comments/Concerns:

____
____
____
____

Please complete this form and bring it to your child's next session. Thank you!

APPENDIX IV

Safe/Calm Place Protocol for Children Worksheet

SAFE/CALM PLACE PROTOCOL FOR CHILDREN WORKSHEET

Image: ____

____

____

Positive emotions: ____

____

____

Physical sensations (location and description): ________________

____

____

Cue word(s): ____

____

____

Minor disturbance for cuing/self-cuing practice: ______________

____

____

Safe/Calm Place Abbreviated Instructions

Step 1: Describe image.

Step 2: Describe emotions and positive sensations (including location).

Step 3: Enhance imagery and affect with soothing tones.

Step 4: Introduce short sets of eye movements (two to four saccades).

- If positive outcome, continue with several more short sets.
- If minimal or neutral outcome, try alternative direction of eye movements.
- If intrusions or negative response, explore solutions (i.e., containment of negative material, add more protective features to safe place) or switch to a different safe place or comforting resource image.

Step 5: Identify cue word(s). Guide child in holding cue word(s) and Safe/Calm Place together, as several sets of eye movements are added.

Step 6: Have child practice self-cuing, focusing on image and word(s) without eye movements.

Step 7: Have child bring up a minor disturbance. Therapist cues Safe/Calm Place.

Step 8: Have child bring up a minor disturbance. Child cues Safe/Calm Place.

APPENDIX V

Mapping Targets for EMDR Processing

Appendix V is included in section 11 of *EMDR and the Art of Psychotherapy With Children Treatment Manual.* The Mapping and Graphing tools were designed by the authors to help organize the EMDR protocol especially with children and can be integrated into the eight- phase protocol from the beginning with Client History and Treatment Planning.

INTRODUCTION TO MAPPING AND GRAPHING

Mapping and Graphing are tools for organizing targets, resources, and mastery experiences for children. We created these techniques in order to assist clients in their ability to grasp the concepts associated with EMDR through art therapy in a tangible clinical process. Throughout EMDR treatment, Mapping and Graphing are tangible ways to conceptualize the work to be done in treatment and then to re-evaluate treatment progress and outcomes. Both techniques teach children to self-assess and enhance their metacognitive skills or their ability to think about their thoughts and feelings while having new tools to explain their experiences. Finally, both Mapping and Graphing can be used as containers where children can have any distressing memories or emotions stick to the paper until the disturbance can be resolved.

INSTRUCTIONS TO THE THERAPIST FOR MAPPING

Mapping targets for EMDR is a technique utilized to organize the information collected when preparing for processing a client's issues with EMDR. Initially mapping was used to organize the child client's trauma history in order to identify targets for EMDR; however, after using the process on a regular basis we found that Mapping targets is an effective tool for utilization when proceeding with the full EMDR protocol for clients of all ages. This protocol is written specifically for children but can also be used very effectively with adults. The therapist can use Mapping for case conceptualization beginning during the Client History and Treatment Planning Phases and continue through the entire eight phases of the EMDR protocol. Mapping integrates with the specific steps of the protocol and helps clients understand the conceptualization that the therapist might consider. Mapping helps to elucidate how EMDR works in a tangible manner for even the youngest clients.

As the therapist begins to explore the parameters of the problem based on parent input and discussion with the child, data regarding the client's trauma history begins to arise and the therapist explains to the client that this is all important information that we need to pay attention to in order to help their brain fix the problem. The therapist can suggest to the child that talking about this information may bother them a little; therefore, with their assistance the therapist would like to create a map where they can put all the important parts about their worries or fears. The therapist can suggest to the child that by putting their worries on the paper, they might not have to worry as much, because the map can be used as a container. The therapist shows the child that they are going to use a piece of paper and pen to begin to make a map of things that bother them and the therapist needs the child's help to get the map correct. The therapist suggests that the child can help with the map or do it entirely by himself or herself.

After completing the map, explain to the child that the map can be changed at any time if something has been forgotten or if something changes. Finally, it is important to encourage the child to take ownership of the map and explain that he or she is in charge of what happens next with the map.

SESSION PROTOCOL FOR MAPPING

1. The therapist greets the child and parent in the waiting room and escorts them to the therapist's office.
2. The therapist reviews the previous session and answers any questions from the child and parent.
3. The therapist assesses general functioning since the previous session. The therapist reviews the current status of any symptoms identified in the previous session and explores any new

symptoms. *"Has anything changed since our last session?"* Ask both the child and the parent. (Refer to the book for detailed instructions.)

4. The therapist reviews any notations from the parent on the Child/Adolescent Symptom Monitoring Form.
5. The therapist reminds the child of the Safe/Calm Place and Stop Signal.
6. The therapist interviews the parent about identifying possible targets for EMDR.
7. The therapist then interviews the child about identifying targets for EMDR and compares with parents' responses.
8. The therapist explains Mapping to the child.
9. The therapist and child then begin drawing the map by having the child pick single words to put in the figure on the map that will help to identify what worry is in each shape.
10. The therapist may need to review Safe/Calm Place or use Cognitive Interweaves as needed if the child becomes anxious while identifying targets.
11. The therapist teaches the child how map entries can also be used as containers where targets stay stuck to the map.
12. The therapist needs to remind the child that the map can be added to or changed at any time.
13. The therapist then directs the child to help rank the targets on the map.
14. The therapist then asks the child to estimate a SUD for targets on the map.
15. The therapist then reviews the SUD as compared to the ranking.
16. The therapist then explains how targets get connected in the brain. The therapist and child can draw lines between targets on the map and show the strength of the connection by the thickness of the line.
17. The therapist then asks the child to identify the bad thought for each target.
18. The therapist then asks the child to identify the good thought for each target.
19. The therapist then asks the child to identify the assess the VoC for each target.
20. The therapist then asks the child to identify the feeling associated with each target.
21. The therapist then asks the child to identify the links between targets and feelings for the child.

22. The therapist then asks the child to explore for feeder memories that are associated with the same feeling.
23. The therapist then asks the child to choose a target to start with and point out associations with other targets including similar feelings and body sensations.
24. The therapist then works with the child to desensitize targets and reevaluate the map.
25. The therapist and the child continue working with the next target.

SCRIPT FOR MAPPING TARGETS

Per the protocol and scripts already included in this book, start with Client History and Treatment Planning. Focus on attunement with the child and listening for negative cognitions and possible targets for EMDR processing. It is helpful for the therapist to make notes of the client's negative cognitions and potential targets.

In the Preparation Phase the therapist explains EMDR to parents *and* to children.

Then the therapist assesses the parent's current stability and ability to participate in the EMDR process with the child.

Teach Safe/Calm Place to the child. During this process allow the child to experiment with the different types of bilateral stimulation: tapping, drumming, stomping, using the buzzies, and so on.

Teach the Stop Signal.

Interview the parent about identifying possible targets for EMDR.

Interview the child about identifying targets for EMDR and compare with parents' responses.

Explain Mapping to the child. *"I would like you to help me create a map where we put all of your worries, owies, etc. Do you know what a map is?"* If the child knows what a map is, continue with the Mapping process. If not, explain what a map is to the child. *"Today we will start your map that shows where the things that bother you or the worries that you have are, just like in your head* (therapist can point to his or her own head and the child's head). *Today we are starting with the map, but we can change it or add worries to it at anytime. Remember that it is your brain that will fix your worries and that I can teach you a way to help your brain shrink the worries and even make the worries go away."*

With large drawing paper and pen or pencil, draw a large odd shape in the middle of the paper and ask the child to identify his or her biggest worry to start the map. *"On this paper, I want us to start drawing your map by picking the biggest worry that you have or the thing that is bothering you the most right now."* Help the child to write his or her biggest concern or symptom in the shape in order to begin the map. Have the child pick single words to put in the figure on the map that will help to identify what worry is in each shape.

"When we make the map you might feel a little bit scared or worried, but remember you're safe here in my office and if you get too scared you can always practice using your safe place like we learned before. Do you remember how to use your safe place to feel better?" If needed, review Safe/Calm Place or continue identifying targets.

In addition to Safe/Calm Place, you can teach the child to use the figures on the map as containers. *"Do you see this big worry here on your map? What do we need to do to keep that worry locked into that shape on the map so it won't bother you?"* Usually children are very creative and come up with many ideas, but you can assist as necessary. You might want to suggest to the child that the shape on the map can have steel walls with lasers to keep anything from escaping the shape. You can also add, *"When we put your worry onto the map, we're sealing it into the shape so it won't come off and bother you. It will stay stuck on the map until we take it off to shrink it. Is that ok with you?"* Continue to collect targets by asking the child to identify more things that bother them, and suggest things that the child's parents may have identified as well. For instance, you may say to Johnny, *"Your mom thinks that you get in trouble a lot in school because you are mad about your daddy leaving. Do you think this is something we should put on your map?"* Continue by asking Johnny if there are things that his mom doesn't understand or know about that should also be on his map. Continue with mapping all of the child's worries by adding to the drawing. You can add additional pieces of paper as needed to identify all of the child's worries. Sometimes this process proceeds very quickly and you can move to the next phases of the EMDR protocol, while other times this process takes an entire session. If you note that the child is becoming agitated in completing the mapping, you can offer cognitive interweaves, suggest that the child practice his Safe/Calm Place, or stop and conduct a resource installation in order for the child to cope with mapping targets. See chapters on cognitive interweaves for children and resource installation for children. Throughout the remainder of this process, try to become attuned with the child and use the child's language regarding how the child labels whatever problems or worries he or she has.

Continue to identify other worries to add to the map. Engage the child in helping you create the map or let the child create the map as appropriate for the child's developmental level and understanding.

Explain to the child that you will also be writing notes, because what she or he says is very important and you want to make sure you remember it correctly. "*I am writing down what you are telling me because it is very important and I'm old and I don't want to forget what you are telling me. Is that OK with you?*"

When the child has identified all the worries that he or she wants to put on the map for the day, remind the child that he or she can add to the map at any time. "*Remember we can change the map at any time if we've forgotten something or something changes.*"

Next ask the child to help rank the targets on the map. "*Now I want you to help me know which worry or target is the biggest or bothers you the most. Would you show me which one is the biggest or worst?*" Proceed with the ranking process from worst or bothers me the most until littlest worry or "*It doesn't bother me hardly at all.*"

After completing the ranking process, explain SUDS to the child and ask the child to identify an SUDS for each target on the map. "*I want us to be able to tell how much something bothers you so when I ask you to tell me how much something bothers you, we can use numbers or you can show me with your hands like this.*" The therapist demonstrates SUDS based on the distance between the therapist's hands. The therapist then says, "*Is it this big, this big, or this big?*" The therapist can also use other measurements for the SUDS. SUDS can be bigger than the whole world or universe or deeper than the ocean, or the therapist can ask the child to tell what the biggest thing is that he or she can imagine. After that the therapist asks the child for the smallest thing they can imagine. Then the therapist asks the child to tell how big each worry is for each target on the map and this is noted on the map. "*What's the biggest thing you can think of in the whole world?*" Whatever the child answers, the therapist explains, "*That tells me that your worry would bother you a lot if it's as big as* _______ (repeat child's answer)." The therapist then asks the child, "*What's the smallest thing you could imagine?*" Whatever the child answers, the therapist says, "*That tells me that your worry doesn't bother you at all if it's as small as* ________ (repeat child's answer)." "*That's how we will both know how much something bothers you.*"

When I do this process, because I'm (R.T.) already working with a map Metaphor, sometimes I will ask the child to show me how big the worry is on the map or globe. I will say things like "*Is it as big as Arizona or bigger?*" (We live in Arizona.) If it's bigger than Arizona, I say, "*Maybe it's as big as the whole United States or bigger?*" If it's bigger than the whole United States we continue with as big as the whole world, the whole universe, or "infinity and beyond." Be creative and help the child feel validated in how big the worry is for them.

After completing the SUDS, review the SUDS compared to the ranking. The therapist notes if the SUDS and ranking do not match as a way to assure that the child is understanding the concept of assessing how distressful the target is for them.

After completing SUDS, the therapist also uses the map as a way to explain how worries or memories get connected in our brains. *"In our brains sometimes memories or worries get connected. Like you told me that when you think about your dad you are sad and when you think about your dog dying you get sad. On your map let's show how strong you think the connection is between the worries."* The therapist demonstrates to the child how to draw lines between the worries and then can make the line very thick or thin depending on how big the child thinks the connection is between the two targets. This serves to help the child understand how his or her brain works and why when feeling sad the child thinks of his or her dad and his or her dog. In addition to being educational for the child, we are also creating links that will ideally assist in linking the two memories when we proceed with desensitization.

After the SUDS, ask the child to help the therapist understand what the bad thought is that goes with the memory. *"When you think about that worry, what's the bad thought that goes with that worry?"* If necessary offer suggestions or use the "Kids List of Cognitions." Then ask the child what he or she would like to think instead or *"What's the good thought?"*

After identifying NC and PC, assess for a VoC. The therapist can use the example of the VoC Bridge by saying, *"If we put your bad thought here* (put bad thought on the left side of the paper) *and your good thought here* (write the good thought on the right side of the paper) *and we make a bridge with seven steps from your bad thought to your good thought* (therapist draws seven steps on an imaginary bridge between the bad thought and the good thought), *where do you think you are right now?"*

After the VoC, ask the child to tell the therapist what the feeling is that goes with the target. Sometimes the therapist may need to offer words for feelings to assist the child. *"When you think of that thing that bothers you and the bad thought, what feelings do you have about that?"*

Once we've identified feelings for the particular memory, look for links between targets for the child. Explain to the child that sometimes things bother us more than we expect because the feeling is connected to something else that bothered us before. For example, if Johnny has identified anger as a feeling associated with one of his targets, ask Johnny to identify other targets where he also might have felt angry and ask if he thinks those are connected to each other. Finally, this may also assist in identifying other feeder memories that are associated with feeling sad, mad, or other feelings.

After identifying the feeling, the therapist then asks the child where they feel that feeling in their body. Sometimes the child can point and tell the therapist where they feel the worry, while other times we need to take a break and teach mindfulness. "*When you think about that thing that bothers you and the ________ feeling, where do you feel that in your body? Some people feel it in their heads, some people feel it in their hearts, some people feel it in their tummies, and some people feel it in their legs and feet.*" The therapist can point to different parts of their body to demonstrate where the child might feel the disturbance.

Once the child has identified the body sensation, the therapist can then explain, "*This map helps to tell us what we need to work on to help you with* ______ (repeat child's concerns, symptoms, or behavioral problems). *Each time we work together we will choose something on your map to work on until we can cross all of these off of your map. Do you have any questions?*" Wait for response. "*Let's pick the first thing we want to work on today or next week*" (depending on the amount of time remaining in the session).

Each session the therapist can check in with the child to ask if any changes have occurred that would suggest something or should be added or removed from the map.

APPENDIX VI

Graphing EMDR Targets or Symptoms

Graphing is also included in Section 11 of *EMDR and the Art of Psychotherapy With Children Treatment Manual.*

INSTRUCTIONS TO THE THERAPIST FOR GRAPHING

Graphing is a multifaceted technique for elucidating various steps in the EMDR protocol. Graphing involves the therapist teaching the child to use a simple bar graph for identifying and assessing mastery experiences, targets, or symptoms; or evaluating progress in treatment; and/or as a container. The purpose for graphing is to help the child develop the observer self and to have a concrete technique for understanding and documenting the pieces of the EMDR treatment protocol.

Graphing for mastery experiences is used for the purpose of identifying resources, activities, abilities, and experiences that have created a positive experience for the child. For example, Riley feels good about how far he hit the ball in his baseball game. Riley would then note hitting the baseball as a mastery experience on his graph. The use of identifying and graphing mastery experiences provides the child with positive associations to the EMDR process, as well as developing a positive internal scaffolding in preparation for the desensitization phase.

For target and symptom identification, graphing helps the child create a list of his problems, worries, or "bothers" through drawing them in a concrete, visual manner. The purpose of graphing targets assists both the therapist and the child in selecting which targets should be reprocessed first.

As an evaluation tool, graphing can be used at the end of the session or for reevaluation in the following session. After the child has identified either resources or targets, the child and therapist can measure the strength of the resource or the level of competency over the target and then reevaluate progress. Graphing is not used as a SUDS scale.

Graphing can also be used as a container during or at the end of the session if the child is flooded by disturbing emotions. The therapist can instruct the child to have worries or bothers stay on the paper like a container.

The therapist can have the child make different graphs for each type of graphing technique, or some of the graphs can be combined. Graphing is a fluid and ongoing part of the treatment protocol in EMDR.

SESSION PROTOCOL FOR GRAPHING

1. The therapist greets the child and parent in the waiting room and escorts them to the therapist's office.
2. The therapist reviews the previous session and answers any questions from the child and parent.
3. The therapist assesses general functioning since the previous session. The therapist reviews the current status of any symptoms identified in the previous session and explores any new symptoms. "*Has anything changed since our last session?*" Ask both the child and the parents. (Refer to the book for detailed instructions.)
4. The therapist reviews any notations from the parent on the Child/Adolescent Symptom Monitoring Form.
5. The therapist reminds the child of the Safe/Calm Place and Stop Signal.
6. Interview the parents about identifying possible targets for EMDR.
7. Interview the child about identifying targets for EMDR and compare with the parent's responses.
8. Explain graphing to the child using the following script to identify first resources and then mastery experiences.
9. Use graphing to identify targets using the script. If necessary, remind the child of Safe/Calm Place if the child becomes anxious while identifying targets.
10. Pick one target to continue with the Assessment Phase of EMDR (see chapter 3 of this book) using the pieces of the protocol.
11. At the end of the session use graphing for assessing progress in treatment and remind the child that the graph can also serve as a container.
12. Review the mastery graph as a resource for the child to use between sessions as needed.
13. At the next session, review the mastery graph before moving to the target graph to continue with the EMDR protocol.

SCRIPT FOR GRAPHING

First the therapist explores whether the child understands the concept of a graph. Often children as young as 6 years old have already learned about simple bar graphs in school. Many times, even a 4-year-old can draw a rudimentary graph with a therapist's help. If the child has not heard of a graph, educate him or her to the idea by saying something like, *"I'm going to show you how to draw a graph. A graph is a way to measure things. Today we are going to measure things that you feel good about and things that you think are problems or worries or bothers."*

The therapist demonstrates what a graph is by drawing a large *L* with a crayon on a piece of drawing paper. The therapist divides the vertical line with 10, small, evenly spaced lines to indicate percentages. At the bottom of the vertical line the therapist puts a 0 and, in increments of 10 at each line, writes 10%, 20%, and so on, with the top of the line showing 100%. *"This line is how we can measure things with numbers where 0 is we don't feel good about them at all and 100 is where we feel really good about something."*

On the bottom horizontal line the therapist can write or draw examples of either mastery experiences/activities or problems and worries that a child might identify for the graph.

For mastery the therapist says, *"We are going to make a list of the things that you feel good about on the bottom so we can measure them. Can you tell me something you feel really good about?"* The Mastery (or Good Things) Graph can be used in every session. To make a Mastery Graph you ask the child to tell you something that they feel like they do well, or something that makes them feel good about themselves, and list those items at the bottom of the horizontal line in one- or two-word descriptions. *"Can you tell me something else that makes you feel good?"* After collecting mastery experiences, the therapist then asks the child to draw and color in a line vertically that goes up to or as close to 100% as possible. *"Can you draw a line that shows how good you feel about that thing? Ten percent is you feel a little bit good and 50% is you feel pretty good, and 100% is you feel the best about that thing."* The 100% represents how good they feel about the experience or activity. For instance, if Phoebe feels good about her drawing and art, we draw a line from the bottom of the horizontal line all the way up to 100%, meaning she feels as good as she can about her drawing. Then we identify several other activities that she feels positive about and she draws the line somewhere from 0 to 100%, demonstrating how good Phoebe feels about those positive experiences.

Then we install the mastery experience by having the child choose one of these positive experiences and enhance the good feelings in his or her body with bilateral stimulation, similar to the abbreviated RDI protocol. The therapist says to the child, *"So I want you to think about how good that* (mastery experience) *feels in your body and hold on to the buzzies for a second."* The therapist can use whatever type of BLS the child had chosen to install the mastery experience.

When completing a Targeting (or Worries and Problems) Graph, use a separate piece of paper and again have them make an L-shaped graph with percentages on the vertical axis, and list on the bottom the child's reported problems, worries, or bothers. The child then draws a bar or line that represents how much better or more competent the child feels regarding that target, with 100% demonstrating that the problem is resolved and/or the child feels competent to handle the problem or issue. Zero means that the child feels unable to handle the problem at all. *"Now we're going to make a worries or problems graph and we're gonna put all your worries or things that bother you on the bottom and this is how we're going to measure how good you feel about that problem. When it gets to the top or 100% you know you can handle the problem. It's kind of like a report card where we know you can handle that thing and it doesn't bother you or worry you anymore."*

The therapist can then refer back to targets on the graph at the end of a session, to assess the target. *"Ok, so we've worked on this problem, and where do you feel you are with handling that problem now?"* The child can draw the bar upward toward 100%, showing how much better he or she feels regarding the target. Often when one target is resolved, the child will spontaneously report that other targets are resolved. The child can then draw lines on the graph representing how much better they feel about each target.

The graph is also very useful to use in the next session to reevaluate the targets. The therapist says, *"Well, do you remember what we worked on last time? Let's take out our graph and look at it now. So with that problem we worked on, where are you now?"* The child may have increased feelings of competency with handling the problem and the percentage goes up, or occasionally the child is more worried about the problem, so the therapist can give the child a black crayon or marker to show that his or her feelings of competency over the problem actually went down. Children often feel empowered by the process of graphing because they can see their progress.

The Targeting Graph can also be used as a container at the end of sessions to assist the child in not having strong emotions or acting out behaviors between sessions. The therapist can simply say, *"This is your worry or bother graph and we're leaving them here on this paper in my office today. If for any reason these problems bother you when you go home, then you can imagine putting them back on the graph in my office and leaving them here."*

There are variations on graphing and we encourage you to use your own ideas to adapt the graph to your own client's needs after you have practiced the basic concept.

APPENDIX VII

Recent Event Protocol for Children

1. Obtain a narrative from the child through verbal, art, or play therapy. Sometimes obtaining the narrative can be overwhelming for the child, and the therapist may need to do a Safe/Calm Place. If the child is able to create a coherent narrative, we find that by having the child draw a series of pictures of the event, the child creates a book or movie about the incident.
2. The therapist then targets the worst part of what the child remembers. The child can pick a picture that represents the worst part or create the worst part in the sand tray.
3. The therapist then targets the remainder of the narrative in chronological order. For children, this can be relatively short if the child does not become avoidant and begin to distract himself or herself by bringing up other issues. The memory network for the child can be relatively short, and if the child does not flood, this is actually a very quick process in our experience.
4. The therapist then has the child visualize the entire narrative of the event by running the movie with his or her eyes closed, and if anything disturbing arises, the therapist then targets that disturbance for reprocessing with each step of the protocol but omits the body scan. This continues until the child can run the entire narrative with no disturbance.
5. The therapist then has the child visualize the entire narrative with his or her eyes open, and then the therapist installs the positive cognition that arose during Step 4, or the PC that appears to be the most prominent and resonate for the child. The therapist has the child conclude with the body scan and address present stimuli, if needed.

APPENDIX VIII

Scripts for Assessment, Desensitization, Installation, Body Scan, Closure, and Reevaluation

PHASE 3: ASSESSMENT

Therapist Instructions to the Child

What we're gonna do is we're going to the _________ [BLS] on that thing _________ [target], and I'm going to it for a while, and then I'm going to stop and tell you to blank it out and take a breath, and then we'll talk a little about it. Sometimes things will change, and sometimes they won't. There is no right or wrong answer. What you think or feel is exactly what I want to know, and you can tell me anything.

Review Stop Signal

If at any time you feel you want to stop, remember what you told me that you would do: _________ [stop signal previously identified].

Review and Check Safe Place and Resource Images

Briefly review the safe place and resource images established in earlier sessions.

Remember that safe place we talked about before [therapist names the safe place and offers descriptive cues]? *We can use that safe place when we are talking about what you remember, if you need to. I also want to make sure you remember what you told me about* _________ [therapist describes the resource images and associated feelings, qualities, or capacities, if needed]. Optional: *Do any of these* __________ [resources] *feel like they could really help us right now? Do you think there are any people, pets, or objects that you would want sitting with you who could help you feel better when we talk about that thing that happened?*

Target Identification

Therapist decides, in collaboration with the child and parent, what to target based on the list of traumatic experiences/targets established during client history and treatment planning process (traumatic experiences). (Often, children's targets are more current. What the child identifies as the trauma may not be what the parent identifies as the trauma.) When choosing a target to reprocess, the therapist should select the target most associated with the current active symptoms the child is experiencing. The child may have multiple traumas, but the trauma that is triggering the worst of the current symptoms should be targeted first. This can be determined during the history-taking portion of the preparation phase. This should be accomplished by first asking the parent (separately from the child) and later asking the child. Then the therapist should proceed by asking the child, *Can you remember a time when you felt like this before?*

This is still addressing the current target but tracing the channel to the past to see if there is an associated memory. Children frequently stay with the current target, which is fine. Frequently, children will say, "No, I don't remember another time, even if there was." If they have no previous associated memory, target the current one. When you choose the target connected to the worst of the current active symptoms, you may also have a generalized desensitization effect on other traumas. A child may have a previous incident of molestation or physical abuse that may get completely reprocessed by targeting the current trigger or trauma. The therapist should use drawing, clay, sand tray, and other techniques to elicit the trauma. This requires that the therapist have patience and become attuned to the child because the target may be expressed in nonverbal ways. As a last resort, if the therapist assesses that the child is completely unable to access the memory networks that are believed to be associated with the current symptoms, the therapist can request that the parent provide suggested targets along with possible negative and positive cognitions.

Picture/Image

For the most disturbing picture or image, the therapist asks, *What's the worst/yuckiest part of the picture?* If no picture, the therapist asks, *When you think about that thing, what happens now?*

Negative Cognition (NC). *When you think about that thing/picture, what words go with that?* Or you can say, *What's the bad thought that goes with that?*, especially with younger children who may again need education. We have changed the language to "what's the bad thought" and "what's the good thought." Even little children can grasp that concept, but the NC may be more trauma-specific. Also, the NC that the child identifies may not be what the parent thinks the NC is for the child. It is important that the NC resonate for the child. Depending on a child's development, the child may not always use *I* statements. The child may speak in third person, such as, "David hurt," with a PC of "David feel better." These all relate to the child's current level of cognitive development or language acquisition level. Sometimes the cognition is concrete, like, "Jeff bad" versus "Jeff good." Or the child may use fantasy to express thoughts about himself or herself. Sometimes you get the PC first and then work backward to get the NC. Just like with adults, the NC and the PC should resonate for the child. When it resonates, the child may tell you in a variety of ways; the child can make eye contact, say it, change his or her body language, change his or her play, or otherwise indicate. (We have included a handout on NC and PC for kids.)

Positive Cognition (PC). *When you think about that thing/picture, what words would you rather say to yourself instead?* Or you can say, *What's the good thought that you want to tell yourself instead?*

Validity of Cognition (VoC). *When you say those words* _________ [repeat PC], *how true do those words feel right now, from 1, which means it's not true at all, to 7, which means it's really true?* (Therapist can use distance between hands or other types of measures to which the child relates that are developmentally appropriate to demonstrate disturbance.)

Emotions/Feelings. *When you bring up that picture [or incident] and the words* __________ [NC], *what do you feel* now? (If the child needs further explanation, the therapist can use the feelings chart or some other type of educational tool to help the child identify emotion. Explore the emotions that the child feels in the present.)

SUDS. *From 0 to 10, where 0 is "it doesn't bother you at all" and 10 is "it bothers you a lot," how much does that thing bother you right* now? (Therapist can use distance between hands or other type of measure to which the child relates.)

Location of Body Sensation. *Where do you feel it in your body?* (If the child is not initially able to answer, the therapist teaches child mindfulness of body sensations by pointing to body parts as the therapist says, *Sometimes people feel it in their head, or their tummy, or their feet. Where do you feel it in your body?*)

PHASE 4: DESENSITIZATION

1. *I'd like you to bring up that picture* [label and describe using client's word] *and the words* [repeat the NC in client's words], *the _________ feeling, and notice where you are feeling it in your body and* _________ [therapist uses whatever BLS was previously identified].
2. Begin the BLS. (You established the BLS method and speed during the introduction to EMDR.)
3. At least once or twice during each set of BLS, or when there is an apparent change, comment to the client, *That's it. Good. That's it.* With children, the type of BLS may need to be changed often to assist the child in sustaining attention.
4. If the child appears to be too upset to continue reprocessing, it is helpful to reassure the child and to remind the child of the Metaphor identified with the child prior to processing. *It's normal for you to feel more as we start to work on this. Remember, we said it's like* _________ [Metaphor], *so just notice it. It's old stuff.* (Only if needed, if child is upset.)
5. After a set of EM, instruct the child by saying, *Take a deep breath.* (It is often helpful if the therapist takes an exaggerated breath to model for the child, as the therapist makes the statements to the child.)
6. Ask something like, *What did you get* now? or *Tell me what you got.* Or if the child needs coaching, say, *What are you thinking and feeling? How does your body feel, or what pictures are you seeing in your head?*
7. After the child recounts his or her experience, say, *Go with that,* and do another set of BLS. (Do not repeat the child's words or statements.) As an optional phrasing, you can say, *Think about that.*
8. Again, ask, *What do you get now?* If new negative material presents itself, continue down that channel with further sets of BLS.
9. Continue with sets of BLS until the child's report indicates that the child is at the end of a memory channel. At that point, the child may appear significantly calmer. No new disturbing material is emerging. Then, return to the target. Ask, *When you think about that thing we first talked about today, what happens now?* (Remember that children may not show affect and may often process very quickly. So there may be no more disturbing material for the child to access or describe about the target memory.) After the child recounts his or her experience (kids may verbalize or draw or otherwise demonstrate through play therapy what they have experienced), add a set of BLS.

10. If positive material is reported, add one or two sets of BLS to increase the strength of the positive associations before returning to the target. If you believe the child is at the end of a channel, that is, the material reported is neutral or positive, then ask, *When you go back to that first thing we talked about today* [therapist references the picture, sand tray, or whatever was used by the child to identify the original target], *what do you get now?* Whatever the child reports, add a set of BLS.
11. If no change occurs, check the SUDS. Ask the child, *When you think about that thing, from 0 to 10, where 0 is "doesn't bother you at all" and 10 is "bothers you a lot," how much does that thing bother you right now?* (Therapist can use one of the alternate ways of checking the SUDS described in the Assessment Phase.)
12. If the SUDS is greater than 0, continue with further sets of BLS, time permitting. If the SUDS is 0, do another set of BLS to verify that no new material opens up. Then proceed to the installation of the PC. (Remember: only proceed to installation after you have returned to target, added a set of BLS, no new material has emerged, and the SUDS is 0.)

PHASE 5: INSTALLATION

Installing the PC is about linking the desired PC with the original memory/incident or picture:

1. *Do the words* _________ [repeat the PC] *still seem right, or are there other positive words that would be better now?*
2. *When you think about that thing we talked about at the beginning and you say those words* _________ [repeat PC], *how true do those words feel right now, from 1, "it's not true at all," to 7, "it's really true"?*
3. Say, *Now think about that event and say those words,* _________ [repeat PC], *and follow,* then do a set of BLS.
4. Then check the VoC again. *When you think about that thing we talked about at the beginning and you say those words* _________ [repeat PC], *how true do those words feel right now from 1, "it's not true at all," to 7, "it's really true"?*
5. Continue doing sets of BLS as in Step 2, as long as the material is becoming more adaptive. If the child reports a 7, repeat Step 3 again to strengthen, and continue until it no longer strengthens. Then go on to the body scan.

6. If, after several sets of BLS, the child still reports a 6 or less, check the appropriateness of the PC, and address any blocking belief (if necessary) with additional reprocessing.

PHASE 6: BODY SCAN

Close your eyes; concentrate on that thing you told me about and the words _________ [repeat the final PC], *and notice your whole body, from the top of your head to the bottom of your feet, and tell me where you feel anything.* If any sensation is reported, do a set of BLS. If a discomfort is reported, reprocess until discomfort fully subsides. Then do the body scan again to see if there are still any negative sensations. If a positive or comfortable sensation is reported, do BLS to strengthen the positive feeling. If a sensation of discomfort is reported, do BLS to strengthen the positive feeling.

The therapist then does several BLS to help the child assimilate the information and develop a positive template for future action.

Future Template or Closure

Sometimes a therapist will not have enough time to complete this future template process all in one session. If time is limited, the therapist should omit the future template at this point and proceed with closure to complete the session. If the future template is omitted, the therapist should return to the future template process in the next session immediately after completing reevaluation.

Instructions to the Therapist. This is different than the future template for adults in that children need immediate and current positive behavioral actions to take because it is empowering to them. Therefore, once earlier memories and present triggers and symptoms are adequately resolved regarding the specific target, the therapist explores how the child would rather feel and act in the future. The therapist may have to teach the skills to the child (e.g., social skills, assertiveness, anger management).

Future Template Script

Target. *What would you like to be able to do?* (positive behavior like "sleep in my own bed").

NC/PC/VoC. *When you think about that thing you'd like to be able to do, what's the bad thought?* (Therapist identifies new NC for future action.) Therapist then asks the child, *What would you rather tell* *yourself instead?*, or therapist explains, *What's the good thought?* Then therapist elicits VoC for new PC by asking, *When you think about that thing you want to be able to do and those words* _________ [therapist repeats PC], *how true does that seem to you right now, from 1, being completely false or not true, to 7, being completely true?*

Emotion. Therapist continues by identifying emotion by saying to the child, *When you think about that thing you want to be able to do, what's the feeling that goes with that?*

Subjective Units of Disturbance. Therapist continues by identifying subjective units of disturbance (SUDS) by saying to child, *How disturbing does that feel?*

Body Sensation. Therapist then identifies body sensation by asking, *Where do you feel that in your body?* (Therapist can use examples of body sensations, as discussed previously.)

Once the therapist has elicited a future target, NC/PC, VoC, emotion, SUDS, and body sensation for future desired behaviors/actions/feelings, therapist continues by saying, *Sometime in the next day or so, I want you to think about* _________ [the desired positive behavior, e.g., sleeping in my own bed alone, handling anger in an appropriate way] *with those words* _________ [say the new PC] *with all the* _________ [elicit positive visual cues], _________ [positive sounds], *and* _______ [positive kinesthetic sensations]. Therapist processes future template with BLS: 24 saccades. If something negative comes up, then process the negative through with whatever comes up as the target. If the adaptive resolution continues in a positive direction, continue as follows:

> *Now, I want you to imagine (or pretend) in three nights from now with the same* _________ [desired positive behavior].
>
> Do BLS.
>
> *Now, in 1 week, . . .* [same words and scenario].
>
> Do BLS.
>
> *Now, in 1 month, . . .* [same words and scenario].
>
> Do BLS.
>
> *Now, let's pretend we are seeing yourself when you're bigger and one time when you would need* _________ [desired behavior]. *Imagine the* _________ [positive behavior] *and* _________ [PC].
>
> Do BLS.

You can have the child draw a picture, use the sand tray, or create a clay sculpture at any point. Stay attuned to evaluate any negative associations or distortions that may emerge. The child should feel emotionally, physically, and cognitively comfortable with the anticipated event.

PHASE 7: CLOSURE

Closure/Debriefing the Experience

Say to the child, *Well, we've done a lot of work today, and you're awesome. Before I see you next time, you may think about stuff, so would you draw me a picture or write something down or tell your mom and dad if you have any thoughts, dreams, or feelings that you want to remember to tell me or would be good for me to know?*

Procedure for Closing Incomplete Sessions

An incomplete session is one in which a child's material is still unresolved, that is, the child is still obviously upset, or the SUDS is above 1 and the VoC is less than 6. The following is a suggested procedure for closing down an incomplete session. The purpose is to acknowledge the child for what he or she has accomplished and to leave the child well grounded before he or she leaves the office:

1. Explain the reason for stopping, and check on the child's state. *We need to stop and clean up now because it's time to go. How're you doing after the thing we talked about today?*
2. Give encouragement and support for the effort made. *We worked hard today, and you're awesome. How are you doing right now?*
3. *Let's stop and do our container and our safe place one more time before we go. Remember your safe place? I want you to think about that place. What do you see? What do you smell? What does it feel like to be there? Where do you notice it in your body?* (Therapist uses process to access containers and safe place for client to close the desensitization process.)

PHASE 8: REEVALUATION

At the start of every session after EMDR has been introduced, the therapist assesses the treatment progress and resolves previously activated traumas:

1. *Remember what we worked on last time? Did you think about it at all? Was there anything that you wanted me to know since our last session?*
2. Ask the parent if there have been any changes since the last session (i.e., changes in symptoms, new behaviors, etc.).

3. The therapist reevaluates the degree of processing of the previous target to determine whether or not the target has been resolved (SUDS = 0, VoC = 7). SUDS of more than 0 or VoC of less than 7 is only acceptable if ecologically valid. The therapist reevaluates SUDS as the child focuses on the target from the previous session. If not, what remains disturbing as the client holds the target in his or her awareness (image, cognition, emotion, sensation)? *When you go back to what we worked on last time, what do you get now?* After the child answers, the therapist responds, *When you think about that* _________ [client's answer], *how much does it bother you now?* (Therapist elicits SUDS.) Therapist continues by asking the child, *And when you think about the thing we worked on and the thought* _________ [therapist repeats client's PC from the previous session], *how true does that feel for you right now, from 1, "not true at all," to 7, "totally true"?* (Therapist can use hand distance or other measure previously utilized with the specific client.)
4. Therapist continues with reprocessing, with all targets associated with current symptoms, until all the necessary targets have been reprocessed.

APPENDIX IX

Kids' List of Cognitions

KIDS' LIST OF COGNITIONS

Bad thoughts (NC)	Good thoughts (PC)
I'm bad	I'm good
I'm in a fog	I'm in clear place/I'm in sunshine
I'm going to blow	I'm calm
I'm going to explode	I'm calm
I'm hot	I'm cool (as a cucumber)
I don't belong	I do belong
I am stupid	I'm smart
I am dumb	I'm smart
I'm sick	I'm all better
I can't do it	I can do it
I'm hurt	I'm better
I don't understand	I do understand
I can't get help	I can get help
I messed up	I did the best I could
I don't know nothing	I do know
I'm dying	I'm alive
I'm hungry	I'm satisfied
I'm not lovable	I'm lovable
I'm fat	I'm just right
I'm lost	I found my way
I almost drowned and I got very scared and that made me hold my breath.	I tell myself, you should be glad you could hold your breath that long.
I couldn't come out from under the water.	I'm glad I can swim.
I didn't get to go the hospital with dad.	I get to go to the hospital with dad.
I'm not comfortable	I am comfortable
I am uncomfortable in my skin	I fit in my skin
I'm not safe	I'm safe now
I can't protect myself	I can protect myself
I don't have control	I do have control
I can't trust	I can trust

Note. Therapists can choose to organize NCs and PCs into categories of safety, responsibility, and choice; however, oftentimes, kids' cognitions are so concrete that it is difficult to determine the specific category into which the NC or PC falls.

APPENDIX X

EMDR Fidelity Questionnaire

Phase 1: Client History and Treatment Planning

Did you identify a client history and treatment planning process? ☐ Yes ☐ No

Phase 2: Preparation

Did you identify aspects of the therapist preparing the client for additional phases of the EMDR protocol? ☐ Yes ☐ No

Phase 3: Assessment

Did you identify aspects of the therapist conducting assessment of the client in anticipation of proceeding with Phase 4, desensitization? ☐ Yes ☐ No

Did the therapist identify a specific memory or picture and then identify the worst part? ☐ Yes ☐ No
If yes, please describe the target. ____________________

Did you identify a NC? ☐ Yes ☐ No
If yes, please describe the NC. ____________________

Did you identify a PC? ☐ Yes ☐ No
If yes, please describe the PC. ____________________

Did you identify a VoC? ☐ Yes ☐ No
If yes, what was the initial VoC? ____________________

Did you identify an emotion? ☐ Yes ☐ No
If yes, what was the emotion identified to be? ____________________

Did the therapist get a SUDS? ☐ Yes ☐ No

Did you identify a body sensation? ☐ Yes ☐ No
If yes, what body sensation was identified? ____________________

Phase 4: Desensitization

Did the therapist desensitize the target to SUDS of 0 and VoC of 7?
☐ Yes ☐ No

If no, did the therapist proceed with desensitization and process the incomplete session? ☐ Yes ☐ No

Phase 5: Installation

Did you identify the therapist utilizing an installation process?
☐ Yes ☐ No

Phase 6: Body Scan

Did you identify the therapist proceeding with the body scan process?
☐ Yes ☐ No

Phase 7: Closure

Did you identify the therapist implementing a closure process?
☐ Yes ☐ No

Phase 8: Reevaluation

At some point in the client's treatment, did you identify a reevaluation process utilized with the client?
☐ Yes ☐ No

Three-pronged protocol:

1. Was there evidence that the therapist assessed processing in the present? ☐ Yes ☐ No
2. Was there evidence of the therapist's application of the future template by guiding the client through application of new skills to a future event? ☐ Yes ☐ No

References

Adler-Tapia, R. (2001). *Traumatic stress symptom checklist for infants, toddlers, and preschoolers.* (Unpublished, available from the author).

Adler-Tapia, R. L., & Settle, C. S. (2008). *EMDR and the art of psychotherapy with children.* New York City, NY: Springer Publishing.

Adler-Tapia, R. L., & Settle, C. S. (2008). *EMDR and the art of psychotherapy with children treatment manual.* New York: Springer Publishing.

Ahmad, A., Larsson, B., & Sundelin-Wahlsten, V. (2007). EMDR treatment for children with PTSD: Results of a randomized controlled trial. *Nordic Journal of Psychiatry, 61*(5), 349–354.

Alpern, G. (2007). *Developmental profile—III.* Los Angeles: Western Psychological Services.

American Psychiatric Association. (2000). *Diagnostic and statistical manual of mental disorders* (4th ed., Text Rev.). Washington, DC: Author.

American Psychiatric Association. (2004). *Practice guidelines for the treatment of patients with acute stress disorder and post-traumatic stress disorder.* Arlington, VA: Author.

Armstrong, J. G., Carlson, E. B., & Putnam, F. W. (1997). Development and validation of a measure of adolescent dissociation: The adolescent dissociative experiences scale. *Journal of Nervous & Mental Disorders, 185*(8), 491–497.

Axline, V. M. (1964). *Dibs: In search of self.* New York: Ballantine Books.

Bowlby, J. (1999). *Attachment and loss* (Vol. 1, 2nd ed.). New York: Basic Books.

Brazleton, T. B. (1992).*Touchpoints: Your child's emotional and behavioral development.* Reading, MA: Perseus Books.

Brazleton, T. B., & Cramer, B. G. (1990). *The earliest relationship: Parents, infants, and the drama of early attachment.* New York: Addison Wesley.

Brazleton, T. B., & Sparrow, J. D. (2006). *Touch points: Birth to 3: your child's emotional and behavioral development (Touchpoints).* Cambridge, MA: Perseus Books Group.

Bretherton, I. (1992). The origins of attachment theory: John Bowlby and Mary Ainsworth. *Developmental Psychology, 28, 759–775.*

Brett, D. (1986). *Annie's stories.* New York: Workman.

Bricker, D., & Squires, J. (1999). *Ages and Stages Questionnaires (ASQ): A parent-completed, child-monitoring system* (2nd ed.). Baltimore: Brookes.

Briere, J. (1996). *Trauma symptom checklist for children: Professional manual.* Florida: Psychological Assessment Resources Inc.

Chemtob, C., Nakashima, J., & Carlson, J. (2002). Brief treatment for elementary school children with disaster-related posttraumatic stress disorder: A field study. *Journal of Clinical Psychology, 58*(1), 99–112.

Clarke, J. I., & Dawson, C. (1998). *Growing up again.* Center City, MN: Hazelton.

Cocco, N., & Sharpe, L. (1993). An auditory variant of eye movement desensitization in a case of childhood post-traumatic stress disorder. *Journal of Behavior Therapy and Experimental Psychiatry, 24*(4), 373–377.

Cohen, J., Deblinger, E., Mannarino, A. P. Wilson, C., Taylor, M., & Ingleman, R. (2007, May). *Trauma focused cognitive behavioral therapy: Addressing the mental health of sexually abused children.* Child Welfare Information Gateway. Retrieved February 3, 2008, from www.childwelfare.gov/pubs/trauma

Donovan, F. (1999). *Looking through hemispheres.* Fran Donovan Productions sold through EMDR Humanitarian Assistance Program, Hamden, CT.

Dworkin, M. (2005). *EMDR and the relational imperative: The therapeutic relationship in EMDR treatment.* New York: Brunner-Routledge.

Edmond, T., Sloan, L., & McCarty, D. (2004). Sexual abuse survivors' perceptions of the effectiveness of EMDR and eclectic therapy. *Research on Social Work Practice, 14*(4), 259–272.

EMDR Humanitarian Assistance Programs. (2007, Winter). *What's happening now . . . IV*(2). EMDR Humanitarian Assistance Program, Hamden, CT.

Fernandez, I., Gallinari, E., & Lorenzetti, A. (2004). A school-based eye movement desensitization and reprocessing intervention for children who witnessed the Pirelli Building airplane crash in Milan, Italy. *Journal of Brief Therapy, 2*(2), 129–135.

Foa, E. B., Cashman, L., Jaycox, L., & Perry, K. (1997). The validation of a self-report measure of PTSD: The Posttraumatic Diagnostic ScaleTM (PDSTM). *Psychological Assessment, 9*(4), 445–451.

Foa, E. B., Johnson, K. M., Feeny, N. C., & Treadwell, K. R. H. (2001). The Child PTSD Symptom Scale: A preliminary examination of its psychometric properties. *Journal of Clinical Child Psychology, 30,* 376–384.

Goleman, D. (1995). *Emotional intelligence.* New York: Bantam.

Gomez, A. (2007). *Dark bad day go away.* Phoenix, AZ: Author.

Greenwald, R. (1994). Applying eye movement desensitization and reprocessing (EMDR) to the treatment of traumatized children: Five case studies. *Anxiety Disorders Practice Journal, 1*(2), 83–97.

Greenwald, R. (1999). *Eye movement desensitization and reprocessing (EMDR) in child and adolescent psychotherapy.* Northvale, NJ: Jason Aronson Press.

Harcourt Assessment. (2003). *Wechsler Intelligence Scales for children* (4th ed.). San Antonio, TX: Author.

Hughes, D. (1997). *Facilitating development attachment.* Northvale, NJ: Jason Aaronson Inc.

Hughes, D. (1998). *Building the bonds of attachment: Awakening love in deeply troubled children.* Northvale, NJ: Jason Aaronson Inc.

Hughes, D. (2007). *Attachment focused family therapy.* New York: W. W. Norton & Co.

International Society for the Study of Dissociation Task Force on Children and Adolescents. (2004). Guidelines for the evaluation and treatment of dissociative symptoms in children and adolescents. *Journal of Trauma and Dissociation, 5*(3), 119–150.

Jaberghaderi, N., Greenwald, R., Rubin, A., Dolatabadim, S., & Zand, S. O. (2002). A comparison of CBT and EMDR for sexually abused Iranian girls. *Clinical Psychology and Psychotherapy, 11,* 358–368.

Jarero, I., Artigas, L., & Hartung, J. (2006). EMDR integrative group treatment protocol: A postdisaster trauma intervention for children and adults. *Traumatology, 12*(2), 121–129.

Jarero, I., Artigas, L., Mauer, M., Alcala, N., & Lupez, T. (1999, November). *EMDR integrative group treatment protocol and the butterfly hug.* Paper presented at the annual meeting of the International Society for Traumatic Stress Studies, Miami, FL.

Jernberg, A. M. (1979). *Theraplay.* San Francisco, CA: Jossey-Bass, Inc.

Jernberg, A. M., & Booth, P. B. (1999). *Theraplay: Helping parents and children build better relationships through attachment-based play.* San Francisco, CA: Jossey-Bass, Inc.

Jones, R. T. (2002). *The child's reaction to traumatic events scale (CRTES): A self-report traumatic stress measure.* Blacksburg: Virginia Polytechnic University.

Jones, R. T., Fletcher, K., & Ribbe D. R. (2002). Child's Reaction to Traumatic Events Scale-Revised (CRTES-R): A self-report traumatic stress measure. (Available from the author, Dept. of Psychology, Stress and Coping Lab, 4102 Derring Hall, Virginia Tech University, Blacksburg, VA 24060).

Korkmazlar-Oral, U., & Pamuk, S. (2002). Group EMDR with child survivors of the earthquake in Turkey (*ACPP Occasional Papers Series No. 19*). Academy of Child & Adolescent Psychiatry (1998). *Journal of the American Academy of Child & Adolescent Psychiatry, 37*(10 Suppl.), 4S–26S.

Korn, D. L., & Leeds, A. M. (2002). Preliminary evidence of efficacy for EMDR resource development and installation in the stabilization phase of treatment of complex posttraumatic stress disorder. *Journal of Clinical Psychology, 58*(12), 1465–1487.

Korn, D. L., & Spinnazola, J. (2001). *EMDR treatment manual research protocol.* Unpublished manuscript.

Kranowitz, C. S. (2005). *The out-of-sync child: Recognizing and coping with sensory processing disorder* (Rev. ed.). New York: Perigee.

Leeds, A. (1998). Lifting the burden of shame: Using EMDR Resource Installation to resolve a therapeutic impasse. In P. Manfield (Ed.), *Extending EMDR, A case book of Innovative Applications* (pp. 256–282). New York: W. W. Norton.

Lovett, J. (1999). *Small wonders: Healing childhood trauma with EMDR.* New York: The Free Press.

Moustakas, C. E. (1959). *Psychotherapy with children: The living relationship.* New York: Ballantine.

Muris, P., Merckelbach, H., Holdrinet, I., & Sijsenaar, M. (1998). Treating phobic children: Effects of EMDR versus exposure. *Journal of Consulting and Clinical Psychology, 66*, 193–198.

Muris, P., Merckelbach, H., van Haaften, H., & Mayer, B. (1997). Eye movement desensitization and reprocessing versus exposure in vivo: A single-session crossover study of spider-phobic children. *British Journal of Psychiatry, 171*, 82–86.

Oras, R., Cancela De Ezpeleta, S., & Ahmad, A. (2004). Treatment of traumatized refugee children with eye movement desensitization and reprocessing in a psychodynamic context. *Nordic Journal of Psychiatry, 58*, 199–203.

Perry, B. (2006). Applying principles of neurodevelopment to clinical work with maltreated and traumatized children. In N. B. Webb (Ed.), *Working with traumatized youth in child welfare* (pp. 27–52). New York: Guilford Press.

Popky, A. J. (2005). DeTUR, an urge reduction protocol for addictions and dysfunctional behaviors. In R. Shapiro (Ed.), *EMDR solutions: Pathways to healing* (pp. 167–188). New York: W. W. Norton.

Puffer, M., Greenwald, R., & Elrod, D. (1997). A single session EMDR study with twenty traumatized children and adolescents. *International Electronic Journal of Innovations in the Study of the Traumatization Process and Methods for Reducing or Eliminating Related Human Suffering, 3*(2), Article 6. Retrieved February 3, 2008, from http://www.fsu.edu/~trauma/v3i2art6.html

Putnam, J. (1997). *Dissociation in children and adolescents: A developmental perspective.* New York City, NY: Guilford Press.

Reynolds, C. R., & Kamphaus, R. W. (2002). *Behavioral Assessment Scale for Children (Second Edition).* Bloomington, MN: Pearson Education, Inc.

Reynolds, C. R., & Kamphaus, R. W. (2006). *Behavioral assessment for children—II.* Bloomington, MN: Pearson's Assessment Group.

Roid, G. H. (2003). *Stanford–Binet Intelligence Scales for children* (5th ed.). Ithasca, IL: Riverside.

Rubin, A., Bischofshausen, S., Conroy-Moore, K., Dennis, B., Hastie, M., Melnick, L., et al. (2001). The effectiveness of EMDR in a child guidance center. *Research on Social Work Practice, 11*(4), 435–457.

Shapiro, F. (1989a). Efficacy of the eye movement desensitization procedure in the treatment of traumatic memories. *Journal of Traumatic Stress, 2*(2), 199–223.

Shapiro, F. (1989b). Eye movement desensitization: A new treatment for post-traumatic stress disorder. *Journal of Behavior Therapy and Experimental Psychiatry, 20,* 211–217.

Shapiro, F. (1995). *Eye movement desensitization and reprocessing: Basic principles, protocols, and procedures.* New York: Guilford Press.

Shapiro, F. (1995–2007). *EMDR part 1 training manual.* Watsonville, CA: EMDR Institute.

Shapiro, F. (2001). *Eye movement desensitization and reprocessing: Basic principles, protocols, and procedures* (2nd ed.). New York: Guilford Press.

Shapiro, F. (2007). EMDR and case conceptualization from an adaptive information processing perspective. In F. Shapiro, F. W. Kaslow, & L. Maxfield (Eds.), *Handbook of EMDR and family therapy processes* (pp. 3–34). Hoboken, NJ: John Wiley.

Shapiro, F., Kaslow, W., & Maxfield, L. (Eds.). (2007). *Handbook of EMDR and family therapy processes.* Hoboken, NJ: John Wiley.

Siegel, D., & Hartzell, M. (2003). *Parenting from the inside out.* New York: Penguin.

Soberman, G., Greenwald, R., & Rule, D. (2002). A controlled study of eye movement desensitization and reprocessing (EMDR) for boys with conduct problems. *Journal of Aggression, Maltreatment and Trauma, 6*(1), 217–236.

Tinker, R. H., & Wilson, S. A. (1999). *Through the eyes of a child: EMDR with children.* New York: W. W. Norton.

Tufnell, G. (2005). Eye movement desensitization and reprocessing in the treatment of preadolescent children with post-traumatic symptoms. *Clinical Child Psychology and Psychiatry, 10*(4), 587–600.

U.S. Department of Veterans Affairs and U.S. Department of Defense. (2004). *VA/DoD clinical practice guideline for the management of post-traumatic stress.* Washington, DC: Authors.

Vygotsky, L. S. (1978). *Mind in society.* Cambridge, MA: Harvard University Press.

Wilson, S., Tinker, R., Hofmann, A., Becker, L., & Marshall, S. (2000, November). *A field study of EMDR with Kosovar-Albanian refugee children using a group treatment protocol.* Paper presented at the annual meeting of the International Society for the Study of Traumatic Stress, San Antonio, TX.

Wolfe, V. V., Gentile, C., Michienzi, T., Sas, L., & Wolfe, D. A. (1991). The children's impact of traumatic events scale: A measure of post-sexual abuse PTSD symptoms. *Behavioral Assessment, 13,* 359–383.

Zaghrout-Hodali, M., Alissa, F., & Dodgson, P. W. (in press). Building resilience and dismantling fear: EMDR group protocol with children in an area of ongoing trauma. *Journal of EMDR Practice and Research.*

Zero to Three. (2005). *Diagnostic classification of mental health and developmental disorders of infancy and early childhood* (Rev. ed., Report No. DC:0-3R). Washington, DC: Author.

Internet Resources

Adler-Tapia, R., & Settle, C. EMDR Kids (Author's Web site), Retrieved February 17, 2008, from www.emdrkids.com

American Academy of Child and Adolescent Psychiatry. (1998). *Practice parameters for the assessment and treatment of children and adolescents with posttraumatic stress disorder.* Retrieved February 17, 2008, from http://www.aacap.org/galleries/Practice Parameters/PTSDT.pdf

Association for the Study and Development of Community. *Measures of child social–emotional, behavioral, and developmental well-being, exposure to violence, and environment.* Retrieved September 26, 2007, from http://www.capacitybuilding.net/Measures%20of%20CEV%20and%20outcomes.pdf

Child and adolescent trauma measures. (2007). Retrieved February 8, 2008, from http://origin.web.fordham.edu/images/academics/graduate_schools/gsss/catm%20-%20introduction.pdf

Dr. Bruce Perry's Web site. Retrieved February 17, 2008, from www.childtrauma.org

Emotional Literacy workbooks for kids with free downloads. Retrieved February 17, 2008, from http://www.kidseq.com/activity.php

International Society for the Study of Dissociation. (2004). Guidelines for the evaluation and treatment of dissociative symptoms in children and adolescents. *Journal of Trauma & Dissociation, 5*(3), Article 10.1300/J229v05n03_09. Retrieved February 8, 2008, from http://www.isst-d.org/education/ChildGuidelines-ISSTD-2003.pdf

National Alliance on Mental Illness. Retrieved February 17, 2008, from www.nami.org

National Center for PTSD. www.ncptsd.va.gov/ncmain/information/

http://www.nami.org/Content/Microsites191/NAMI_Oklahoma/Home178/Veterans3/Veterans_Articles/9childrenofveteransandadultswithPTSD.pdf (This is a handout on children of veterans and adults with PTSD).

PTSD and Dissociative Measures for Children. (This site includes all the measures to assess trauma and dissociation for children with free, downloadable copies of the forms.) http://www.podcastforteachers.org/childrenfirstwebsite/cfresources/ptsd_dissociative_measures_201.pdf

Steiner, C. (2002). *Emotional literacy: Intelligence with a heart.* Retrieved February 8, 2008, from http://www.claudesteiner.com/ Training for emotional literacy. http://www.claudesteiner.com/2000_i.htm; Follow links to Steiner's book, *A Warm Fuzzy Tale.*

World Federation for Mental Health. N.I.C.E. Guidelines for treating PTSD. http://www.nice.org.uk/nicemedia/pdf/CG026fullguideline.pdf

Zero to Three Website. Website for information on infant toddler development with handouts for parents. www.zerotothree.org

Assessment Tools for Evaluating Children

Researchers will need to determine which assessment tools to use in the study; however, we suggest the CPSS and CRTES be used at minimum for pre/postmeasures of outcome from the group protocol.

A-DES: Adolescent–Dissociative Experiences Scale (Armstrong, Carlson, & Putnam, 1997). Retrieved from http://www.energyhealing.net/pdf_files/a-des.pdf

BASC-2: Behavioral Assessment Scale for Children (2nd ed.) (Reynolds & Kamphaus, 2002). This form must be purchased.

CDC: Child Dissociative Checklist (CDC), Version 3 (Putnam, 1997). Retrieved from http://www.energyhealing.net/pdf_files/cdc.pdf

Child/Adolescent Behavioral Monitoring Form (Adler-Tapia & Settle, 2008).

CITES: Children's Impact of Traumatic Events Scale (Wolfe et al., 1991). Retrieved from http://www.swin.edu.au/victims/resources/assessment/ptsd/cites-r.pdf

CPSS: Child PTSD Symptom Scale (Foa, Cashman, Jaycox, & Perry, 1997; Foa, Johnson, Feeny, & Treadwell, 2001). Requests for use of this measure must be made to Dr. Edna Foa.

CRTES: *The Child's Reaction to Traumatic Events Scale–Revised* (CRTES-Revised) (Jones, 2002; Jones, Fletcher, & Ribbe, 2002).

TSCC: Trauma Symptom Checklist for Children (Briere, 1996).

TSSC: Traumatic Stress Symptom Checklist for Infants, Toddlers, and Preschoolers (Adler-Tapia, 2001). Retrieved from www.emdrkids.com

Index